Assistive Devices for Persons with Hearing Impairment

RELATED TITLES OF INTEREST

Handbook of Auditory Evoked Responses
James W. Hall III
ISBN: 0-205-13566-8

Principles and Applications in Auditory Evoked Potentials
John T. Jacobson (Editor)
ISBN: 0-205-14846-8

Audiometric Interpretation: A Manual of Basic Audiometry, Second Edition
Harriet Kaplan, Vic S. Gladstone, and Lyle L. Lloyd
ISBN: 0-205-14753-4

Hearing Disabilities, Third Edition
Jerry L. Northern
ISBN: 0-205-15226-0

Toward a Psychology of Deafness
Peter V. Paul and Dorothy W. Jackson
ISBN: 0-205-14112-9

Understanding Digitally Programmable Hearing Aids
Robert E. Sandlin (Editor)
ISBN: 0-205-14845-X

Orientation to Deafness
Nanci A. Sheetz
ISBN: 0-205-13438-6

Mechanisms of Tinnitus
Jack A. Vernon and Aage Moller (Editors)
ISBN: 0-205-14083-1

Assistive Devices for Persons with Hearing Impairment

EDITED BY

Richard S. Tyler
The University of Iowa

Donald J. Schum
The University of Iowa

Allyn and Bacon
Boston • London • Toronto • Sydney • Tokyo • Singapore

Assistive devices for
persons with hearing

Series Editor: Kris Farnsworth
Editorial Assistant: Christine M. Shaw
Editorial-Production Service: Walsh Associates
Cover Administrator: Linda Knowles
Composition Buyer: Linda Cox
Manufacturing Buyer: Louise Richardson

Copyright © 1995 by Allyn & Bacon
A Simon & Schuster Company
Needham Heights, Mass. 02194

Library of Congress Cataloging-in-Publication Data

Assistive devices for persons with hearing impairment / edited by
  Richard S. Tyler and Donald J. Schum.
      p.   cm.
    Includes blbliographical references and index.
    ISBN 0-205-15126-4
    1. Hearing aids.   2. Hearing impaired—Rehabilitation.   3. Self-help
  devices for the disabled.   I. Tyler, Richard S. II. Schum, Donald J.
  RF298.A85   1994
  617.8'9—dc20   94-26290
                                                            CIP

Printed in the United States of America
10   9   8   7   6   5   4   3   2   1   00   99   98   97   96   95

Contents

Foreword   ix

Preface   xi

Acknowledgment   xii

About the Editors   xiii

Contributing Authors   xv

1   Impact of the Americans with Disabilities Act
on Audiologists   1
by Jo Williams and Ann L. Carey
Introduction   1
The Role of Assistive Technology   3
Implications for Audiologists   7
References   9

2   An Overview of The Food and Drug Administration's Medical
Device Amendments   10
by Celeste F. Bové
Introduction   10
Assistive Listening Devices   15
Hearing Aid Regulation   18
Implications for Audiology   19
References   20
Glossary   21
Additional Contacts   23

3   Interfacing with the Telephone System   24
     by Ronald D. Slager
     The Carter Decision   26
     The Telephone Transmission System   27
     Telephone Assistive Devices and Their Applications   33
     What Does the Future Hold?   64
     Conclusion   64
     Appendix 3-1: Telephone Technology Resources   65

4   Clinical Procedures for Evaluating Telephone Use and
     Need for Related Assistive Devices   66
     by Nancy Tye-Murray and Lorianne K. Schum
     Informal Evaluation   67
     Formal Evaluation   68
     Conclusions   78
     Final Remarks   78
     References   79
     Appendix 4-1: Description of the Test Site   80
     Appendix 4-2: Description of Cochlear Corporation TLP-102
          Telephone Adapter   81
     Appendix 4-3: Conversational Test Items, Organized by
          Conversational Goal   82
     Appendix 4-4: Script Used for QUEST?AR Task   83

5   Alerting and Assistive Systems: Counseling Implications
     for Cochlear Implant Users   86
     by Lorianne K. Schum and Nancy Tye-Murray
     Introduction   86
     Needs Assessment and Counseling   89
     Alerting Systems   95
     Assistive Listening and Visual Support Systems   99
     Final Remarks   104
     Conclusions   106
     References   107
     Appendix 5-1   109
     Appendix 5-2   110
     Appendix 5-3   121

6   Television Viewing for Persons with Hearing
     Impairment   123
     by Donald J. Schum and Lynn Vance Crum
     Introduction   123
     The Problem   124
     Assisted Listening for Television Viewing   125

Captioning   136
The Role of Counseling   139
References   140

7   The Importance of Room Acoustics   142
      by Carl C. Crandell and Joseph J. Smaldino
      Introduction   142
      Reverberation   143
      Noise   145
      Noise and Reverberation   151
      Speaker-Listener Distance   152
      Methods to Improve Classroom Acoustics   155
      Conclusions   160
      References   160

8   Orientation to the Use of Frequency Modulated Systems   165
      by Dawna E. Lewis
      Frequency Modulation Devices in Classrooms   165
      Summary   181
      References   181

9   Orientation to the Use of Induction Loop Systems   185
      by Robert A. Gilmore
      How Conventional Loop Systems Work   185
      Telecoil-Equipped Induction Receivers   191
      Advantages and Limitations of Conventional Loop Systems   192
      3-D Loop Systems   194
      Loop System Standards   195
      Recommended Readings   196

10   Alerting Devices for the Hearing-Impaired   197
      by Dean C. Garstecki
      The Sensing Stage   198
      The Transmitting Stage   201
      The Alerting Stage   202
      Summary   205
      References   206

11   Integrating Assistive Devices into the Hospital Setting   207
      by Helene Frye-Osier and Donald J. Schum
      Introduction   207
      Needs Assessment   208
      Services and Equipment   210

Staff Training   214
Administration   220
Conclusion   222
References   222

12   Selecting What's Best for the Individual   224
by Cynthia L. Compton
Audiologic/Communication Needs Assessment   226
Fire Signaling Devices   234
Counseling   235
Hearing Aid/Assistive Devices Evaluation   236
Use of Hearing Aids with the Telephone   236
Use of Hearing Aids with Assistive Devices   239
Follow-up/Aural Rehabilitation   247
The Role of the Professional   247
Summary   248
References   248
Appendix 12-1: Resources   249

13   Increasing Consumer Acceptance of Assistive Devices   251
by Glen Sutherland
Introduction   251
Meeting Consumer Needs   252
Individual Information/Training Sessions   252
Group Information/Training Sessions   255
Use of Volunteers as Trainers   256
Educational Materials   257
Public Awareness and Public Accessibility   259
Summary   261
Appendix 13-1: Recommendations to Make Public Places
       Accessible to Deaf and Hard of Hearing People   262

14   Assistive Device Research Needs   267
by Dean C. Garstecki
Product Research   268
People Research   274
Summary   275
References   275

Index   277

Foreword

BY SENATOR TOM HARKIN
March 19, 1993

Unless it was a work of fiction, the book you now hold in your hands wouldn't have been possible five years ago, for one simple reason: There wasn't much of a story to tell. Sadly, neither technology nor laws quite matched the potential and the promise of people with hearing impairments.

But today, all that has changed. In the past five years, we have crossed more frontiers for people with hearing impairments than we have in the entire 216-year history of the United States.

When I was growing up, people like my brother Frank, who is deaf, had limited opportunities. Back in the 1940s, Frank was told that he could be one of three things: a printer's assistant, a cobbler, or a baker. But today, as Gallaudet University President I. King Jordan said in a recent speech, "the world is open to (students who are deaf and hard of hearing). Students come to Gallaudet knowing they want to be attorneys, computer system designers, entrepreneurs, educators, actors, and even politicians."

More than ever before, Americans today are beginning to understand that people who listen with their eyes and speak with their hands are just as able to achieve the American Dream as their non-disabled peers. And now, through the implementation of the Americans with Disabilities Act, 43 million Americans with disabilities have the opportunity to become fully integrated into the economic and social mainstream of American life.

The ADA is landmark civil rights legislation that prohibits discrimination on the basis of disability in private sector employment, services provided by state and local government, public and private transportation, public accommodations, and telecommunications.

Among other things, the ADA requires that employers provide "reasonable accommodations"—qualified interpreters, amplified telephones, TDDs, or job restructuring—to employees who are deaf or hard of hearing. Employers are finding that these accommodations represent minor costs compared to the contributions of talent, energy, and creativity that these individuals bring with them.

I was recently told of a bank that invested in equipment similar to a TDD to provide reasonable accommodations for a teller who is deaf. The bank was happy to report that this accommodation not only brought the bank a hard-working and dedicated employee, it also helped business and improved its ability to serve customers who are deaf.

As the ADA is implemented, doors will be opened, barriers will be broken down, and basic human rights will be extended to all people with disabilities. But as I've often said, you can't just pass a law and expect to change attitudes overnight. Discrimination is no longer protected under the law, but there's still a lot of work to do.

That's part of the reason for this book. Assistive technology can help individuals of all ages, and in all areas of life—including recreation, education, independent living, and other community activities. This book will serve as a guide to tens of thousands of Americans with disabilities who have yet to realize the promise of assistive technology. What's more, it also dispenses vital and accurate information to millions of Americans who must meet the requirements of the ADA.

In the end, the pages before you are not so much a book as they are a blueprint to a Brave New World—a world where the ladder or ramp of opportunity is left down for every American to ascend; where all our citizens are treated with dignity and respect; and where every American has a fair shot at the American Dream. The first chapters have been written, the groundwork has been laid, and the plot is unfolding—but it's up to all of us to make sure that this story has a happy ending.

Preface

With the passage of the Americans with Disabilities Act, providing assistive devices for hearing-impaired persons will appropriately receive much attention in the upcoming years. The technology available to provide both simple and sophisticated assistive devices to hearing-impaired individuals has increased substantially in the last five years. However, we suspect that many important aspects of this technology are poorly understood by designers, distributors, audiologists, and consumers. On June 11–14, 1992 we held an "Assistive Devices for the Hearing Impaired" conference at the University of Iowa to provide tutorials, discuss applications, and present recent research. Although not the conference proceedings, this book is a direct product of the conference.

Assistive Devices for Persons with Hearing Impairment can serve as a textbook for courses and seminars on assistive devices for hearing-impaired people. However, it is intended both for students and practicing audiologists. It should also be of interest to manufacturers, product designers, distributors, and possibly some consumers. The book is intended to be a tutorial, providing both general information and specific practical suggestions. In each chapter, the authors have provided conceptual and technical background information that should be helpful for some time.

In Chapter 1, the impact of the Americans with Disabilities Act on audiologists is discussed by Jo Williams and Ann Carey. It is vital to understand the implications of this act on services for people with hearing loss. The Act could have the greatest effect on audiology since the dispensing of hearing aids became professionally acceptable. In Chapter 2, Celeste Bové explains the involvement of the Food and Drug Administration with hearing impairment and associated assistive devices. This unique contribution provides an important perspective on government regulations.

In Chapter 3, Ronald Slager explains the electroacoustics of telephones and their interface with assistive devices. Chapter 4, Clinical Procedures for Evaluating Telephone Use and Needs for Related Assistive Devices, by Nancy Tye-Murray and Lorianne Schum, provides some useful strategies for understanding problems experienced on the telephone. In Chapter 5, Lorianne Schum and Nancy Tye-Murray discuss alerting and assistive systems for cochlear implant users. Chapter 6 reviews television for persons with hearing impairment. Donald Schum and Lynn Vance Crum provide important suggestions for providing hearing assistance during this common pastime.

In Chapter 7, the importance of room acoustics to assistive devices is discussed by Carl Crandell and Joseph Smaldino. Dawna Lewis reviews (Chapter 8) the application of frequency modulation devices in classrooms. Chapter 9 provides an orientation to the use of induction loop systems. Robert Gilmore discusses the basic principles and some new technology. In Chapter 10, Dean Garstecki reviews a broad spectrum of alerting devices. Chapter 11 provides a plan for integrating assistive devices into the hospital settings. Helene Frye-Osier and Donald Schum share their experiences in two different hospital settings.

In Chapter 12, Cynthia Compton provides a general framework for selecting what is best for the individual. Glen Sutherland describes a variety of approaches to increase consumer acceptance of assistive devices (Chapter 13). The book concludes (Chapter 14) with a discussion of assistive device research needs by Dean Garstecki.

ACKNOWLEDGMENT

We would like to sincerely thank Regina Tisor for the many hours she contributed in the preparation of this book.

About the Editors

Richard S. Tyler received an M.Sc. in Audiology from the University of Western Ontario, and a Ph.D. in Psychoacoustics at the University of Iowa. He was Scientist in Charge of the Clinical Outstation at the Institute of Hearing Research in Nottingham, United Kingdom, before becoming Professor and Director of Audiology in the Department of Otolaryngology at the University of Iowa. He has a joint appointment in the Department of Speech Pathology and Audiology. Dr. Tyler's interests include hearing aids, tinnitus, aural rehabilitation, and cochlear implants. He is co-director of a cochlear implant research project supported by the National Institutes of Health.

Donald J. Schum is an assistant professor in the Department of Otolaryngology—Head and Neck Surgery at The University of Iowa Hospital. His primary responsibility is to direct the clinical and research activities in the Hearing Aid Laboratory. He received his B.S. in speech and hearing science from the University of Illinois in 1982, his M.A. in audiology from the University of Iowa in 1984, and his Ph.D. in audiology from Louisiana State University in 1988. His primary research interests are in the areas of speech perception and the role of amplification for persons with hearing impairment.

► Contributing Authors

Celeste Bové came to the Food and Drug Administration in 1987 after fifteen years of clinical audiology experience in a federal psychiatric setting. She received her masters degree in audiology from Memphis State University in December 1971 and is currently pursuing a doctoral degree in Public Administration through Nova University, Fort Lauderdale, Florida. She previously worked in the Office of Device Evaluation of the FDA as a scientific reviewer, and as Executive Secretary to the Ear, Nose, and Throat Devices Advisory Panel. Currently, she is Deputy Director, Division of Planning, Evaluation, and Information Services of the Office of Management Services, Center for Devices and Radiological Health of the FDA.

Ann Carey, Ph.D., CCC-A, SLP, is Professor of Speech Pathology and Audiology at Southern Illinois University at Edwardsville. Long active in professional affairs, she is a former Legislative Councilor, Vice President for Professional and Governmental Affairs, and was 1992 President of the American Speech-Language-Hearing Association.

Cynthia Compton is Director and co-founder of the Assistive Devices Center at Gallaudet University's Department of Audiology and Speech-Language Pathology. A noted authority on assistive technology, Ms. Compton has published, lectured, and consulted extensively on the topic.

Carl C. Crandell graduated from Vanderbilt University and is currently affiliated with the Department of Communication Processes and Disorders at the University of Florida. Dr. Crandell's research activities concern the effects of environmental distortions on the speech perception of hearing-impaired, pediatric, and elderly listeners.

Lynn Vance Crum received her B.A. in communication studies at the University of Iowa in 1987. She is currently a master's candidate in the Department of Speech Pathology at the University of Iowa. She is also the coordinator of the assistive device display center in the Department of Otolaryngology at the University of Iowa Hospitals and Clinics.

Helene Frye-Osier, Ph.D., is the Director of Audiology at Williams S. Middleton Memorial Veterans Affairs Hospital, Madison, Wisconsin. Dr. Frye-Osier has been involved with direct hearing aid and assistive device selection and dispensing for more than fourteen years. As part of the Veterans Affairs Hearing Loss Management program, she has conducted a series of workshops for agency audiologists on strategies and techniques to advance the use of assistive device technology with the Veterans Affairs Medical Centers.

Dean C. Garstecki, Ph.D., is a professor and head of the Audiology and Hearing Sciences Program, professor of Otolaryngology-Head and Neck Surgery, and director of the Hugh Knowles Center for Clinical and Basic Science in Hearing and its Disorders at Northwestern University with over twenty years experience as a certified and licensed audiologist.

Robert A. Gilmore, M.S., CCC-A, is president and director of research and development at American Loop Systems in Milford, Massachusetts. Mr. Gilmore received his M.S. degree from Gallaudet University. Gilmore was research audiologist on grant projects resulting in the TACTAID 7, the CHORUS Universal Listening System, and the 3-D Loop System.

Dawna E. Lewis received her M.A. in Audiology from the University of Tennessee. She works as a clinical audiologist at Boys Town National Research Hospital in Omaha, NE. Ms. Lewis' clinical/research interests include pediatric audiology and amplification, particularly FM systems.

Lorianne K. Schum, M.A., CCC-A, is a certified clinical audiologist, presently employed as an assistant research scientist in the Department of Otolaryngology-Head and Neck Surgery, at The University of Iowa Hospital, Iowa City, Iowa. Her research experience includes device programming and aural rehabilitation with adult cochlear implant recipients. Ms. Schum's past work experiences have included clinical audiology in hospital-based and private otolaryngology settings, as well as clinical supervision in the Department of Communication Disorders at Louisiana State University. She received a B.A. in Speech and Hearing Science (1981) and a M.A. in Audiology (1983), both from the Department of Speech and Hearing Sciences at the University of Illinois.

Ronald D. Slager is currently Vice President, Hearing Aid Center of Kalamazoo and HARC Mercantile, Ltd., Divisions of HAC of America, Inc., a manufacturer/distributor of hearing aids and related products for the hearing impaired and deaf. Slager is also an ADA consultant and lecturer.

Joseph Smaldino graduated from the University of Florida and is currently a professor of audiology and department head in the Department of Communicative Disorders at the University of Northern Iowa. Dr. Smaldino is interested in the effects of amplification systems on speech, and the development of rehabilitative procedures to maximize speech perception.

Glen Sutherland received his Communicative Disorders degrees from the University of Western Ontario. He has worked as a Speech-Language Pathologist and an Audiologist. While working at the Canadian Hearing Society he was Director of the Technical Devices and Audiology departments. Presently he is employed by VOICE For Hearing Impaired Children.

Nancy Tye-Murray directs the aural rehabilitation and speech production program for cochlear implant adults and children at the University of Iowa Hospital. This hospital is one of the largest cochlear implant centers in the United States. Dr. Tye-Murray has made numerous contributions to the literature in the areas of aural rehabilitation, speech science, speech perception, and cochlear implants.

Jo Williams, M.Aud., CC-A, has extensive background with the Americans with Disabilities Act (ADA) and audiology practice issues. Her responsibilities at the American Speech-Language-Hearing Association (ASHA) include directing ASHA's U.S. Department of Justice ADA grant, providing ADA technical assistance, and commenting on proposed ADA regulations.

▶ 1

Impact of the Americans with Disabilities Act on Audiologists

JO WILLIAMS
American Speech-Language-Hearing Association

ANN L. CAREY
American Speech-Language-Hearing Association

INTRODUCTION

The passage of the Americans with Disabilities Act (ADA) represents a major shift in public policy regarding people with disabilities, their constitutional rights, and their quality of life. For the most part, the burden has been on people with disabilities to access American society. The ADA has shifted responsibility from the individual to society. The ADA provides (a) new protections in both the public and private sectors where no laws prohibiting discrimination based on disability existed before, and (b) expands protections in those programs and services covered by other laws and regulations. The stage is set for a radically improved way of life, now and in the future, for the millions of Americans of all ages who have disabilities among whom are the people audiologists serve: the more than 26 million Americans with auditory, vestibular, and communication-related impairments. Audiologists can and must play a pivotal role in the challenge ahead—putting policy into everyday practice.

History and Scope of the ADA

The Americans with Disabilities Act of 1990 is comprehensive civil rights legislation for people with disabilities. Much of the ADA is derived from the Rehabilitation Act

1

of 1973, which prohibits discrimination based on disability in federal agencies or institutions receiving federal funds. However, for a number of reasons, including lack of codification, the Rehabilitation Act has been ignored, for the most part, and has not resulted in significantly improved access for people with disabilities. In addition, the Rehabilitation Act paid little attention to communication issues and the needs of people with communication disabilities.

During the 20 years leading up to the ADA, the disability-rights community and its allies have evolved and learned about the steps necessary to effect change in society. In order to ensure enforcement and swift implementation of the ADA, legislation required regulations to be developed and enacted within a short time period. Although the ADA is directed primarily at preventing discrimination in the private sector, public programs and services, such as 911 emergency services, not covered under the Rehabilitiation Act are covered by the ADA.

The disability community and advocates also have become broader based. The ADA goes beyond physical/mobility access issues to include the interests of people of all ages with a range of physical and mental disabilities. One of the most significant accomplishments of the ADA was a change in national policy regarding the role and importance of communication in everyday life, and the high standard required of facilities and programs to provide access for people with hearing, speech, and cognitive language impairments.

The ADA in turn has impacted the Rehabilitation Act. Interestingly, the attention and publicity generated by the ADA has led to new interest and recognition of the Rehabilitation Act. Facilities and programs seeking information about their ADA obligations are discovering that they should have been providing access for the past 15 years (and are now scrambling around to come into compliance). The Rehabiliation Act was brought up to the higher requirements of the ADA, such as those for communication access, during recent reauthorization and amendment activities (1992).

At this point in time, between the ADA and other disability laws, people with communication and other disabilities are ensured equal opportunities and access to benefit from, participate fully in, and enjoy all aspects of American society—employment, traveling, telecommunications, shopping, dining out, public assembly and entertainment activities, social and public services, and health care services. For people with communication disabilities, the ADA offers important new safeguards in matters involving informed consent and civil liberties, which typically involve complicated and important information exchange. Public and private programs and services, such as law enforcement agencies, health care providers, and judicial systems, will be held to a high standard of ensuring effective communication, including providing appropriate assistive technology and services.

ADA Regulations

The ADA was signed into law on July 26, 1990. The following year, 1991, comprehensive regulations for implementing the ADA were developed in record time, and in January 1992, the regulations started to become effective.

TABLE 1–1 **ADA Regulations, Statutory Deadlines, and Responsible Agencies**

Title I Employment

July 26, 1992 - Employers with 25 or more employees
July 26, 1994 - Employers with 15 to 24 employees

Equal Employment Opportunity Commission
1801 L Street, NW
Washington, DC 20507
800-669-EEOC (V)
800-800-3302 (TDD)

Title II State and Local Government Services

January 26, 1992 (Date varies for transportation)

Title III Public Accommodations and Commercial Facilities

January 26, 1992

U.S. Department of Justice	U.S. Department of Transportation
P.O. Box 66118	400 Seventh Street SW
Washington, DC 20035-6118	Washington, DC 20590
202-514-0301 (V)	202-366-9305 (V)
202-514-0383 (TDD)	202-755-7687 (TDD)

Title IV Telecommunications

July 26, 1993

Federal Communications Commission (FCC)
1919 M Street, NW
Washington, DC 20554
202-632-7260 (V)
202-632-6901 (TDD)

There are five ADA titles. The key ADA regulatory areas (and their respective titles) are Employment (Title I), State and Local Government Services, including public transportation (Title II), Public Accommodations, including private transportation (Title III), and Telecommunications (Title IV). Title V contains miscellaneous provisions, such as state immunity. Regulations vary in their effective dates and responsible federal agency. Table 1–1 provides the effective date for each regulation, as well as the corresponding agency responsible for implementation and enforcement.

THE ROLE OF ASSISTIVE TECHNOLOGY

Assistive technology plays a key role in all regulatory areas of the ADA: as a means of accommodation for employees, effective communication with customers and citizens, communication accessibility in programs and facilities, and telecommunications accessibility. The types of technology and services that can be used include low-tech to high-tech strategies and the range of assistive listening, alerting, and signaling devices; visual communication technologies; environmental modification techniques; and telecommunication technologies (See Slager, Chapter 3; Schum & Crum, Chapter 6; Crandell & Smaldino, Chapter 7; Lewis, Chapter 8; Gilmore, Chapter 9; Garstecki, Chapter 10; Schum & Frye-Osier, Chapter 11; Compton, Chapter 12).

Although the types of assistive technology and services used for accommodations and accessibility are similar across regulatory areas, selection criteria will vary. The Title II and Title III regulations address accessibility for the public at large. The Title I employment regulation focuses on the individual. Accordingly, selection of assistive technology will depend on whether it is for an employee or for the public, and, in some cases, for both employees and the public.

Assistive Technology in Employment

Employers are prohibited from discriminating against applicants and existing employees on the basis of hearing disability throughout the full range of employment opportunities—from hiring and promotions to fringe benefits. Employers are required to determine if reasonable accommodation would permit a qualified person with a hearing disability to perform necessary job functions, and to provide that accommodation unless an undue hardship (significant difficulty or expense) or fundamental alteration in the nature of the business services or operations would result. Employers also are to provide any necessary accommodations for pre-employment activities such as interviews and examinations.

Accommodations for employees with hearing impairments include providing assistive devices and communication services (e.g., amplified telephones, assistive listening devices, visual signaling and alerting devices); modifying the work environment (e.g., reducing electrical and acoustic noise levels); modifying the way the job is done (e.g., using the text telephone/voice telephone relay system); and training co-workers and supervisors in effective ways to communicate with employees who have hearing impairments. Accommodations may be necessary for employees to enjoy the full range of employment benefits and activities. For example, in order for an employee with hearing impairment to participate fully in staff meetings and training seminars, it may be necessary to provide assistive listening systems, preferential seating, computer-assisted notetaking, interpreters, or other services. Each job, each individual, and each employment setting have to be looked at on a case-by-case basis (See Compton, Chapter 12).

Employers are prohibited from basing employment decisions on stereotypes or prejudices about what someone with a hearing impairment is able to do. Qualification standards, such as hearing ability, that tend to screen out people with hearing disabilities, must be job-related and consistent with business necessity. For example, if the requirements for the position of security guard state that hearing must be within "normal limits," the employer must be able to show that this criterion is based on valid data and necessary for the individual to perform the essential functions of the job.

And, if a certain level of hearing ability is a legitimate standard, the individual with a hearing impairment must be assessed with respect to accommodations or devices (e.g., hearing aids) that would allow him or her to meet this criterion.

A person who poses a direct threat to self or others can be denied employment. However, direct threat means that there is significant risk of substantial harm. Slightly increased possibility of harm occurring because of the person's disability does not meet the test of a direct threat. Decisions about whether a person with a hearing loss poses a safety risk must be made on an individual basis using the best objective evidence or the opinion of a professional with expertise in the disability area (e.g., audiologist), not on supposition or stereotypes. And, direct threat also must be assessed in terms of accommodations, such as hearing aids or visual alerting devices, that could reduce the likelihood of serious harm occurring below a significant level (eliminating the risk entirely is not required).

Assistive Technology in Private Facilities and Public Programs

Title II and III regulations require facilities, services, and programs in the private and public sectors to take steps to ensure effective communication with customers and citizens who have communication disabilities. These steps include providing any necessary auxiliary aids and services without a surcharge to the individual with the hearing disability requesting or needing the aid/service, unless an undue burden (significant difficulty or expense) or fundamental alteration in the nature of the program or activities would result.

What devices and services are necessary for effective communication will vary with the type of facility, the clientele, and the type of communication. Although the public sector must give primary consideration to the individual's specific request for an aid or service, and the private sector is strongly encouraged to do so, the facility/program has the final decision regarding whether devices and services are necessary. The aids or services provided do not have to be the best available, but they must be effective for the individual and the particular communication activity.

If the provision of a particular aid or service would constitute an undue burden or fundamental alteration, then an alternative aid or service that would be effective and would not cause an undue burden or fundamental alteration must be provided, if one is available. For example, if oral interpreter services are requested but cannot be provided because no interpreters are available on that date, alternatives might be computer-aided notetaking services or a written transcript.

As a general rule of thumb, the need for assistive aids/services for communication to be effective becomes greater as the information to be communicated increases in complexity, length, and importance. Written note exchanges with someone who has a hearing impairment may be effective for a simple sales transaction or simple traffic violation. However, the use of an assistive listening device or interpreter services will usually be necessary for more complex interactions such as informed consent procedures, police questioning, or big ticket purchases such as a car or hearing aids.

Facilities that customarily provide their patrons with telephones to make outgoing calls must provide telephone access for patrons with hearing disabilities. For example, public pay telephones must include hearing aid compatible telephones with adjustable volume control, and text telephone access may need to be provided. Hospitals and lodging facilities must provide telephone and text telephone access in sleeping accommodations for people with hearing impairments (See Slager, Chapter 3; Schum & Frye-Osier, Chapter 11). Access to the full range of facility services, such as room service and housekeeping, must be available to hotel guests who use text telephones. Caption decoders or some means of caption decoding must be provided upon request in hotels and hospitals that offer television in the rooms.

Lodging facilities also must provide alerting and signaling devices in designated accessible sleeping rooms (See Garstecki, Chapter 10). Newly constructed places of lodging are required to have 8 percent of the guest rooms equipped with visual signaling devices for telephone/text telephone calls, fire/smoke alarms, and door knocks (4 percent of these rooms must be fully accessible). Existing facilities also are to meet this 8 percent standard unless an undue burden would result. Vibrotactile alerting devices, although not mandated in the current regulations, are strongly encouraged for the sleeping accommodations of people with hearing impairments.

Places of assembly and entertainment, such as convention centers, auditoriums, courtrooms, and theaters, where communication is an integral part of the facility's or room's function, must provide the communication aids and services necessary for effective communication in group settings. These aids and services may include assistive listening systems, real-time captioning/transcription, and computer-assisted notetaking. In assembly areas where there is fixed seating for 50 or more people or an audioamplification system, an assistive listening system with receivers for 4 percent of the seats (no fewer than two receivers) is required (See Crandell & Smaldino, Chapter 7).

Those public sector programs and agencies (such as public aid offices or information services of state and local governments), a significant portion of whose contact with the public is via the telephone, must make sure these services are accessible to people with hearing impairments. Public services are strongly encouraged to provide direct text telephone services. If the relay system is used, then staff members are to be appropriately trained in handling and responding to relay calls. Emergency communication services and 911 systems are required to provide direct access for users of text telephones and computer modems; they cannot rely on relay systems or third-party operators. Television and videotape programs of state and local governments must be accessible to people with hearing impairments. For example, captioning telecasts of city council meetings might be necessary.

Communication Barriers and Accessibility

Structural communication accessibility also is addressed by the ADA. In the private sector, structural communication barriers in existing facilities are to be removed, if readily achievable (i.e., easily and inexpensively accomplished given the facility's overall resources). Examples of communication barriers and readily achievable removal strategies include installing sound buffers to reduce noise and reverberation levels and installing visual signal devices for audible emergency alarms. If barrier removal is not readily achievable, then an alternative method to provide access is required. For example, partitions between customers and staff that block speech sounds are considered a barrier. If, because of security or other reasons, these barriers cannot be removed, an alternative might be to provide an assistive listening device at the counter or have staff come from behind the counter to communicate with patrons.

With an eye to the future, new construction and alterations in publicly owned facilities and in privately owned places of public accommodation and commercial facilities must follow accessibility guidelines. Eventually all facilities will be accessible. Facilities should follow the guidelines for new construction to help identify communication barriers and develop a plan for removing barriers.

Telecommunications Accessibility

The fourth regulatory area addresses telecommunications accessibility. Not all businesses or facilities are required to have text telephones. Customers and citizens who use text telephones now should have access to all of these services and programs. As of July 1993, the Title IV regulation required establishment of an intra- and interstate text telephone/voice telephone relay system to be available 24 hours a day, seven days a week. One of the features of this system is the Voice and Hearing Carry-Over service. That is, with voice carry-over, someone who has good speech but can't hear can request the operator to let the other party hear his or her voice. Only the voice information going to the person with the hearing impairment would be sent via the text telephone.

IMPLICATIONS FOR AUDIOLOGISTS

Each of these regulatory areas has implications for audiologists as professionals, as employees/employers, and as service providers. Professionals have legal obligations and responsibilities. As such, audiologists must examine their policies and practices, evaluate their program/facility accessibility, and their employment policies with respect to the ADA.

At a different level, professionals can play an important role as consultants to communities, businesses, and consumers. Each facility and program is unique in its specific communication activities and accessibility needs. Each employment setting, each job, and each employee with a hearing (or auditory-related) impairment is unique in terms of specific job requirements and accommodation needs (See Compton, Chapter 12). In addition, rapid advances in assistive technology and services continue to expand the accessibility solution options available. Determining what is most appropriate, cost-effective, and reasonable must be done on a case-by-case basis. The public and employers know little about hearing impairment, what communication accessibility means, or what appropriate accommodation strategies are available. Audiologists have the knowledge and expertise to determine cost-effective compliance strategies.

The biggest impact of the ADA on audiologists is in the area of client assessment and management. The ADA can open a new world to people with hearing disabilities. Audiologists have an obligation to inform clients about their rights and privileges under the ADA. Assessment and management strategies should take into account the person's total communication needs and should promote independent function and the highest possible quality of life at work, at home, and in the community (see Compton, Chapter 12; Sutherland, Chapter 13). Professionals who work with children must be aware of the implications of the ADA for school services, the need for advocacy in effecting necessary changes, and of the need to educate children on how to gain full participation in community and employment opportunities.

Audiologic assessment approaches need to address functional assessment. The ADA regulations for employment are based on the concept of functional ability. Disability is defined under the ADA as a substantial limitation in ability—not acuity. Determining the need for and type of accommodation requires analysis of how the individual is able to function with respect to specific job tasks. Hearing criteria for employment decisions must be based on the relationship of hearing ability to essential job functions. The determination of direct threat must consider the particular individual's abilities in the context of the specific work environment and conditions.

Audiologists are the *only* professionals capable of determining an individual's functional hearing ability, with or without assistive devices or other accommodations. This is an area where audiologists can and must assert their professional role and autonomy. Other professionals, with no expertise, have been setting criteria and making determinations about ability: for example, physicians using a "whisper test" to determine candidates' suitability as police officers.

The ADA offers a new professional challenge to audiologists. It will require us to rethink our clinical approaches, find new ways to use the assessment tools we currently have, and to develop new assessment tools. For example, how can the real-life experiences encountered by the employee be simulated in order to determine his or her ability to localize to sound or to hear speech in noise. Not all of these measures will be obtainable in a sound booth situation. Assessment will often require going to the job site and performing job task analysis. (See also Compton, Chapter 12; Garstecki, Chapter 14.)

Audiologists also should be taking a systems approach in determining the assistive devices and services, including hearing aids, that would offer the most benefit to the individual (See Compton, Chapter 12). Hearing aid and assistive device selection must consider options and features, such as telecoil switches, that provide clients with maximum communication accessibility in their community, school, and work environments.

For audiologists and people with hearing impairments, the greatest challenge and most important work lies ahead. The ADA has meaning only if it works in everyday life; if it really succeeds in changing public attitudes, policies, and practices; if it actually ends discrimination against people with disabilities in all aspects of their life; and if it makes communities and services accessible and usable for all. The comprehensiveness of ADA and the sheer number of employers and entities affected makes putting ADA into practice a monumental task. The Title III regulation alone affects more than 5 million places of public accommodation in the private sector.

To accomplish this task and assume a leadership role, audiologists must become familiar with ADA regulations and applications of state-of-the-art assistive technology and services. One source of information for audiologists is the American Speech-Language-Hearing Association (ASHA). ASHA offers ongoing ADA technical assistance and materials on ADA communication requirements. A videotape, "Communication Means Business," and written materials on ADA Titles II and III regulations developed as part of a grant from the U.S. Department of Justice are available. Other support includes the special ADA issue of Asha (June/July 1992) and a videotape, "Putting the ADA to Work For You," to educate the business community about the ADA and the services of rehabilitation professionals.

For audiologists and ASHA, our efforts must focus on implementing the ADA as smoothly and as quickly as possible; fostering the necessary partnership among consumers, the public sector, and the business community; educating our clients about their rights and opportunities; offering technical support and training; disseminating accurate ADA information; acting as consultants for business and the community; and working with consumers in advocacy.

As rehabilitation professionals, audiologists have special responsibilities related to ADA—to be leaders and role models—to go beyond the letter of the law to its spirit.

REFERENCES

Asha. (June/July 1992). The Americans with Disabilities Act. American Speech-Language-Hearing Association. Rockville, MD.

Equal Employment Opportunity Commission. (1992). *The Americans with Disabilities Act: Title I Technical Assistance Manual.* Washington, DC: Author.

Equal Employment Opportunity Commission and U.S. Department of Justice. (1991). *Americans with Disabilities Act Handbook.* Washington, DC: U.S. Government Printing Office.

Nondiscrimination on the basis of disability in state and local government services. 28 CFR Part 35.

Regulations to implement the equal employment provisions of the Americans with Disabilities Act. 29 CFR Part 1630. Appendix to part 1630—Interpretive guidance on Title I of the Americans with Disabilities Act.

U.S. Department of Justice. (1992). *The Americans with Disabilities Act: Title II Technical Assistance Manual.* Washington, DC: Author.

U.S. Department of Justice. (1992). *The Americans with Disabilities Act: Title III Technical Assistance Manual.* Washington, DC: Author.

▶ 2

An Overview of The Food and Drug Administration's Medical Device Amendments

CELESTE F. BOVÉ
Center for Devices and Radiological Health,
Food and Drug Administration

INTRODUCTION

Historical Background

The Commonwealth of Massachusetts enacted the first general food law in the United States in 1784. Other states passed similar legislation, and by 1906 almost all states had food laws. During the 1890s bills to regulate interstate commerce in foods and drugs were introduced in the Congress, but failed to pass. Dr. Harvey W. Wiley, who became Chief Chemist of the Department of Agriculture in 1883, pursued research in food and drug adulteration. In 1902, Dr. Wiley began experiments with preservatives that received wide publicity. He actually fed various preservatives to a young group of volunteers from his own staff and a nearby medical school. Journalists called these volunteers the "poison squad" and widely publicized Wiley's experiments in the press. Consequently, Theodore Roosevelt recommended food and drug legislation, and passage seemed assured. Finally, in 1906 a law was enacted to be effective the following year.

The opinions or assertions presented are the private views of the author and are not to be construed as conveying either an official endorsement or criticism by the U.S. Department of Health and Human Services, the Public Health Service, or the Food and Drug Administration.

The Food and Drugs Act of 1906 provided definitions of adulterated and misbranded foods and drugs and included provisions for seizure and criminal prosecution. After the distribution of Elixir Sulfanilamide, a drug that resulted in the death of over 100 persons, a new drug safety provision was added to the bill. Spurred by the tragic "Elixir" event, Congress enacted the Food, Drug and Cosmetic Act in 1938, but it did not include medical devices.

After World War II, many innovative developments occurred in the field of biomedical technology that resulted in the introduction of a wide variety of complicated medical devices such as cardiac pacers, artificial vessels, heart valves, new electronic hearing aid designs, intraocular lens, and surgical implants. Medical technology continued to advance, and by 1960, the Food and Drug Administration recognized that along with medical device manufacture came device failures and hazards.

Over time, the need for more comprehensive authority to regulate medical devices was recognized by Presidents Kennedy, Johnson, and Nixon. In late 1969, under President Nixon's direction, a medical device study group, the Cooper Committee[1], was convened to investigate the issue. The Cooper Committee completed its report in 1974. The report underscored the existence of problems with medical devices and stated that a predictable increase in device complexity and sophistication required action to prevent the emergence of even more serious problems in the future. The Cooper Committee recommended that legislation be enacted to address the quality of medical device usage as well as the quality of medical devices.

Medical Device Amendments

On May 28, 1976, President Gerald R. Ford signed Public Law 94-295, the Medical Device Amendments to the Food, Drug and Cosmetic Act. President Ford stated that the Amendments would eliminate outdated constraints on Food and Drug Administration authority, and enable the agency to deal with "laser age" problems in order to provide protection for the individual citizen that was otherwise unobtainable. The 1976 Amendments defined a medical device in a manner that clearly distinguished it from a drug. A medical device is:

Any instrument, apparatus, or other similar or related article, including component, part, or accessory, which is:

- recognized in the national formulary, the U.S. Pharmacopoeia, or any supplement to either;
- intended for use in the diagnosis of disease or other conditions, or in the cure, mitigation, treatment, or prevention of disease in man or other animal;

[1]The Cooper Committee, chaired by Dr. Theodore Cooper, was composed of experts in medicine and technology. Dr. Cooper was at that time the Director of the National Heart and Lung Institute and subsequently became Assistant Secretary of Health.

- intended to affect the structure or any function of the body of man or other animal; and that
- does not achieve its primary intended purpose through chemical action within or on the body of man or other animal, and which is not dependent upon being metabolized for achievement of any of its principal intended purposes.

Classification

The Food and Drug Administration regulates over 1700 generic types of medical devices. The range is broad and diverse, including simple devices such as a thermometer or toothbrush, and more complicated devices such as a cochlear implant, cardiac pacemaker, or DNA Probe and Recombinant DNA Test Kits. The Amendments enable the Food and Drug Administration to classify and regulate devices according to the risks they present based on a three-tier system. The Food and Drug Administration must classify all medical devices intended for human use into one of three regulatory categories (class I, II, or III), based on the extent of control necessary for assuring safety and effectiveness as shown below.

- Class I -   Subject to general controls
- Class II - Subject to general and special controls which may include performance standards
- Class III - Subject to premarket approval

Of the generic medical devices the Food and Drug Administration has finally classified, 40 percent are class I, 50 percent are class II, and 10 percent are class III. Class I is the least stringent regulatory category. Devices placed in this class are subject to general controls, that is, pre-existing controls that prohibit adulteration or misbranding, and additional controls from the 1976 Amendments: (1) registration of establishments and listing of products; (2) authority to ban devices; (3) requirements with respect to premarket notification and repair, replacement, or refund; (4) requirements to keep records and make reports; and, (5) requirements with respect to good manufacturing practices (GMPs). Some examples of audiological devices in class I include: acoustic chamber for audiometric testing, earphone cushion for audiometric testing, and conventional air conduction hearing aids. Fifty percent of class I devices are exempt from premarket clearance requirements.

Class II devices are products for which general controls are insufficient to assure safety and effectiveness, and which need special controls to provide such assurance. Devices placed in this category may be required to meet an applicable performance standard as prescribed by the Food and Drug Administration. Examples of class II audiological devices include bone conduction hearing aids, audiometers, auditory impedance testers, hearing aid calibrator and analysis systems, and group hearing aids or group auditory trainers.

Class III devices are those that are life-supporting or life-sustaining, are of substantial importance in preventing impairment to health, or, as a function of their potential for failure, present an unreasonable risk of illness or injury. New class III devices require premarket approval by the agency before they can be legally marketed in the United States. They are subject to the most restrictive regulation; many are designed to be implanted. An example of a class III audiological device is a cochlear implant. Such class III devices may be categorized as investigational devices (unapproved devices used on humans to collect safety and effectiveness data); transitional devices (regulated as drugs before May 28, 1976 and now regulated as class III devices requiring premarket approval); critical devices (defined in the GMP regulation as life-supporting, life-sustaining, or intended for surgical implantation, requiring additional provisions under the GMP regulation); or custom devices (not generally available or offered for commercial distribution and intended for use with a specific patient by physician/dentist).

Most medical devices have already been classified. If a device has not been classified, the Commissioner refers the device to the appropriate classification panel, which reviews the device for safety and effectiveness. Each classification panel is comprised of persons who are qualified by training and experience to evaluate the devices and who, to the extent feasible, possess skill in the use of, or experience in the development, manufacture, or utilization of, such devices. In reviewing evidence concerning the safety and effectiveness of a device, the panel requires valid scientific evidence. Safety is defined in Title 21 of the Code of Federal Regulations §860.7 (d)(1) as reasonable assurance that a device is safe when it can be determined, based upon valid scientific evidence, that the probable benefits to health from the use of the device for its intended uses and conditions of use, when accompanied by adequate directions and warnings against unsafe use, outweigh any probable risks. Effectiveness is also defined in Title 21 of the Code of Federal Regulations §860.7 (e)(1) with the statement that there is reasonable assurance that a device is effective when it can be determined, based upon valid scientific evidence, that in a significant portion of the target population, the use of the device for its intended uses and conditions of use, when accompanied by adequate directions and warnings against unsafe use, will provide clinically significant results.

Advisory Panels

For the classification of medical devices, the Food and Drug Administration has enlisted, and continues to enlist, the aid of sixteen advisory panels of experts. Each panel consists of eight members appointed by the agency for three years. An individual advisory panel has its own executive secretary, who is a full-time employee from the Office of Device Evaluation, within the Center for Devices and Radiological Health. The Executive Secretary oversees the function of the panel and is responsible for selecting panel members, setting agendas, and publishing results of panel meetings. The panel has six voting members selected from research and medical fields and two non-voting members, one from industry and one representing consumer interests.

The panels are responsible for: (1) classifying old devices, i.e., those on the market prior to the 1976 Amendments; (2) reviewing premarket approval applications for new devices; (3) reviewing petitions for reclassification; (4) assisting in the review of premarket approval applications or investigations device exemption (IDE) submissions; and (5) reviewing product-development protocols. *Ear, nose, and throat* medical devices are the responsibility of one of the current 16 advisory medical panels:

1. anesthesiology and respiratory therapy devices
2. clinical chemistry and clinical toxicology devices
3. circulatory systems devices
4. dental devices and products
5. ear, nose, and throat devices
6. gastroenterology-urology devices
7. general and plastic surgery devices
8. general hospital and personal use devices
9. hematology and pathology devices
10. immunology devices
11. microbiology devices
12. neurology devices
13. obstetrics-gynecology devices
14. ophthalmic devices
15. orthopedic and rehabilitation devices
16. radiology devices

Division of Small Manufacturers Assistance

As indicated by the large number of advisory panels, the medical device industry is very diverse in both the extent and types of manufacturers represented, which range from large conglomerates to small garage operations. In recognition of the unusual character of the medical device industry, the Amendments mandated an identifiable office to provide technical and other non-financial assistance to small manufacturers of medical devices to assist them in complying with the requirements of the Food, Drug and Cosmetic Act.

Consequently, the Food and Drug Administration founded the Division of Small Manufacturers Assistance in response to the requirement. The Division of Small Manufacturers Assistance has a toll-free telephone number (1-800-638-2041/within Maryland, 301-443-6597) which medical device establishment personnel may call for information or advice to assure compliance with the Food, Drug and Cosmetic Act. The Division of Small Manufacturers Assistance also conducts workshops on a nationwide basis to address premarket and good manufacturing practices topics.

Safe Medical Devices Act of 1990

The 1976 Medical Device Amendments have been modified, and some new provisions added, with the enactment of Safe Medical Devices Act and Medical Device Amendments of 1992, signed into law on November 28, 1990 and June 16, 1992, respectively. The new provisions were added to better assure that devices entering the market are safe and effective, that the Food and Drug Administration can learn quickly about serious device problems, and that the Food and Drug Administration can more easily remove defective devices from the market.

Under the Safe Medical Devices Act, enforcement authority, the Food and Drug Administration, can: 1) order manufacturers to cease distribution of a device immediately and/or to notify health professionals/facilities to cease use; 2) temporarily suspend premarket application approval; and 3) assess civil penalties.

The Safe Medical Devices Act and the 1992 Amendments provided the Food and Drug Administration with new regulatory controls in the following areas: 1) classification; 2) premarket approval; 3) registration and listing; 4) good manufacturing practices; 5) inspections (Section 704); 6) biennial inspections (Section 510[h]); 7) detention; 8) banning; 9) repair or replacement of, or refund for, a defective device; 10) restriction of devices; and, 11) presumption of interstate commerce.

The Safe Medical Devices Act premarket regulations require applicants to submit summaries of adverse safety and effectiveness data for class III pre-Amendments devices still under premarket notification 510(k) provisions, and also require summaries of safety and effectiveness for 510(k) products. The Safe Medical Devices Act postmarket provisions require: 1) medical device user facilities to report incidents that reasonably suggest that a device has contributed to a death, serious injury, or serious illness of a patient; 2) distributors to report under Medical Device Reporting (MDR), that is, report when information suggests that one of their marketed devices may have caused or contributed to a death, serious injury, or serious illness; 3) manufacturers, distributors, and importers to certify the number of Medical Device Reporting incidents submitted to the Food and Drug Administration; 4) manufacturers, distributors, and importers to report removal and corrections to the Food and Drug Administration; 5) manufacturers to establish procedures for tracking devices; and 6) manufacturers to conduct postmarket surveillance studies on devices introduced after January 1, 1991, that are permanent implants or life-sustaining, life-supporting devices used outside a health facility (studies on other types of devices can be required at the Agency's discretion).

ASSISTIVE LISTENING DEVICES

On October 26, 1990, the Food and Drug Administration Advisory Panel for Ear, Nose, and Throat Devices met to consider and recommend classification for nine medical devices, one of which was an assistive listening device. As part of the deliberative process for the classification and definition for assistive listening devices for hearing-impaired individuals, the Advisory Panel for Ear, Nose, and Throat Devices reviewed all of the classification regulations and some of the previously promulgated definitions for other audiological medical devices. Those definitions are given below, and are presented as they were originally published in the *Federal Register* on November 6, 1986; they also can be found in Title 21 of the Code of Federal Regulations Part 874—Ear, Nose, and Throat Devices. If these "identifications" appear somewhat dated, remember that the device definitions were originally generated during the late 1970s.

Definitions

§ 874.3300 Hearing aid.
   (a) Identification. A hearing aid is a wearable sound-amplifying device that is intended to compensate for impaired hearing. This generic type of device includes the air-conduction hearing aid and the bone-conduction hearing aid, but excludes the group hearing aid or group auditory trainer, master hearing aid, and tinnitus masker.
   (b) Classification. (1) Class I for the air-conduction hearing aid. (2) Class II for the bone-conduction hearing aid.

§ 874.3320 Group hearing aid or group auditory trainer.
   (a) Identification. A group hearing aid or group auditory trainer is a hearing aid that is intended for use in communicating simultaneously with one or more listeners having hearing impairment. The device is used with an associated transmitter microphone. It may be either monaural or binaural, and it provides coupling to the ear through earphones or earmolds. The generic type of device includes three types of applications: hardwire systems, inductance loop systems, and wireless systems.
   (b) Classification. Class II.

Advisory Panel Recommendations

On October 26, 1990, as part of the Food and Drug Administration process of classification, the Ear, Nose, and Throat Advisory Panel recommended that the device category be renamed to that of "assistive devices for the hearing-impaired," which would include the category of assistive listening devices. The panel discussed the definition at length and considered several approaches to defining this broad device category.

   In view of the wide disparity of products categorized as assistive devices, members of the advisory panel expressed concern that purchasers of such devices understand what they are buying and the benefits they can hope to gain from them. The panel agreed that these concerns would be best addressed via labeling.

   Among the labeling recommendations proffered by the panel was a warning that maximum sound pressure level exceeding 132 decibels may result in hearing damage. The panel also noted that the sound pressure level of 132 decibels may be too high and needs examination.

Recommended Definition and Classification

The advisory panel voted to recommend the following device definition for an assistive device for the hearing-impaired:

> Assistive devices not elsewhere classified that deliver signals to hearing-impaired persons to mitigate problems associated with hearing loss. Some types of assistive devices may be used in conjunction with personal hearing aids. Assistive device products come in many forms and may include the following:

- Signaling devices.
- Listening devices (used to deliver sound to the hearing-impaired listener's ear and overcome the problems of background noise and distance; devices have personal use and a wide area of applications and consist of such things as induction loop systems, personal amplifiers with microphones and receivers, and infrared and frequency modulated [FM] transmitters and receivers).
- Telecommunication devices (used for telephone communication, including such things as amplified handsets, portable telephone amplifiers (acoustic and electromagnetic), and telecommunication devices for the deaf.
- Television devices (e.g., closed captioning devices).
- Hearing aids and vibrotactile devices are excluded.

The panel chairperson appointed a subcommittee of advisory panel members and consultants to work with the Food and Drug Administration and to examine any devices in this category in need of additional labeling pertaining to distribution.

The advisory panel unanimously recommended that an "assistive device for the hearing-impaired" be placed in class I. Why is it important whether a device is classified into class I or class II? There are two main considerations: 1) Class I indicates that general controls are sufficient to assure safety and effectiveness, that is, technical or performance specifications are not necessary, whereas class II devices need special controls (e.g., performance standards or technical specifications) to provide assurance of safety and effectiveness; and 2) every registered establishment engaging in the manufacture, preparation, propagation, compounding, or processing of a drug or a device classified in class II or III shall be inspected at least once in the two-year period beginning with the date of registration of such establishment, and at least once in every successive two-year period thereafter (Food, Drug and Cosmetic Act §510.[360](b)-(h)). In comparison, class I device manufacturers, although still subject to inspection, have no mandated inspection schedule. Therefore, it is very important to have device labeling requirements that will assure the safety and effectiveness of these devices.

HEARING AID REGULATION

Since assistive listening devices and hearing aids are both types of amplification devices, it is important to be aware of current hearing aid regulatory actions. Beginning in April 1993, the Food and Drug Administration sent warning letters to hearing aid manufacturers concerning misleading and unsubstantiated advertising claims involving user benefit, especially the ability to understand speech in noisy listening environments. Subsequently, David A. Kessler, M.D., Commissioner, Food and Drug Administration, publicly stated that the current hearing aid dispensing system was not working, and that the Agency is taking steps to revise and update the 1977 hearing aid regulations (21 CFR §801.420 and .421) in order to improve patient care.

The proposed revised regulation would govern the sale and distribution of hearing aids and would improve patient care by establishing a new regulatory framework to correct two major shortfalls in the current regulation:

1. The current regulation permits an adult purchaser to waive the requirement to see a physician for a hearing evaluation prior to the sale of a hearing aid (this waiver has been widely used and has resulted in too many hearing aid purchasers not being properly evaluated prior to hearing aid purchase and use); and,
2. The regulation limits the authority to conduct the hearing evaluation to physicians (who may or may not be competent) to conduct the appropriate battery of tests.

In addition, the proposed revised hearing aid regulation would improve patient care by doing away with the medical waiver (there would be no exemptions or exceptions) and by requiring:

- The establishment of minimum qualifications for a comprehensive diagnostic hearing assessment in order to establish hearing aid candidacy, and
- The establishment of minimum qualifications for hearing aid evaluation, i.e., selection, fitting, and/or dispensing.

The proposed revised regulation states that the hearing aid professionals must be state licensed. Therefore, the regulation will be designed to give the states the licensing responsibility of deciding which health care professionals are qualified to conduct a comprehensive hearing assessment to determine hearing aid candidacy and which professionals are qualified to conduct a hearing aid evaluation to select, fit, and dispense a hearing aid.

On November 10, 1993, FDA announced a public hearing on an advance notice of proposed rule making that outlined the agency's intention to revise the federal hearing aid regulation. At the public hearing on December 6–7, FDA solicited comments on all aspects of the 1977 hearing aid regulation and also asked for comment on eight specific issues involving hearing aid assessment, purchase, and consumer access:

1. The minimum components of a comprehensive hearing assessment;
2. The minimum qualifications that health professionals should possess to perform a comprehensive hearing assessment;
3. Any waiver conditions;
4. Mail order purchase of hearing aids;
5. Prohibition of hearing aid sale by person performing pre-purchase evaluation;
6. Licensure requirement;
7. Current number of persons qualified to perform pre-purchase examinations and geographic distribution; and
8. Impact of proposed regulation on consumer access to hearing aid distributors.
* In addition, any information documenting consumer use of the pre-purchase medical waiver.

The time period to comment on the proposed hearing aid regulations closed on January 10, 1994. Since then, FDA has been busy reviewing all of the written information and the public hearing testimony (FDA received over 3000 written comments). Next, FDA completes a summary of the comments and the public hearing testimony, drafts its response to the comments for the proposed rule, and completes a "draft" proposed rule. Subsequent to various clearances, including clearance from the Office of Management and Budget, FDA will publish the proposed rule and give a 90-day comment period.

It is important that audiologists take an active role in the development of future hearing aid regulations. These regulations will cover hearing aids, but there needs to be a recognized definition for a hearing aid that differentiates it from an assistive listening device, perhaps by intended use or design. Audiologists, both as part of professional organizations and as individuals, need to address the need for clear device and assessment definitions.

IMPLICATIONS FOR AUDIOLOGY

As of this writing, The Food and Drug Administration has not yet published proposed regulations classifying an assistive device for the hearing-impaired. How does all of this impact audiology? Hearing aids are a restrictive device, that is, analogous to prescriptive devices where there are federal regulations that place specific restrictions on the sale of hearing aids. However, there are also devices resembling personal hearing aids that are sold through the mail or over-the-counter that do not have to adhere to any conditions for sale, because they are sold as assistive devices. Are auditory trainers that are no longer just used in the classroom, but used as a full-time personal amplification devices, still auditory trainers or hearing aids or assistive devices?

Some hearing health care professionals consider a hearing aid to be a "prescriptive" or "custom" device that is fitted to an individual's specific auditory abilities and intended for full-time use, while an assistive device is designed for the hearing-impaired population in general, and for use on an occasional or less than full-time basis. Others have stated that if the amplification device is worn somewhere on the body, it is a hearing aid and should be regulated under the more stringent hearing aid labeling and conditions for sale regulations. Audiologists and hearing aid dispensers fit both types of devices, and some of the assistive devices are also sold over the counter.

The terminology for varying and overlapping amplification situations (conditions of use) often creates problems for health care professionals and insurance companies. It has been documented that some audiologists fit patients with assistive devices for use at home and not just in educational or training settings; some even fit individuals with normal hearing with assistive devices to help with listening tasks in certain situations.

What should delimit a device's name or conditions for sale? Should the acoustical specifications of the instrument, the location on the body, or the intended use of the instrument define its name and conditions of sale? The definition given earlier for the determination of a device's effectiveness is when, in a significant portion of the target population, the use of the device for its intended uses and conditions of use, when accompanied by adequate directions and warnings against unsafe use, will provide clinically significant results. It is impractical to think that a manufacturer would have to submit information to cover all of the possible intended uses and the device could be regulated accordingly. This situation will not be simple to resolve.

It is important to emphasize that the issue here is not whether assistive devices for the hearing-impaired are medical devices—*they are medical devices*—but how to properly identify the devices, the labeling that should be required to accompany each device, and the conditions for sale. When the Food and Drug Administration requests comment regarding the hearing aid regulations, this will be an opportunity to provide input regarding the following issues:

- The difference between a hearing aid and an assistive listening device for the hearing-impaired (including a definition of an assistive listening device for the hearing-impaired);
- The difference between an auditory trainer, an assistive listening device, and a hearing aid; and
- Sample labeling (including user brochure and conditions for sale information) which should accompany a hearing aid, an assistive listening device, and an auditory trainer.

As part of the federal rulemaking process, written comments may be submitted to:

Dockets Management Branch (HFA-305)
Food and Drug Administration, Room 1-23
12420 Parklawn Drive
Rockville, Maryland 20857

REFERENCES

Code of Federal Regulations, Food and Drugs, Section 21, Parts 800 to 1299. Revised as of April 1, 1992.

Federal Register. Department of Health and Human Services, Food and Drug Administration, Medical Devices; Ear, Nose, and Throat Devices, Final Rule, Proposed Rule and Withdrawal of Proposed Rules. Vol. 51, No. 215, Thursday, November 6, 1986, pp. 40377-40397.

Food and Drug Administration, U.S. Public Health Service. Summary Minutes of the Thirty-fifth Meeting of the Ear, Nose, and Throat Devices Panel, October 25-26, 1990.

Food and Drug Administration, prepared by Office of Training and Assistance, Division of Small Manufacturers Assistance. Highlights of the Safe Medical Devices Act of 1990 (Public Law 101-629), FDA 91-4243, August 1991.

GLOSSARY

Terms and Definitions

Component   (21 CFR 820.3) Any material, substance, piece, part, or assembly used during device manufacture which is intended to be included in the finished device.

Medical Device   Any instrument, apparatus, or other similar or related article, including component, part, or accessory, which is:

- recognized in the national formulary, the U.S. Pharmacopoeia or any supplement to either;
- intended for use in the diagnosis of disease or other conditions, or in the cure, mitigation, treatment, or prevention of disease in man or other animal;
- intended to affect the structure or any function of the body of man or other animal; and that
- does not achieve its primary intended purpose through chemical action within or on the body of man or other animal, and which is not dependent upon being metabolized for achievement of any of its principal intended purposes.

FD & C Act   (21 CFR 52.3, 54.3, 58.3, 110.3, 210.3) The Federal Food, Drug and Cosmetic Act, as amended (§ 201–902, 1040 et seq., as amended), (21 USC 321–392), also referred to in the text as the "act".

Finished Device   (21 CFR 820.3) A device, or any accessory to a device, which is suitable for use, whether or not packaged or labeled for commercial distribution.

Labeling   All labels and other written, printed, or graphic matter upon any article or any of its containers or wrappers, or accompanying such article.

Manufacturer   Any person, including any repacker and/or relabeler, who manufactures, fabricates, assembles, or processes a finished device. The term does not include any person who only distributes a finished device.

Misbranding   If an article is alleged to be misbranded because the labeling or advertising is misleading, then in determining whether the labeling or advertising is misleading there shall be taken into account (among other things) not only representations made or suggested by statement, word, design, device, or any combination thereof, but also the extent to which labeling or advertising fails to reveal facts material in light of such representations or material with respect to consequences which may result from the use of the article to which the labeling or advertising relates under the conditions of use prescribed in the labeling or advertising thereof or under such conditions of use as are customary or usual.

HEARING AID REGULATION CHRONOLOGY

In the *Federal Register* of February 15, 1977 (42 FR 9286), FDA promulgated a regulation that established the provisions for the sale and distribution of hearing aids. The regulation (21 CFR 801.420 and .421) prescribed the types of information that must be included in the labeling; ensured that health professionals have adequate information to select, fit, and repair a hearing aid for a patient; and restricted the sale of a hearing aid to patients who have undergone a medical evaluation within the past six months. The regulation also allowed any informed adult, eighteen years of age or older, to waive the medical evaluation requirement by signing a written statement. Several events developed that caused FDA to reevaluate the regulatory framework governing the sale and distribution of hearing aids.

Vermont Petition

- *July 21, 1989*   The state of Vermont submitted an application requesting exemption from federal preemption for one provision (§ 3283a) of a state statute (Act No. 60) that requires a physician evaluation for all first-time purchasers of hearing aids; no waiver option allowed. Vermont requested the exemption based on results of a state survey of hearing aid dispensers that suggested abuse of the medical waiver.
- *April 9, 1991*   FDA held a public hearing on hearing aids. Testimony indicated that the use of medical waivers for hearing aid sales was being abused. During the hearing, FDA's Boston District presented findings from its January 1991 survey of hearing aid sales by Vermont dispensers. Results indicated that there were no waivers or physicians' statements for 60 percent of first time hearing aid users.
- *October 14, 1993*   FDA sent a letter to Vermont indicating agreement on the medical waiver issue, but that the pre-purchase hearing evaluation should not be limited to physicians (no exemption was granted).

Revising the Hearing Aid Regulations

- *April 16, 1993*   Based on information that hearing aid manufacturers were making unsubstantiated user-benefit performance claims that mislead the public by creating unrealistic expectations about hearing aid performance, FDA sent warning letters to hearing aid manufacturers. The warning letter directing the hearing aid industry to review and correct their promotional literature and advertising.

- *July 2, 1993* Dr. Kessler held a meeting to brief the hearing aid industry and the hearing health care professional organizations concerning recent and proposed action involving hearing aids. During the meeting he discussed the recent warning letters that FDA sent to the hearing aid industry concerning misleading and unsubstantiated advertising. He also said that in the future FDA would propose revisions to the hearing aid regulation to improve patient care.
- *November 10, 1993* The Advanced Notice of Proposed Rule Making (ANPRM) announcing the agency's plan to revise the Federal hearing aid regulation and notice of the Part 15 Public Hearing was published in the *Federal Register*. The major components of the ANPRM included improvements for regulating hearing aid devices: (1) a clear requirement for a hearing evaluation before the purchase of a hearing aid to determine hearing aid candidacy, (2) a requirement that both the hearing evaluation for hearing aid candidacy and the hearing aid assessment for selecting/dispensing a hearing aid be conducted by a qualified health professional, and (3) the requirement that the health professionals who conduct the evaluations would be licensed by the states.
- *December 6 and 7, 1993* FDA conducted the Part 15 Public Hearing on hearing aids in Rockville, MD. An FDA panel listened to testimony presented by manufacturers, audiologists, physicians, dispensers, consumers, and consumer interest groups.
- *January 10, 1994* The comment period to the ANPRM closed. FDA received and reviewed over three thousand comments. After review of the ANPRM background information, comments received on the ANPRM, and testimony from the public hearing, the agency decided to revise the hearing aid regulations. FDA has stated that imposing more stringent requirements will not be preempted if the agency's proposed regulations become final. The final proposed rule is tentatively due out of the Center by Fall, 1994.
- *June 27 and 28, 1994* FDA's Ear, Nose, and Throat (ENT) Devices Advisory Panel convened in Silver Spring, MD, to discuss a proposed protocol for the clinical trials of hearing aids to substantiate manufacturers' user-benefit claims. The draft protocol is intended to give guidance for gathering clinical data to substantiate claims for improved hearing in background noise. Manufacturers would develop their own protocols for other types of user-benefit claims. The advisory panel recommended that the term "acclimatization effects" should not be included in the protocol; the term should be replaced with "learning effects." The meeting did not address in what situations and with what types of substantiation a 510(k) premarket notification is required.

Acknowledgements

I want to thank the Division of Small Manufacturers Assistance staff, especially Ronald P. Parr, for providing information on the Safe Medical Devices Act.

I also want to acknowledge the use of historical and glossary information from the Food and Drug Administration's Basic Food and Drug Law Course manual of 1988.

▶ 3

Interfacing with the Telephone System

RONALD D. SLAGER
*Vice President, Hearing Aid Center of Kalamazoo
and HARC Mercantile, Ltd.*

By root definition, the word TELEPHONE means sending a sound over distance. Tele = Distance; Phone = Sound.

The need to communicate ranks third in the list of basic human desires; third behind the will to live and the need for sustenance, food and water. The human ability to communicate over great distances has been unique among the various species, and has contributed to the dominance of humans over other animals.

Over the years the scheme remained the same; only technology changed.

In the Romans' quest to conquer the world, swift communications from the battlefields to or from one battle force to another were essential. As the empire grew, its *modus communicus* could not keep pace. The distances and terrain stretched the communications network beyond its limits. As the Romans' lines of communication broke down, so did their lines of supply.

The need for communications from home to the front was not just for tactical advantages: That link to home played an important psychological role in the morale of the ranks. So Rome failed in its quest for the world. Since then other cultures have tried and failed; each, however, reaching further out as communication capabilities improved, expanding the envelope of civilization.

As Britain expanded its kingdom across the oceans, it lost its rapid communicative interchange and had to give up its claim to the new territories, such as the colonies in North America and Australia. With the advent of the telegraph, which allowed the transmission of messages via wires using simple unmodulated electric impulses, vast expanses of land were tied together. With the development of transoceanic telegraph lines, the British Empire could again expand; this time with a communications lifeline stretching across the waters.

In 1876, 100 years after the United States became independent from British rule, Alexander Graham Bell was granted a United States patent (Figure 3-1) for the telephone. Little did he know what importance his invention would have on the world. The technology Bell used in his telephone would be used by him later to develop the first electric hearing aid. This was said to have been his quest from the start in an effort to help his profoundly hearing-disabled mother.

The telephone would mark the beginning of what was to become two of the world's largest and most powerful companies. About the same time as Bell's inven-

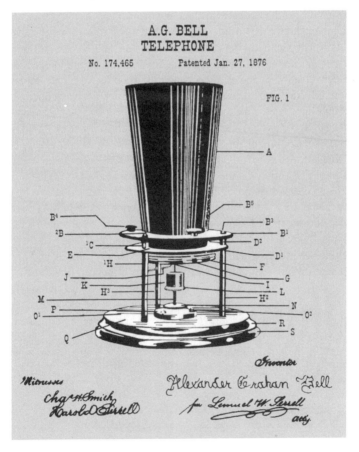

FIGURE 3-1   **A.G. Bell's original telephone patent**

(Courtesy HARC Mercantile, Ltd.)

tion was gaining momentum in the United States, Germany's Werner Von Siemens was developing the telephone for most of Europe. Today both companies reign as the leaders in telecommunications and other high-tech electrical equipment. Both companies have built, or still build, hearing aids. Bell/Western Electric dropped out of the hearing aid manufacturing business in the 1950s. Siemens is today one of the world's largest hearing aid manufacturers.

Bell's original telephone company grew not only to build and specify equipment but also to control the service of signal distribution (the actual call). During this company's reign, the telephone grew to become the heart of the twentieth century. The 975 million miles of wire strung on some 21 million poles, half a million miles of underground cable, a quarter of a million miles linked by microwave relay stations, and dozens of communication satellites orbiting the earth became its arteries. The telephone company was the pulse of the nation and the world.

As the nation and the world became more dependent on the telephone, a segment of the population gradually became more isolated in a world that was getting even smaller. How could this happen in this day and age? It's quite simple. Just think about it. Those being isolated are persons with hearing and auditory perception problems. The simplest telephone conversation becomes a difficult experience because they cannot hear, or, more importantly, understand the caller. Why is something not being done? The answer is, some things have been done, but only aggressively for less than 25 years.

Before 1968, American Telephone and Telegraph Company (AT&T) had a monopoly on the telecommunications market, allowing only its products to be attached to AT&T lines. It was even forbidden to attach shoulder rests or other nonmechanical items to a phone instrument if they had not been provided by AT&T.

For all intents and purposes, AT&T was the only game in town, even though there were some 1500 independent telephone companies operating in the United States. Most of these independents were small, local, rural companies handling one or two exchanges, and they did not manufacture equipment. They just provided the telephone lines. While products were being created for the masses, and high technology equipment for business and industry, the needs of hearing-impaired people were more or less only a second thought. The hard-of-hearing and deaf marketplace simply was not large enough to warrant much attention or produce much revenue. A token amount of effort was made in some limited areas. For example, the first telecommunication devices for the deaf (TDDs) were old teletype machines formerly used in industry and business as telephone amplifiers, and were hand-me-downs from the noisy office or machine shop.

THE CARTER DECISION

The 1968 Carter Phone Decision changed the face of telecommunications when it allowed products not manufactured by AT&T to be used on AT&T lines, provided proper precautions were taken to protect the integrity of the system. In the aftermath of the decision, the floodgates were opened wide. Now, private industry and special interest groups, such as the hearing-disabled, could pursue the development of products designed for their specific needs, and, more importantly, they could market them independently of the telephone company. Since that decision, there has been a proliferation of products—some acceptable, some excellent, and some not worth mentioning. We have seen a wide array of telephones reach the marketplace, ranging in price from $7.95 to $795.00.

Although the Carter Phone Decision made room for new products to reach the buying public, it also created a market flooded with various new telephones and accessories, many of which were not being built to any specific standards—telephones put in everything from automobiles to shoes, and even telephones that moo. These less-than-quality products are being taken home and installed by less-than-qualified technicians, increasing the potential for degradation of the overall system. The mass market has embraced the new "bells and whistles," but has ignored the established specifications and standards that made the system work so well in the past. The companies providing the wires, poles, and switches, AT&T or one of the "Baby Bell" companies, have lost control of what products are connected to their telephone lines. As a result, there is no way of predicting how the system will perform on a given line in a given exchange or individual phone number. Ultimately, the end user now appears to be responsible for his or her own telephone's performance. This is a difficult task because the lack of an enforceable standard makes it difficult to determine compatibility and performance of new assistive products, that is, telephone amplifiers. In addition, it is hit or miss as to whether a given telephone amplifier will work on a particular telephone in a given area. This is because a telephone's performance could depend on its location.

When clients come in, they should be asked to describe how their telephone sounds and what the perception of their problem seems to be. It must be determined whether they have a problem with only certain telephones, telephones in certain locations, or with telephones in general. The first step may not be amplification; rather a new telephone instrument may be in order.

THE TELEPHONE TRANSMISSION SYSTEM

For the hearing disabled, assistive products or devices include not only products for carrying on a conversation, but also alerting products such as louder ringers, light flashers, or strobes. It only makes sense that a means of carrying on a conversation would not do much good if the phone never got answered because no one knew it was ringing. Before things can be attached to the phone line, a basic understanding and respect of the phone transmission system is required.

Telephone Subassemblies

Every telephone consists of three subassemblies: the speech network, the dialing mechanism, and the ringer. All are capable of independent operation. These parts,

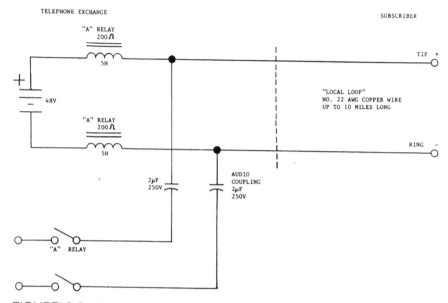

FIGURE 3-2   **Schematic of telephone line**

(Courtesy HARC Mercantile, Ltd.)

together or separately, along with other devices, such as telephone answering machines or modems, all attach to the telephone line (Figure 3-2).

Signal Distribution

All functions of the telephone are handled by a pair of small, twisted copper wires. The ring signal, as well as the voltage to operate the telephone instrument and the voice transmission, are sent down these wires. Two to four additional wires may be used to carry assorted features, such as a second line or a 7-volt direct current (DC) to illuminate the dial on a telephone. This DC power is converted to AC by a transformer, plugged into an electrical outlet somewhere in the subscriber's house. Party lines also use the extra wires to carry the other subscriber's lines. Knowing which two wires the phone is to be attached to is only the start. Another important question is, Is there enough power to actually operate the telephone and any attachments to it?

At the telephone company's local exchange, where the call is switched and routed, 48 volts of DC power are applied to those two small wires that complete the telephone line. These runs of wires from the local exchange are called local loops and vary from 1 to 10 miles in length, the average being 3 miles long. The length of loop greatly affects the available power for a telephone's operation. The longer the loop, the greater the resistance and the less available current there is available for the telephone and its attachments. The telephone company assures that no lower current than about 20 milliamps will be provided, which is about the amount available in a long local loop. By comparison, a short loop will allow a draw of 60 to 80 milliamps, so the difference can be as much as 60 milliamps, or 75 percent less current available in a long loop. This is a dramatic difference. The average loop provides about 35 milliamps. A standard carbon bell telephone can operate with currents as low as 14 milliamps, but not well. For a new solid-state telephone, there is just not enough power to operate when current levels decrease to less than 20 milliamps. In fact, some supposedly "high-gain" amplified replacement handsets tend not to function well, if at all, when connected to a telephone on a long loop, because they require more power to function compared with a regular non-amplified handset. These details are important to remember because they affect the performance of certain amplification devices and are not within the equipment vendor's or the user's control. Knowing this will avoid product performance misrepresentation.

One should be aware that the telephone line's impedance is affected not only by the length of the local loop, but also by the method of delivering the loop (buried cable or aerial delivery). For most applications, the impedance is assumed to be 300 to 900 ohms. If the instrument attached is of the wrong impedance, a mismatch occurs that can result in an echo and a whistling—which owners of cheap telephones, where appearances are more important than electronics, have come to expect.

A telephone line has a balanced feed with each side equally balanced to ground. Any imbalance can introduce hum or noise into a telephone line. This can be annoying to normal-hearing listeners, but it can be a major obstacle to speech recognition for hearing-disabled listeners. If an imbalance or impedance mismatch exists and any kind of amplification device is attached to the telephone, the competing noise will only be made louder.

In summary, there are several factors that may impact on the potential for successful amplification of voice transmission on the telephone. They are (1) length of local loop, (2) telephone type, (3) instrument impedance mismatch between the instrument line, and (4) line balance.

The Speech Network

The speech network's function is twofold: to take the incoming electrical signal from the remote party and convert it to an acoustic signal in the earpiece; and, in turn, to transduce the talker's acoustic signal from the microphone into an electrical signal to be transmitted back down the line.

Before the Carter Decision, a standard network, called the loop compensation (LC) device, was used worldwide. This network utilizes a carbon microphone. However, today, a variety of networks using integrated circuits or discrete transistors have become commonplace. Many telephones no longer use carbon microphones or coil-wound receivers that create the inductive field that allows the coupling of hearing aids with telecoil circuitry.

Whereas the old standard loop compensation network is not voltage sensitive and will continue to operate as voltage is reduced, many newer transistorized telephones cease working as power approaches 3 to 4 volts and seldom pass high enough levels of power through to the handset to enable line-driven amplification. The 48 volts, referred to as the amount of power applied to the line at the local exchange, drops to between 9 and 3 volts, depending on the length of the loop, when the telephone is taken off the hook. If another telephone in parallel is taken off the hook at the same time, the voltage will drop even further.

Original AT&T specifications require that three telephones should work in parallel on a 20 mA loop. Most of today's transistorized telephones tend not to pass this test individually, let alone in parallel with any other instrument.

Telephones utilizing the standard loop compensation network also have a built-in loop compensation feature that adjusts the receiver and transmitter levels to provide a constant intensity level, regardless of variations of voltage levels caused by the length of the local loop. Most solid-state telephones lack this loop compensation feature. They have been designed to provide adequate intensity levels on the average loop only, meaning that they will provide insufficient intensity levels on long loops and excessive intensity levels on short loops (See Signal Distribution).

Another point to remember is that the telephone is designed to produce "side-tone." A certain amount of the caller's voice signal is fed back into the earpiece for voice monitoring purposes. A weak side-tone tends to make the user talk louder; too much makes the user talk softer. Balance is critical. Again, solid-state telephones without loop compensation will affect the perception of side-tone, depending on the current levels, causing problems for the user.

Multiline Systems

The effects of the telephone company's local loop, impedance matching, line balance, and phone construction are of great significance in the application of assistive devices to single-line telephones. Multiline systems, such as those found in most business and institutions, have their own unique set of problems. In these systems, the effect of the power from the local loop is not as much a factor because this "in-house" system or "mini exchange" creates its own local loop with its own power supply and properly matched equipment. In turn, its output is patched into the telephone company's loop by a properly designed matching bridge.

The old-style multiline office telephone system uses mechanical relays and carbon bell telephones, which are easily adaptable for use with telephone assistive listening and alerting devices because the telephones' power supply provides ample power for the ring, buzz, and talk path and provides an analog signal.

The new multiline office telephone system (Figures 3-3 and 3-4), the "digital key system" (computer chip technology), is fully solid state, a true departure from carbon/bell phones, and its key switching unit distributes calls for any number of incoming lines down a single pair of wires to the instrument. It is capable of many functions,

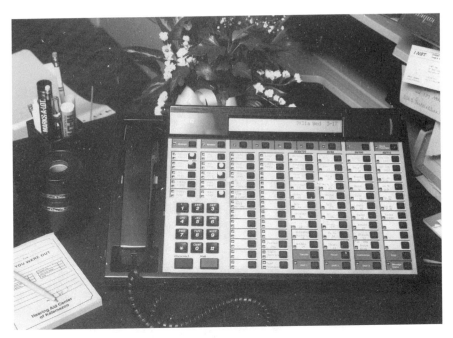

FIGURE 3-3   **Switchboard console for digital key phone system**

(Courtesy HARC Mercantile, Ltd.)

such as speed dialing, which allows a preprogrammed number to be dialed with a single key stroke; teleconferencing, which allows multiple callers to talk to one another; and call forwarding. However, this technology makes the addition of amplification or the direct connection of teletext a nightmare. It also causes problems concerning the compatibility of the system's telephones with hearing aids equipped with telecoils. Some manufacturers of amplification devices provide a listing of what key telephone systems they know their equipment will work with and can be consulted before making a recommendation. Otherwise, it is trial and error to find a workable solution.

Generally, in-line amplifiers, amplification devices that connect between a phone base network and the handset, have their own power source, and tend to work more often on these systems than do "line power" devices, such as replacement receivers, which are dependent on voltage being passed on to the receiver because the amplifier circuit has a consistent source of power.

If the system's telephone receivers are not hearing-aid compatible, and if its design will not allow a hearing-aid compatible receiver to be attached, there are portable, acoustically coupled induction amplifiers available. An induction amplifier increases the strength of the electromagnetic field as opposed to making a sound louder.

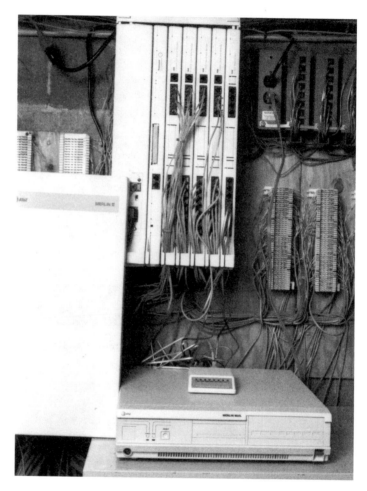

FIGURE 3-4 **KSU and switching network for digital key phone system**

(Courtesy HARC Mercantile, Ltd.)

The digital key system's manufacturer or distributor might be consulted for the availability of modems (Figure 3-5), switchers, or interfaces that would allow the direct connection of a teletext to the system.

The Home Phone or Single Line Phone

Whether a client's need is for a private single-line telephone or for a multiline system, a general understanding of how the telephone system works is important.

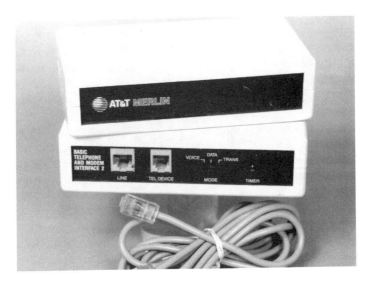

FIGURE 3-5   **Analog modem and interface for digital key phone system**

(Courtesy HARC Mercantile, Ltd.)

TELEPHONE ASSISTIVE DEVICES AND THEIR APPLICATIONS

Also important is familiarity with the various ways a telephone can be made accessible to a hearing-disabled person, despite the inherent problems that exist with today's telephone systems. The following is a general overview of these different classifications of telephone assistive devices and their potential applications.

Alerting Devices

One of the most important areas of telecommunication is alerting the user of an incoming call. Since the late 1970s the U.S. phone companies, headed by AT&T, began a standardization of phone connectors. Post-network phone connectors are coil cords and handsets, Pre-network connectors are line jacks, cords, and phone electronics. The RJ11 jack and plug are now the standard means of attaching telephones, modem, fax, and alerting products to the local loop (Figures 3-6 and 3-7). Most of the products on the market have these direct connection capabilities.

Prior to the Carter Phone Decision, some indirect methods of coupling alerting products were used. Some were sound-activated, triggering a steady light or strobe light when it heard the ring of the phone. This listening or sound-activated method

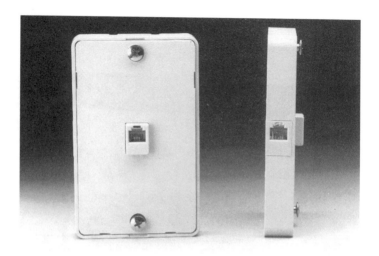

FIGURE 3-6   **RJ11 phone jack**

(Courtesy HARC Mercantile, Ltd.)

tends not to be dependable with many false alarms from extraneous sound (Figures 3-8 and 3-9). Other systems would detect the magnetic activation of the ringer mechanism in the phone, and in turn, sound a horn, buzzer, bell, or flash a light. Those systems also were not 100 percent dependable. Quite often the sensor would fall off or be placed too far away from the electromagnet and not pick up the trigger ring signal.

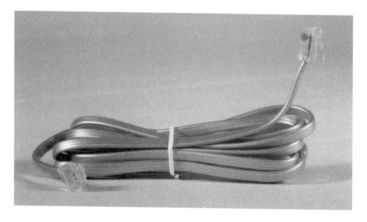

FIGURE 3-7   **RJ11 phone line cord**

(Courtesy HARC Mercantile, Ltd.)

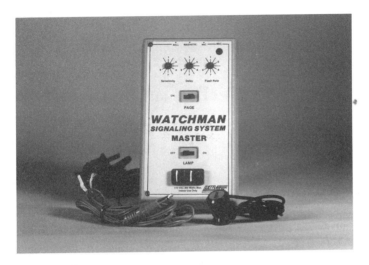

FIGURE 3-8   **Sound-activated phone signaling device**

(Courtesy HARC Mercantile, Ltd.)

The direct connect, connecting the ring signal device directly to the line, is the best method of ring detection. Although typically working well in most situations, direct-connect devices also have limitations. For example, if the line voltage is too low, the signal may not function at all.

Earlier, mention was made that the phone company will guarantee the supply of

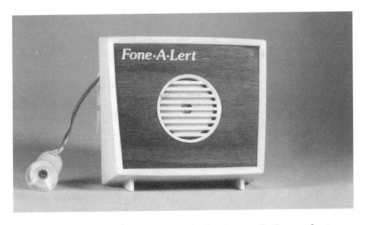

FIGURE 3-9   **Magnetic (inductive) triggered phone alert**

(Courtesy HARC Mercantile, Ltd.)

enough voltage to support the equivalent of three phones. That is the minimum, depending on where the installation is in relation to the local exchange. If too many ring devices are connected to the subscriber loop, the overall performance of all the products will drop, that is, if the loop can support a ringer equivalence of three and there is an equivalent of six attached, they all may ring or flash, but may be difficult to detect audibly or visually.

How does a subscriber know how many phones or auxiliary devices can be supported? There are several ways. The most common (not necessarily recommended) trial and error method is to just keep adding products until performance deficiency is noted, then remove the least desired devices until satisfactory performance is reached.

Option two is to contact the local carrier. In some areas the local phone carrier can be contacted to analyze the individual loop and can tell the subscriber exactly how many "ring" equivalents the local loop can support without degradation. A ring equivalent is the amount of power required to ring one standard carbon bell network phone.

Option three would be to buy or borrow a line tester and see for oneself the adequacy of the loop. (Figure 3-10). It's really quite simple. Today, every legitimate phone device has a ringer equivalency number. This number represents the relationship of the device's efficiency to the standard established of one carbon bell ringing phone. To determine the "load," simply look for the ringer equivalencies and add them up (Figure 3-11). In most cases today, products are less than .9 ringer equivalent, so more devices can be attached, even on the weaker loop. If ringer equivalencies

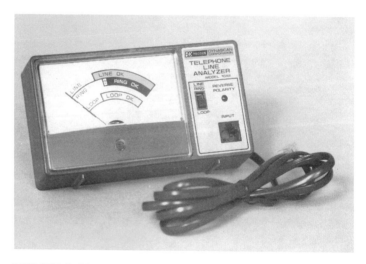

FIGURE 3-10   **Telephone line analyzer**

(Courtesy HARC Mercantile, Ltd.)

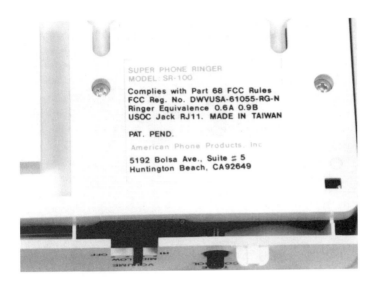

FIGURE 3-11 **FCC ringer equivalence label**

(Courtesy HARC Mercantile, Ltd.)

are not posted on the products, in support literature, or on the carton, use of the product would not be recommended.

How to Connect Auxiliary Alerting Devices to the Phone Line
Alerting devices with RJ11 plugs can be plugged into any available jack. If an empty jack is not available in the area, a two-way, three-way, or five-way adapter may be used, allowing connection to two, three, five phone devices (Figures 3-12, 3-13 and 3-14). Some alerting products have a jack built in, so the use of an adapter would not be required.

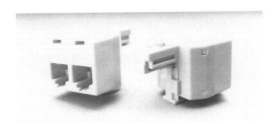

FIGURE 3-12 **RJ11 T-Adapter**

(Courtesy HARC Mercantile, Ltd.)

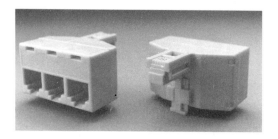

FIGURE 3-13   **RJ11 Three-way adapter**

(Courtesy HARC Mercantile, Ltd.)

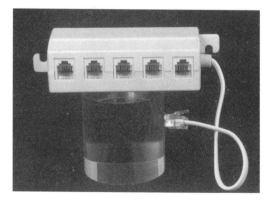

FIGURE 3-14   **RJ11 Five-way tap**

(Courtesy HARC Mercantile, Ltd.)

Types of Alerts

The most common alert is an additional bell or tone signaler. These signals make the ring louder and are for the moderately hearing-impaired (Figure 3-15). Some of the newer electronic tone ringers are good for hearing disabled, because in addition to being louder, the frequency or pitch can be adjusted to the loss of the user (Figures 3-16 and 3-17). However, most of these electronic ringers are in the higher frequencies, so the pitch might not be appropriate for persons with severe high-frequency hearing loss.

Other types of phone alerts connect to the loop in the same way as the audible alert, using the RJ11 plus the basic relay alert by simply flashing a light when the phone rings (Figure 3-18). Some relays can support alert stimuli other than incandescent lamps such as bed shakers, fans, etc. (Figures 3-19 and 3-20). Yet others can trigger a flashing light and a tactile device at the same time. In addition to a simple flashing light, there are also strobe light alerts. (Figures 3-21, 3-22, and 3-23).

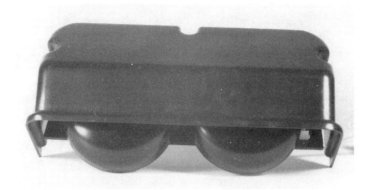

FIGURE 3-15   **Typical exterior telephone bell ringer**

(Courtesy HARC Mercantile, Ltd.)

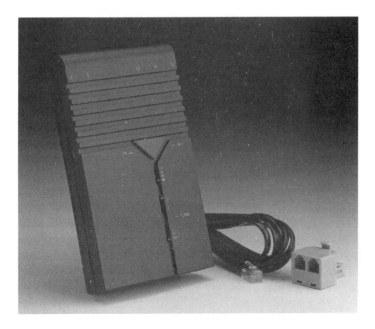

FIGURE 3-16   **Telephone ringer signal with adjustable frequency and volume control**

(Courtesy HARC Mercantile, Ltd.)

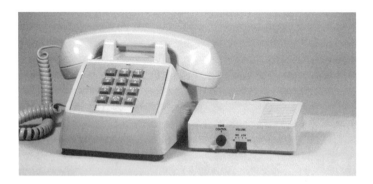

FIGURE 3-17   **Ringer with adjustable tone control and three-position volume control**

(Courtesy HARC Mercantile, Ltd.)

While some devices utilize power from normal means to power the strobe and only need enough ring voltage to trigger the strobe, other alerts work with systems. This means the ring signal is detected by one device and the trigger signal is transmitted by another (Figures 3-24 and 3-25). The most common of these are "line-carried systems" where the activation or trigger signal is detected by a "transmitter" that sends the trigger or flash signal through the household wiring to remote receivers that can flash lights, shake beds, turn on various things—even sound a buzzer (Figure 3-26). Other systems

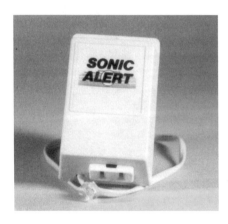

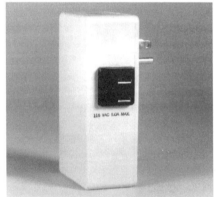

FIGURE 3-18   **Telephone ring light flasher**

(Courtesy HARC Mercantile, Ltd.)

FIGURE 3-19   **Telephone-activated AC relay**

(Courtesy HARC Mercantile, Ltd.)

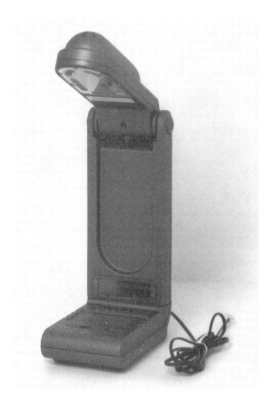

FIGURE 3-20   **Telephone ring signal with flashing light and bed shaker**

(Courtesy HARC Mercantile, Ltd.)

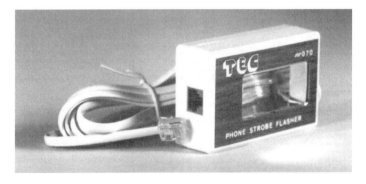

FIGURE 3-21   **Line-powered miniature phone strobe**

(Courtesy HARC Mercantile, Ltd.)

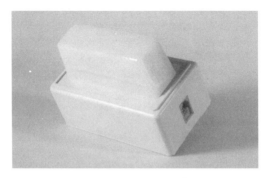

FIGURE 3-22 **Line-powered industrial phone strobe**

(Courtesy HARC Mercantile, Ltd.)

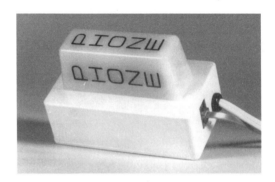

FIGURE 3-23 **AC-powered phone strobe**

(Courtesy HARC Mercantile, Ltd.)

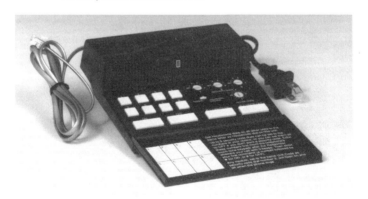

FIGURE 3-24 **Line-carried telephone ring signaler**

(Courtesy HARC Mercantile, Ltd.)

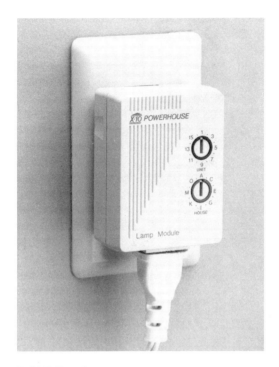

FIGURE 3-25 **Line-carried remote receiver for lamp activation**

(Courtesy HARC Mercantile, Ltd.)

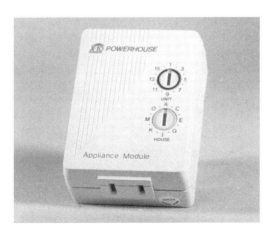

FIGURE 3-26 **Line-carried remote receiver for motor-driven appliances**

(Courtesy HARC Mercantile, Ltd.)

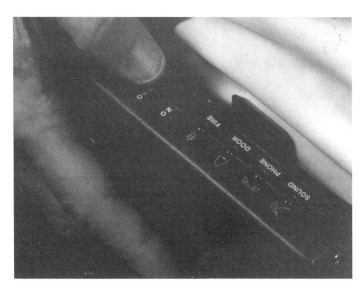

FIGURE 3-27   **Tactile body-worn remote receiver**

(Courtesy HARC Mercantile, Ltd.)

send the trigger or flash via radio waves to remote receivers that can be worn or stationary (Figures 3-27 and 3-28). In turn, these worn receivers can vibrate or sound a beep. The stationary receiver can turn on lights, strobes, shake beds, sound horns, or most anything. User preference will vary and will be determined by what stimulates the user's response.

   Now that the subscriber or client knows when the phone is ringing, how can they carry on a conversation if they have impaired hearing or are deaf?

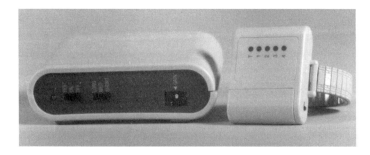

FIGURE 3-28   **Tactile alerting system**

(Courtesy HARC Mercantile, Ltd.)

Telephone Amplification Devices

Replacement Handsets

Amplified replacement handsets are probably the easiest and most efficient means of adding amplification to a telephone. However, replacement handsets can only be added to modular phones—those with detachable receivers. Also they will not work on telephones with dials in the handset, as with Trimline or Trendline models and cordless/wireless telephones. Hardwired telephones may be retrofitted with built-in amplification (usually on the body of the telephone), but this may be more expensive than simply purchasing a new handset-compatible modular phone.

Most replacement amplified handsets are compatible with all carbon bell ring telephones. A carbon bell ringing phone is the style traditionally available from the phone company prior to divestiture—basically, a phone that has a mechanical bell sound as opposed to an electronic sound. New high efficiency telephones or electronic telephones, especially inexpensive imports or "throwaway" telephones, have less power coming to the handset and may not be able to power the amplifier section of the replacement handset.

Replacement handsets come in a variety of matching telephone colors and are available in two styles. The traditional style with a round ear and mouthpiece is referred to as the 500 type or "G" style handset, whereas the modern "K" style handset has a square ear and mouthpiece (Figure 3-29). The actual intensity level that any one receiver will have can vary from telephone to telephone and from location to location. Satisfactory performance also depends on whether or not the handset amplifier's

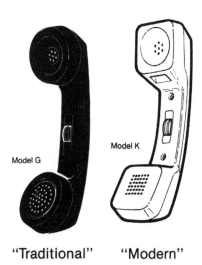

"Traditional"   "Modern"

FIGURE 3-29   **Common styles of telephone handsets: Round, Model G; Square, Model K**

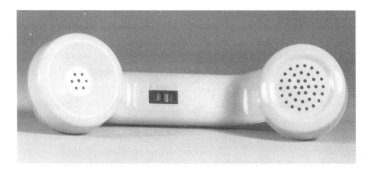

FIGURE 3-30 **Typical G-style rotary volume control handset**

(Courtesy HARC Mercantile, Ltd.)

impedance matches that of the telephone to which it is attached. If it does not, the resulting signal may be too weak or too loud and distorted.

The most common style of handset amplifier has a rotary, sometimes numbered, volume control wheel (Figure 3-30). Once the loudness is set, it is maintained until the volume control is changed, even if the telephone is hung up. When reused, the output is already at the predetermined level; a convenient feature if the same person uses the same telephone frequently.

If the telephone has many different users, it might be prudent to consider a replacement handset that automatically returns to normal volume at hang-up (Figure 3-31).

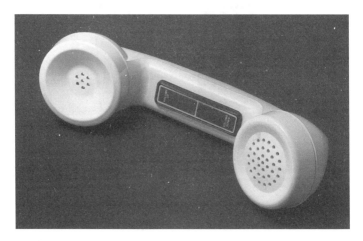

FIGURE 3-31 **G-style touchbar auto reset volume control handset**

(Courtesy HARC Mercantile, Ltd.)

This feature prevents the next caller from being "blasted" because the handset was left in a turned-up position. This particular handset tends to be more expensive than the common rotary type, but this automatic "turn down" feature is well worth it.

Other styles of amplified replacement receivers utilize a discrete, three-positioned slide switch offering normal, medium, and high volume choices. One disadvantage of this style is that the user has to be satisfied with the sound levels at each position and cannot adjust in between.

Since most new phones entering the market are electronic network phones, fewer phones will work with these line power replacement handsets because the network does not pass enough voltage through to the amplifier. This has allowed the development of auxiliary powered amplified handsets. Some require the use of a power supply that works off the main power and is converted by a power module to provide voltage to run the amplifier, yet the volume control is conveniently located in the handset.

Others utilize batteries and have volume and tone controls. Many of these handsets designed for electronic phones work only with electronic phones and do not operate on carbon bell network phones.

Use of a Handset Amplifier in a Noisy Environment

As stated previously, all telephone receiver mouthpieces pick up the caller's voice and direct it to the caller's receiver earpiece (side-tone) for voice monitoring. However, the receiver mouthpiece is a microphone and, as such, can also pick up ambient noise as well, especially when a telephone amplifier is turned up. The listener can reduce this background noise in the following ways:

1. When listening, cover the mouthpiece with the opposite hand (Figure 3-32).
2. Check to see if a replacement handset is available with a "noise-cancelling" mouthpiece.

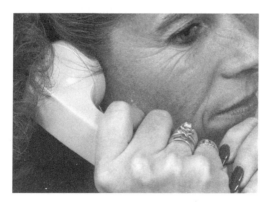

FIGURE 3-32 **Proper use of telephone in noisy environment**

(Courtesy HARC Mercantile, Ltd.)

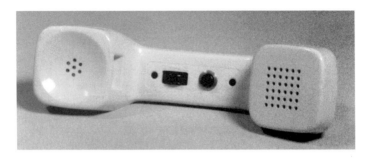

FIGURE 3-33   **K-style push-to-talk rotary volume control handset**

(Courtesy HARC Mercantile, Ltd.)

3. Purchase a replacement receiver that offers a "push-to-talk" button (Figure 3-33).
4. If the competing noise is from a radio or stereo, the use of a device that automatically mutes the audio source when the telephone is taken off the hook might be a feasible solution.

Built-In Amplifiers

In contrast to add-on or replacement handsets, some telephones have amplifiers built into the body of the instrument. The volume control is located somewhere on the top, by the dial, or on the side, near the receiver cord. Frequently, amplification will be added to telephones when they are reconditioned and made ready for their second market. In the past, amplified telephones have been limited to the standard carbon bell desk model phone (Figure 3-34), but now a popular Trimline type is available. On this model, the volume control wheel is located on the back of the handset and also serves to illuminate the dial when pushed in (Figure 3-35). Either style of telephone plugs into an existing RJ11 jack, the reference used for the standard modular line cord connection used on all single-line telephones.

In addition to the carbon bell desk phone and Trimline phones, many of the newer electronic phones say they have volume controls. Most of these amplifiers only increase the signal a few decibels, and by hearing-impaired standards, are not considered adequate.

There are currently a few complete phones designed with the hearing-disabled in mind, having volume controls that deliver significant increases in volume. Some claim to have an enhanced frequency response or dynamic range that compensates for the compression of audio signal quality normally experienced by the sound signal running through the system and the acoustic limitations of standard phone microphones and receiver earpieces. Some of this "expansion" is artificial and some is due to enhanced telephone receiver components (Figures 3-36, 3-37, and 3-38).

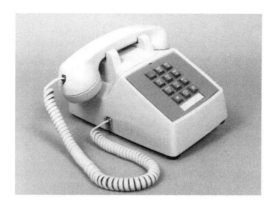

FIGURE 3-34 **Standard carbon bell ringing desk model phone (500 style)**

(Courtesy HARC Mercantile, Ltd.)

One totally specially designed phone for the profoundly hearing disabled is capable of outputs in excess of 100dB and frequency response shaping that can be set or "tuned" by the user. These phones tend to be expensive, but effective (Figure 3-39).

With 75 percent of the hearing-aid-wearing population using in-the-ear or canal-type hearing aids, volume control speaker phones have become quite popular. This allows an in-the-ear hearing-aid wearer to use the phone without taking off the hearing aid.

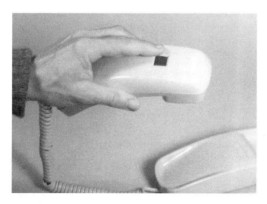

FIGURE 3-35 **Trimline telephone with built-in volume control**

(Courtesy HARC Mercantile, Ltd.)

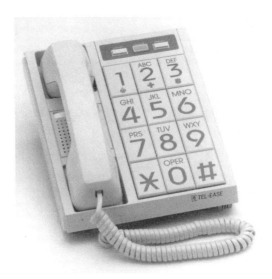

FIGURE 3-36 **Complete telephone with built-in volume control and specially designed phone ringer for the hearing impaired**

(Courtesy HARC Mercantile, Ltd.)

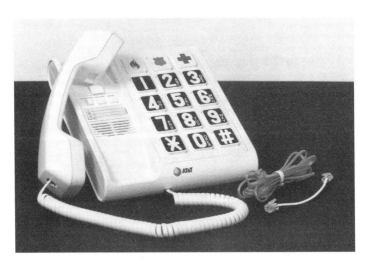

FIGURE 3-37 **Large-button volume control telephone**

(Courtesy HARC Mercantile, Ltd.)

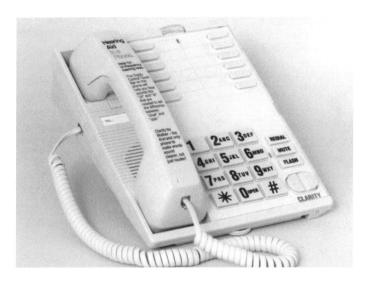

FIGURE 3-38   **Multi-featured volume control telephone for hotels**

(Courtesy HARC Mercantile, Ltd.)

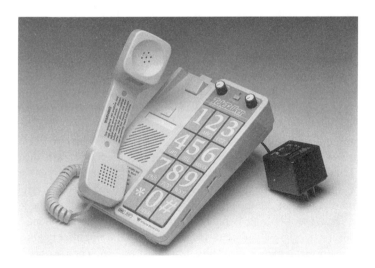

FIGURE 3-39   **Telephone with built-in volume control and frequency adjustment**

(Courtesy HARC Mercantile, Ltd.)

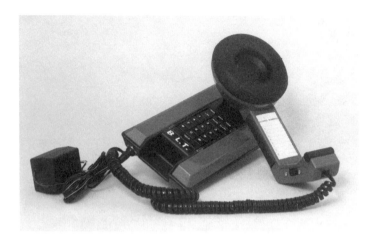

FIGURE 3-40 **Amplified telephone with padded earpiece for in-the-ear hearing aid wearers**

(Courtesy HARC Mercantile, Ltd.)

A new phone on the market is equipped with a rotary volume controlled handset that has a specially designed padded deep well earpiece that can be used easily by an in-the-ear hearing-aid wearer without feedback and still have high enough volume levels to be used without a hearing aid as well (Figure 3-40). As the technology increases, expect to see more complete specialty phones for the hearing disabled.

In-Line Telephone Amplifiers

In-line amplifiers work only with modular phones. In-line amplifiers that receive their operating power from the telephone line itself are referred to as line powered (Figure 3-41). These amplifiers will work on most carbon bell ringing telephones, but they will not work on all styles of electronic telephones.

In-line amplifiers with an external power source, such as batteries or transformers (Figure 3-42), are said to work with all telephones except those with the dial in the handset (Trimline). In fact, no in-line amplifier will work with this type of telephone. The installation of an in-line amplifier is simple. The coiled handset cord is disconnected from the base of the telephone and plugged into the jack on the side of the amplifier. Then, the amplifier is plugged into the base of the telephone where the coiled handset was originally plugged (Figure 3-43). If the amplifier requires external power, a transformer is also plugged into the nearest AC outlet or a battery is installed before attaching the unit to the telephone.

In-line amplifiers are not as convenient as handset or built-in amplifiers, but they tend to be slightly less expensive. The externally powered in-line amplifiers work with many telephones where replacement handsets do not.

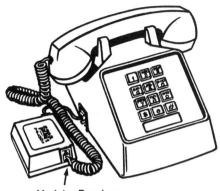

Modular Receiver
Cord Connection

FIGURE 3-41 **Line-powered in-line telephone amplifier**

(Courtesy HARC Mercantile, Ltd.)

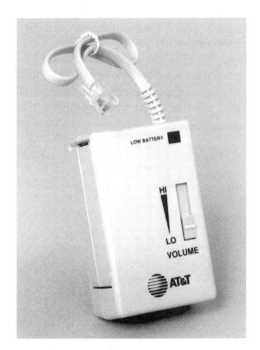

FIGURE 3-42 **Line-powered in-line telephone amplifier**

(Courtesy HARC Mercantile, Ltd.)

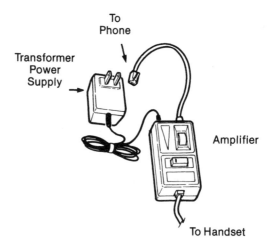

FIGURE 3-43 **Auxiliary-powered in-line amplifier**

Portable Audio Amplifiers

The portable, or strap-on amplifier was, until recently, the only option for a retrofit amplification device (Figure 3-44). However, as telephone instruments became more energy efficient, the portable amplifier became less dependable, due to the fact that most require that the telephones to which they attach be hearing-aid compatible, meaning the telephone receiver, must generate a magnetic field that the amplifier can inductively pick up, reamplify, and convert to sound for the listener.

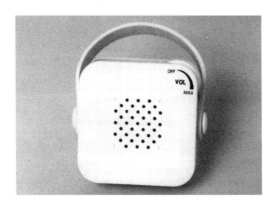

FIGURE 3-44 **Typical strap-on phone amplifier, inductive couple**

(Courtesy HARC Mercantile, Ltd.)

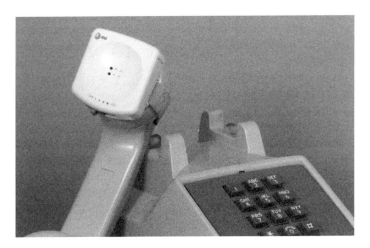

FIGURE 3-45 **Typical strap-on phone amplifier, acoustic couple**

(Courtesy HARC Mercantile, Ltd.)

Fortunately, there are now some strap-on amplifiers that have their own microphone, allowing them to couple acoustically to the telephone receiver, thus guaranteeing the fact that they will work on any telephone, anywhere. This includes cellular phones, which are not classified as telephones, but are radios and because of that do not have to be hearing-aid compatible. The amplifier (Figure 3-45 and 3-46) provides enough gain (approximately 21 to 22dB) to be appropriate for use with mild to moderate losses without the use of a hearing aid. This device has another advantage. It also creates a moderate magnetic field, thereby providing telephone access to those telephone listeners who use a hearing-aid telecoil.

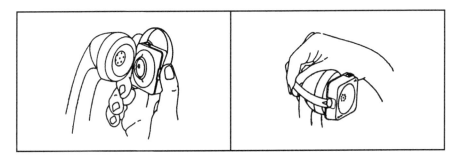

FIGURE 3-46 **Strap-on phone amplifier installation procedure**

Portable Induction Field Adapters

Other portable devices are available that are similar in appearance to strap-on audio amplifiers but that pick up the acoustic output of the telephone and change it into a magnetic field only. These acoustic-to-magnetic devices can only be used with a hearing-aid telecoil (Figure 3-47) and can make any telephone potentially hearing-aid compatible for listeners, provided their hearing aid has an efficient telecoil circuit. These induction amplifiers can create a magnetic field on phones that are not hearing-aid compatible, or on cellular phones, which then would allow the use of the hearing aid's T-coil.

These devices can be ordered with accessories such as plug-in silhouette inductors, enclasps, or direct audio input connections that allow the devices to be used on the telephone with two hearing aids (telecoil or direct audio input mode). They can also be used as remote microphone assistive listening devices for improvement of the signal-to-noise ratio in one-to-one or small group communication as well as television or radio listening.

To review, there are two types of portable telephone devices: (1) audio amplifiers and (2) inductive field adapters. Regardless of which type is used, these devices are ideal for travel because they can easily fit into a pocket or purse to provide dependable telephone access anywhere.

It should be noted here that even pay telephones equipped with handset amplifiers may not necessarily be hearing-aid compatible. If they are, they will usually (though not always) have a blue plastic grommet located where the armored receiver cable enters the receiver (Figure 3-48). Otherwise, the grommet will be black or gray, indicating lack of magnetic leakage. On March 24, 1988, the Federal Communications Commission (FCC), in an extension of the Telecommunications for the Disabled Act of 1982, proposed to expand its services to require that all coin- and

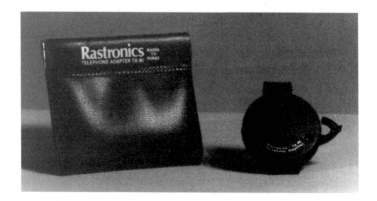

FIGURE 3-47   **Strap-on induction phone amplifier, acoustic couple**

(Courtesy HARC Mercantile, Ltd.)

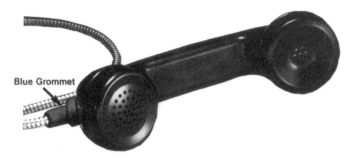

Blue Grommet Denotes Hearing Aid Compatibility on Public Phones

FIGURE 3-48 **Hearing-aid-compatible pay phone**

(Courtesy HARC Mercantile, Ltd.)

credit-card-operated telephones in common areas in workplaces of the hearing impaired be made hearing-aid compatible. This is in addition to the previous requirement that telephones be accessible for hearing-impaired persons in elevators, tunnels, hospitals, convalescent homes, 10 percent of phones in hotels and motels, and places of business or other buildings visited frequently by the public. Special symbols also indicate the presence of specially amplified handsets (Figure 3-49).

Portable amplifiers and adapters are not ideal for permanent installation for the following reasons:

1. Depending on telephone style, the adapter may have to be physically removed and reattached each time the telephone is used because the amplifier's or adapter's size precludes the telephone from being hung up.

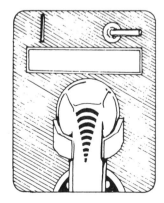
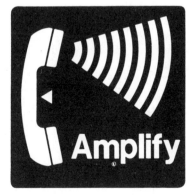

FIGURE 3-49 **Symbols identifying public pay phones equipped with amplification**

2. All portable devices use batteries. If left on, the battery will drain and the device will not function when needed.

Hearing Aid Telecoil

In the past, the telecoil was less dependable than the weather in Michigan, and, as a result, many hearing-aid users and dispensers became disenchanted. However, today's telecoils are much improved and are, for the most part, dependable and efficient. The telecoil's use today far exceeds telephone applications and allows coupling with assistive listening systems. However, with nearly 75 percent of hearing aids being custom in-the-ear (ITE) or custom canal types, fewer hearing aids are being equipped with telecoils.

ITE and mini-canal hearing aids can, and should, be equipped with telecoil circuitry to provide communication access both on the telephone and in various other difficult listening situations. Furthermore, space permitting, the installation of a preamplifier chip can boost the power of the telecoil of an in-the-ear hearing aid to almost match that of its microphone circuit.

When buying a telephone to be used with a hearing-aid telecoil, the client should be instructed to buy only telephones that are clearly identified as being hearing-aid compatible. Even then, each instrument should be tested, because there are no standards for the strength of magnetic leakage from telephones. If the telephone receiver creates too weak a signal or has no inductive field, as in the case with most new solid-state telephones, Trimline models, and those equipped with "L" type receivers, the telecoil will not couple properly and portable induction adapters will be needed.

Telephone Pads

Acoustic coupling of the hearing aid to the telephone often causes feedback due to pressure from the receiver on the ear, which loosens the hearing aid fit. Feedback can also result from the existence of vent in the earmold or shell of the hearing aid. The use of an inexpensive foam telepad (Figure 3-50) often eliminates feedback. An alternative is to simply hold the receiver a short distance form the ear. This may also eliminate feedback, especially if the telephone is equipped with an audio amplifier.

Improving acoustic coupling of the hearing aid to the telephone becomes crucial for those clients fitted with custom ITE (and canal aids) that may be too small for telecoil circuitry.

Teletext (TT)/Telecommunication Devices for the Deaf (TDD)

There are several million persons in the United States who cannot understand speech on the telephone, even with add-on amplification systems. These persons may be deaf, or they may be hard-of-hearing with severely reduced speech recognition ability. There are also persons who have speech impediments preventing them from using the voice telephone. Until recently, these persons have been cut off from a vital form

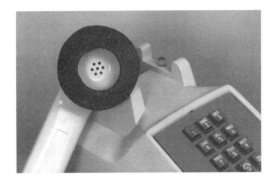

FIGURE 3-50 **Foam pad for telephone receiver to reduce feedback**

(Courtesy HARC Mercantile, Ltd.)

of communication. Today, however, there are visual-based systems that can provide telephone access.

Standard Devices

Based on teletypewriter technology, modern teletexts transmit over regular telephone lines. Each teletext has a typewriter keyboard. Typed communication appears on either a soft light-emitting diode 20- or 40-character display or on paper (Figures 3-51 and 3-52). Teletexts connect to the telephone system either acoustically through a built-in or add-on modem or directly using a standard telephone cord.

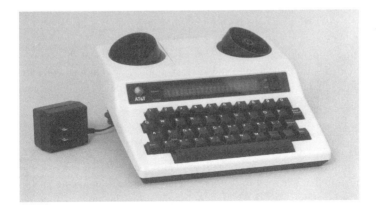

FIGURE 3-51 **Display-only acoustically coupled TDD**

(Courtesy HARC Mercantile, Ltd.)

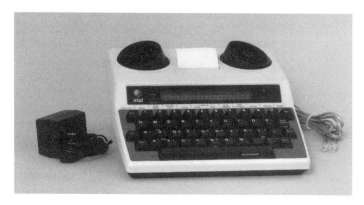

FIGURE 3-52   **Display and printing TDD acoustic couple and direct connect**

(Courtesy HARC Mercantile, Ltd.)

In order for a teletext conversation to take place, both parties to the call must have a teletext unit and each must be compatible with the other.

Standard teletext transmission occurs at 45.5 baud, which is the reference speed in sending and receiving signals. A teletext unit can also communicate with a computer. However, an interface option is required to convert the slow transmission rate of the teletext to the faster computer transmission speed (referred to as ASCII).

Teletexts range in price from $219 to $700, depending on the number of features they contain. Some commonly requested features include: a rechargeable battery pack for travel, extra memory, automatic answering, calculator, and external printer. Some even announce, in synthesized speech, "Hearing-impaired caller, use teletext." For homes and offices where both telephones and teletexts are used, combination voice and teletext answering machines are also available.

Hearing-impaired teletext users can also purchase visual displays that can be connected to the printer ports of some teletexts to provide characters that are ten times larger than a standard teletext display. Finally, braille teletexts can provide telephone access to deaf-blind persons.

Computers and Telecommunication Devices

As already mentioned above, a teletext must have a special ASCII feature that allows it to communicate with a computer. It is also possible to equip a computer with a special modem that allows it to emulate a teletext and communicate in Baudot code, which is the language used in teletext communication. The important point is that the equipment at each end of the communication link must be communicating at the same speed in the same code.

As the cost of personal computers has been dropping, their use throughout the populace has gone up tremendously; so has the availability of teletext programs and modems. IBM's Phone Communicator is the most elaborate system. It is PC-based and uses a full card slot and enough hard disk to allow it to operate as a resident program while utilizing the computer for other functions. The system has full screen view message and storage to disk or paper, synthesized voice for outgoing, and a capability to listen and convert signals from the keypad of a standard touchtone phone to letters and words through a comprehensive dictionary. These systems allow the user to talk to (1) other computers, (2) other teletext units, and (3) normal-hearing people with a touchtone phone, offering almost unlimited communicative possibilities for the profound or deaf user.

Another personal-computer-based system on the market is MicroFlip, which includes a card slot modem and software that can automatically answer and save teletext calls. It has many of the same features as the IBM program, except no voice synthesizer and no touchtone capability, but it is half the cost of the IBM system (Figure 3-53).

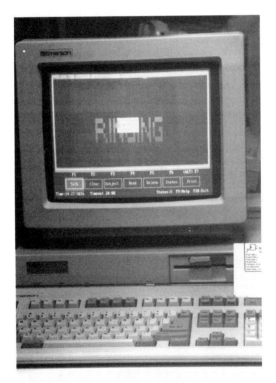

FIGURE 3-53   **Typical display for computer modem TDD**

(Courtesy HARC Mercantile, Ltd.)

Message Relay Systems

Relay services are available for teletext users to converse with anyone who does not have a teletext. The teletext user calls a central number, where a hearing operator places a call to the non-teletext number as specified by the hearing-impaired person. The relay operator acts as an intermediary by typing the spoken message to the hearing-impaired communicant and vice versa. Relay services also permit hearing persons to call hearing-impaired users. Currently, there are a number of states that have their own relay services. However, on March 24, 1988, as part of its proposal to increase telephone access to hearing impaired persons, the FCC ruled for the implementation of an interstate relay system for teletext, users enabling teletext users to make relay calls outside of their local area code or state.

Many 911 and other emergency and government agencies have added TT/TDDs to their communications equipment. Accessibility to these agencies has been mandated by various barrier-free legislation and affirmative action plans.

In 1990, President George Bush signed into law the Americans with Disabilities Act (ADA). It became effective on January 26, 1992, so persons with hearing impairments and other disabilities have new opportunities and benefits.

ADA mandates that public and private telecommunications relay services be available to hearing- and speech-impaired individuals in the United States.

Privately owned places of public accommodation such as hotels, restaurants, theaters, stores, offices, and gyms, as well as transit stations, museums, parks, schools, and social service agencies must not discriminate against individuals with a disability as of January 1992.

One of the telecommunication mandates is that local or regional carriers provide access to the phone systems for all persons. This has spurred on several new relay services in many states. It has also seen the first lawsuit regarding accessibility to 911 by deaf persons using teletext. The City of New York's 911 systems were not accessible by TT/teletext, and they refused a citizen's request to be accessible. A court case ensued in which the city lost. They were given 36 hours to comply or face very large fines.

As the smoke and dust clear from the initial ADA explosion, expect to see several more services for TT/TDD users.

Interfacing Telecommunication Devices
to the Telephone Lines

Earlier, the effect of the length of the loop, impedance, and balance on telephone performance was discussed. If the telephone line is noisy or buzzing, the teletext will not properly "hear" the incoming message. With acoustic coupling, a loose-fitting telephone receiver placed into the teletext coupler can also result in insufficient intensity of the teletext beeps that are sent through the telephone lines. In addition, noise from the room can also enter into the telephone line through the coupler. These problems can result in missed messages or the production of random letters and other symbols, creating a garbled message. For acoustic coupling, a properly fitting telephone handset is essential. Adapters are available to interface round teletext modems to accept square telephone receivers and vice versa. If this does not result in accurate transmission or reception, then oftentimes an amplified handset can be used to solve this problem.

Facsimile Transmission

Another form of communication that has applications for hearing-disabled persons is the facsimile machine or fax (Figure 3-54). This device allows a hand-drawn or typed hard copy message to be sent over the telephone lines to another fax machine. With the increased popularity of this technology in the business world, the cost of hardware has begun to drop, making it more accessible.

In Japan, the fax now is the number one choice for deaf telecommunication because it allows the rapid dispatch of their symbol type language. Also, phone scratch pads, which allow written symbols to be transmitted over phone lines, are gaining momentum in communications. You can expect to see more symbol transmission devices on the market.

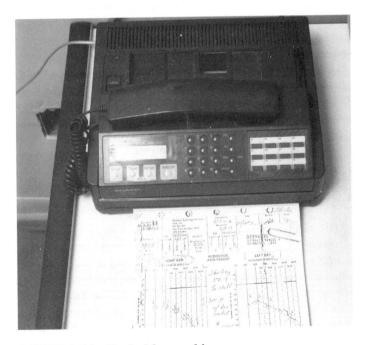

FIGURE 3-54   **Typical fax machine**

(Courtesy HARC Mercantile, Ltd.)

WHAT DOES THE FUTURE HOLD?

What does the year 2001 and beyond hold in telecommunications for the hearing disabled? As technology becomes more sophisticated, we can expect to see devices that will make telephone access to the hearing disabled even more convenient. For example, Bell Communications Research is currently involved in a project using technology to improve telephone relay services for the deaf. It involves the use of a computer that interfaces with a teletext to a regular telephone. Two-way communications are performed by synthesizing text typed from the teletext to the earset of the telephone and utilizing speech recognition to transpose text to the teletext from the mouthpiece of the telephone. Various voice recognition systems and algorithms are being examined for better recognition rates, continuous speech, large vocabularies, and, as the technologies develop, independent speaker recognition.

Currently, still life visual image transmission is available, giving new meaning to the "person-to-person" call. Research is also being done of real time image transmission, which may some day result in a true "video telephone." This device will open further the door of communication to those who depend on visual cues, such as speech reading, cued speech, and sign language.

The future also holds new forms of transmission, such as fiberoptics, which are already being discussed as replacement for the local loop. This will force a standardization of equipment or the equipment will not work.

New projects are under development. One utilizes an electronic glove that transmits an image of hand and finger movement, which allows finger spelling to be sent over the telephone lines and the visual image interpreted.

HARC Mercantile, Ltd. is developing the "Liperator"™ which will work on a type of voice inflection recognition, causing a visual display of lips to move in relation to the phoneme it hears. This lipreading addition to amplification will help hearing disabled better understand phone conversations.

CONCLUSION

With the ADA mandating removal of communication barriers, a demand is created for new technology. This, coming on the heels of the Carter Phone Decision, followed by the subsequent divestiture of AT&T, was a blessing in that innovative products were introduced into the marketplace. However, it was a curse as well. The termination of the monopoly marked the end of the standardization that made the telephone system work so well in the past. In addition, the improvement of technology has, ironically, resulted in less reliable telephone compatibility with the hearing aid and add-on assistive technology.

Fortunately, there are numerous products available to make telephone access possible to the millions of hearing-disabled persons in this country. Although coupling these products to the telephone is not always easy, audiologists can assist clients by gaining a knowledge of the products that are available and what factors must be considered when interfacing them to the telephone system. Until standards for telephones and peripherals are developed, the old trial and error method may be the only choice, especially when dealing with telephone systems with which audiologists and clients are not completely familiar. However, the more we work with these products, the easier our job will become.

Ever since Watson heeded the call of his boss some 100 years ago, the telephone system has become the lifeline to communication. More recently, the development of special auditory and visual products has extended this lifeline to the hearing disabled. It is hoped that, with further technological advances and the development of enforceable standards, it will be easier to extend this lifeline to hearing-disabled persons everywhere.

APPENDIX 3–1: TELEPHONE TECHNOLOGY RESOURCES

For additional information on telephone technology, contact:

AT&T National Special Needs Center
2001 Route 48
Parsippany, NJ 07054
1-800-233-1222 (voice)
1-800-833-3232 (TDD)

HARC Mercantile, Ltd.
P.O. Box 3055
3130 Portage Road
Kalamazoo, MI 49003-3055
1-800-445-9968 (voice/TDD)
1-616-381-3319 (TDD)
1-616-3381-3614 (FAX)

Tele-Consumer Hotline
1536 16th Street, NW
Washington, DC 20036
1-800-332-1124 (voice/TDD)

Telecommunications for the Deaf, Inc.
814 Thayer Avenue
Silver Spring, MD 20910
1-301-589-3006 (voice/TDD)

▶ 4

Clinical Procedures for Evaluating Telephone Use and Need for Related Assistive Devices

NANCY TYE-MURRAY
LORIANNE K. SCHUM
The University of Iowa Hospitals

In the last few years, advances in technology and the passage of the American with Disabilities Act of 1990 (PL 101-336) have created new service possibilities for audiologists. Audiologists now have opportunities to expand their businesses by evaluating and selecting assistive listening devices for their hearing-impaired clients. Along with this opportunity comes responsibility in at least three ways. First, it is incumbent upon audiologists who dispense assistive devices to counsel clients about which devices may and may not be helpful, and (when possible) to provide objective data that support their recommendations. Secondly, if and when insurance health care plans begin to provide coverage for assistive devices, audiologists will need to document needs and benefits in order for clients to receive reimbursement. Finally, some audiologists do not sell assistive devices from an in-house stock, and/or they stock only a limited inventory. In these situations, clients usually cannot try a particular assistive device on a loaner basis. Objective data collected during a formal evaluation

This study was supported by research grant DC00242 from the National Institutes of Health/NIDCD, grant RR59 from the General Clinical Research Centers Program, Division of Research Resources, NIH, and the Iowa Lions Sight and Hearing Foundation. We thank Cheryl Sobaski and Don Schum for their assistance in designing and completing the experiments.

may provide the only basis for an audiologist to encourage a client to make an assistive device purchase. To these ends, objective procedures for selecting, evaluating, and fitting appropriate assistive listening devices must be developed.

In this chapter, we describe objective test procedures that can be used to assess clients' abilities to use the telephone and the benefits that can be derived from telephone assistive devices. Data collected from a group of adults who use the Cochlear Corporation Nucleus multichannel cochlear implant are presented to illustrate how results from the test procedures might be used in a clinical setting (see also Dorman, Dove, Parkin, Zacharchuk, & Dankowski, 1991; Cohen, Waltzman, & Shapiro, 1989).[1]

INFORMAL EVALUATION

Before the formal assessment, information about telephone usage and telephone apparatus can be obtained by asking clients to complete a questionnaire. The questionnaire can be mailed to the client, who then completes it before arriving at the clinic. Alternatively, the client can complete it immediately before the formal assessment begins. There is some advantage to asking the client to complete the questionnaire beforehand. The client can record brand names of the telephone apparatus used in the home or office, and check the telephone ringer settings.

Erber (1985, pp. 47–50) presents one possible questionnaire. His items include questions about communication ability and experience (e.g., "Which method [speech, oral interpreter, code, or TDD] do you use?"), frequency of use (e.g., "How often do you use the telephone?" "Who do you call regularly?"), conversational goals (e.g., "What is a typical reason for a call?"), hearing aids (e.g., "Do you have a microphone/ telecoil switch on your hearing aid[s]?"), telephone apparatus (e.g., "Do you typically use any other supplementary amplification device?"), and confidence (e.g., "When nobody else is nearby, and the telephone rings, how do you respond?").

Clients' responses about telephone usage will indicate their preferred telecommunication method (e.g., conversational speech versus a yes-yes/no code), their subjective impressions of how well they can recognize speech over the telephone, and the frequency with which they use the telephone. This information will alert the audiologist to a client's specific problems and needs. Responses about telephone apparatus will indicate the model or brand of their telephones, their supplementary amplification devices, and their special ringing apparatus. In addition, a client's responses may influence the design of the formal assessment. For instance, if the client uses a particular supplementary amplification device, the audiologist may choose to compare the client's speech recognition skills when using it versus another device. If the client's particular telephone model is available in the clinic, the audiologist might use it while assessing speech recognition skills.

---

[1]The same group of subjects participated in all of the studies reviewed in this report. Each study included between 18 and 20 subjects, so some subjects did not participate in all of the experiments. Audiological and biographical data for the subjects appear in Table 4-3.

FORMAL EVALUATION

Three skills that are typically associated with using the telephone may be assessed during a formal evaluation: 1) detecting the ring, 2) identifying telephone signals, and 3) recognizing speech. In this section, we consider assessment procedures.

Detecting Telephone Rings

The reason for evaluating whether a client can detect a telephone ring is to determine whether or not a telephone ring alerting system would be beneficial. The most straightforward evaluation procedure is to place a client in a room and have a telephone ring on several occasions. The client must then indicate when the rings began and when they end by raising his hand. Since both environmental listening conditions and the amplitude of the rings may change, the audiologist may wish to assess performance in quiet and in the presence of background noise, and with soft and loud telephone rings.

We test clients individually, while they stand at a specified location in the test room. The client's task is to raise his hand when the telephone begins to ring and to lower it when ringing ceases.

We test with a total of four conditions where two variables are altered, background noise and ring amplitude. Clients are tested in quiet and noise, and with a soft and loud ring. In a busy clinical setting, the audiologist might choose to test in only one condition (e.g., in noise with a loud ring).

For the noise condition, an audiovisual recording of a news broadcast is presented at 56 dBA SPL (measured at the level of the subject's aided ear) on a Sony television unit. Three persons with normal hearing have judged this to be a typical and comfortable listening level from the location where the clients are asked to listen. The news broadcast also serves to distract the client's attention from the listening task. Thus, the task in noise resembles a real world situation in that persons are usually engaged in some activity when their telephone rings.

During each condition, the telephone rings three times on three occasions. The three presentations are separated with a varying time interval (20-60 s). A clinician sits behind the client and records whether or not he or she correctly raises and lowers his or her hand.

The size and sound-absorbing characteristics of the room will influence how well the client may detect telephone rings. Thus, if possible, the test room architecture should resemble a room wherein the client most often uses a telephone. Since individuals often use the telephone in their work setting, we test our clients in a room that resembles an office (both in terms of the architectural structure and the furnishings). The room is described in Appendix A. If the client's home telephone is located in a living room, then ideally the test room should be fairly large, and should have carpeting, drapery, and padded furnishings. In the event that only one room is available for testing, it is desirable that its structural characteristics be described. In counseling the client, the audiologist can explain that the test results apply to a room with these characteristics, and suggest how performance might change in different settings.

Not only do rooms vary, so too do the spectral and amplitude characteristics of rings produced by different telephones. When testing, we use a standard office telephone (manufactured by Comdial, Charlottesville, VA) since this is a common instrument. The acoustic spectrum of this telephone ring appears in Figure 4-1. We test with the ring set to its lowest amplitude (56 dBA SPL measured at the level of the client's aided ear) and its highest amplitude (69 dBA SPL). However, the spectrum in Figure 4-1 is specific to only one telephone. Figure 4-2 provides the acoustic spectra of five other telephone rings, which differ significantly in spectral characteristics. It is possible that an audiologic clinic may have a variety of telephones in stock, and the audiologist can select the one that best matches the client's home or office telephone. Otherwise, during counseling, the audiologist can describe how the spectrum of the test telephone ring corresponds to other commonly used telephones that are commercially available.

We have evaluated 19 Nucleus cochlear-implant users' ability to detect soft and loud telephone rings, in quiet and noise. The results appear in Table 4-1. In the quiet condition, subjects almost always detected the rings, regardless of whether they were soft or loud. In the noise condition, subjects always detected the rings when the telephone was set to its loudest ring (69 dBA SPL). Performance showed a marginal decrease in the noise condition when the telephone was set to its softest ring (56 dBA SPL).

On the basis of these results, we now counsel our cochlear-implant candidates that many individuals who use the Nucleus cochlear implant may not require a telephone ring alerting system if they are typically in the same room as their telephone. If they are not usually in the same room, then additional remote ringing devices, a wrist-

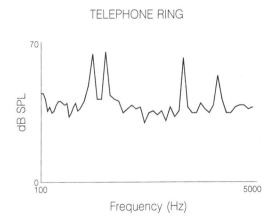

FIGURE 4-1 **Acoustic spectrum of the Comdial telephone ring**

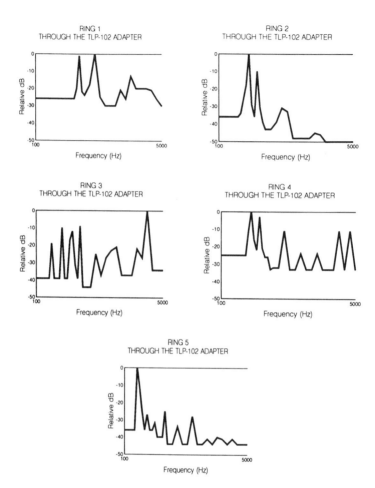

FIGURE 4-2 **Acoustic spectra of five other telephone rings**

TABLE 4-1 **Mean Number of Telephone Rings Detected (out of three possible) (N=19)**

CONDITION	LEVEL	
	LOUD (69 DBA SPL)	SOFT (56 DBA SPL)
Quiet	3.0	2.8
Noise (56 dBA SPL)	3.0	2.5

worn alerting device or a strobe light, may be indicated. After receiving a cochlear implant, the individual client should be tested and questioned individually to determine his or her particular needs.

Identifying Telephone Signals

Identifying telephone signals is such an intrinsic part of using the telephone that we often do not appreciate the importance of this skill. For instance, when an individual picks up the receiver to make a telephone call, he or she must determine whether or not a dial tone is present before beginning to dial. After dialing, the subject will have to decide whether the telephone is delivering a ringing signal or a busy signal. He or she must then recognize when ringing ceases and a voice answers. Finally, he or she must determine whether the voice is someone talking or a recorded message.

Recognizing and identifying the presence or absence of voice may be a particularly important skill for persons who have severe and profound hearing impairments. During telephone communication strategies training, these clients are often encouraged to use a yes-yes/no code (e.g., Castle, 1988; Erber, 1985). The client controls the telephone conversation by asking yes-no questions, and the communication partner indicates an affirmative response by saying "yes-yes" and a negative response by saying "no."

Clients' ability to identify telephone signals can be evaluated systematically. Common telephone signals can be recorded with a cassette tape recorder and then presented through a telephone receiver to the client for identification (see Erber, 1985; Castle, 1984).

We test signal recognition skills with seven common telephone signals: 1) a dial tone, 2) a busy signal, 3) a ring-back signal, 4) an answering machine message, 5) an operator message, 6) silence, and 7) an off-the-hook signal. During recording of the signals, a ¼" microphone was placed at the position of the tympanic membrane on a commercially available replica of the external ear. The telephone receiver was pressed gently against the pinna of the ear replica during recording.

Testing can be performed in one of two conditions, or both. The conditions are *open-set* and *closed-set*. During open-set testing, clients are told that they will hear "common telephone sounds." The telephone signals are played on a cassette tape deck and delivered to a telephone outside of the test room. The signal from this telephone is delivered to a second telephone located inside the test room. The client listens with the receiver held to his or her listening aid microphone. Clients are permitted to adjust their volume control level on their listening aid so that speech is received at a comfortable level. The client is presented with a signal, and then asked to name it.

Closed-set testing proceeds in the same fashion as open-set testing, with one exception. Clients have before them a list of the signals as they listen. When time constraints are present, and only one test condition is possible, we recommend closed-set testing. Closed-set testing may better approximate the real-world listening task because context cues usually limit the possible signals that the client must choose from (e.g., if the client has dialed the telephone, she will expect a ring-back or busy signal).

One purpose of testing might be to determine whether the client could benefit from purchasing a telephone adapter, an amplification device, or a hearing aid telecoil. The audiologist can evaluate the client without and with an assistive device, and then determine the extent to which the device improves the subject's ability to identify telephone signals. Another purpose might be to compare the benefits provided by two different assistive devices. Fikret-Pasa and Garstecki (1993) recently demonstrated that different telephone amplifiers vary in their frequency response spectra, and their volume control linearity. This finding suggests that clients might perform better with one device than another.

As with telephone rings, signals associated with different telephones have different spectral characteristics. Therefore, it is important to describe the spectra of the test signals, and be aware of how well they reflect the signals of other commercially available instruments. The relative electrical spectra of the our test signals appear in Figure 4-3.

We have evaluated 20 Nucleus cochlear-implant users' abilities to identify common telephone signals. Subjects used a Cochlear Corporation TLP-102 telephone adapter (Cochlear Corporation, 1991) during testing. A complete description of this adapter appears in Appendix B. Subjects performed poorly in an open-set condition. On average, they recognized 2.9 signals correctly (SD = 1.1) of the 7 possible. They performed better in the closed-set condition, with an average of 5.2 signals correctly recognized (SD = 1.3).

These data can be used for counseling cochlear-implant and hearing-aid candidates. The poor performance of the 20 subjects, who on average exhibit listening skills comparable to individuals who have severe or profound hearing impairment, also suggests a direction for future product development. A signal identification system for telephones might be useful for clients who have severe and profound hearing impairments. For instance a series of colored light-emitting diodes (LEDs) could be placed near the receiver cradle, with each LED indicating a different telephone signal. The appropriate LED would illuminate when the corresponding signal occurred. The LED paired with voicing could serve a dual purpose: it could signal the presence or absence of speech and also be used in a yes-yes/no communication interaction (Castle, 1977; 1984). To our knowledge, no such system currently exists.

Recognizing Speech

There are at least three reasons why audiologists test how well a client recognizes speech over the telephone. First, test results obtained without a telephone assistive device can be used to counsel the individual about his or her performance. The audiologist can suggest whether or not the client has the potential to benefit from an assistive device, such as a telephone amplifier or a telephone adapter. Secondly, a particular assistive device can be assessed. The client can be tested without and then

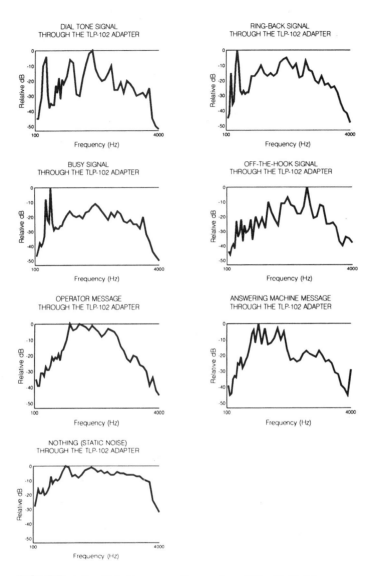

FIGURE 4-3　**Relative acoustic spectra of the 1) dial tone signal, 2) ring-back signal, 3) busy signal, 4) off-the-hook signal, 5) operator message, 6) answering machine message, and 7) silence (static noise) through the TLP-102 telephone adapter**

with the device, and be advised of how much performance improved. This information may help the client decide whether or not to purchase the device. Finally, results obtained from a specific population of subjects, such as cochlear-implant users, can be used to counsel candidates who are considering implantation, or who are considering other services, such as a hearing-aid fitting.

In testing speech recognition skills, we use three different types of speech samples. In a typical clinical setting, the audiologist may have time to test speech recognition using only one of the three samples. A telephone that meets the Bell system acceptable frequency bandwidths for speech should be used for the evaluation. Cohen et al. (1989) note that the acceptable bandwidth is 200 – 3,500 Hz.

The first speech sample contains sentences from a standardized sentence test. Recorded sentences from the *Revised Speech Perception in Noise (SPIN) Test* (Bilger, 1984) are presented to the client through a telephone receiver. The client's task is to repeat the last word of each sentence, which is a common, monosyllabic noun. The SPIN contains two types of sentences, *high-predictability* and *low-predictability*. In a high-predictability sentence, the sentence provides semantic clues about the last word (e.g., *Stir your coffee with a SPOON*). In a low-predictability sentence, the sentence provides little or no semantic clues about the last word (e.g., *Bob could have known about the SPOON*). The sentences have been recorded by a male talker who is experienced in making audio recordings (Kalikow, Stevens, & Elliott, 1977). This sample allows the audiologist to compare a client's test results with those obtained from other clinics, and in other listening conditions (such as an audiometric test booth).

The second speech sample that can be used to assess speech recognition skills with the telephone contains 33 unrelated sentences and questions that one might hear during a telephone conversation (adapted from Erber, 1985). The sentences and questions were designed to meet one of eight conversational goals. For example, one goal of a telephone conversation might be to obtain information, such as, *Is Bill home?* The eight conversational goals and corresponding statements are presented in Appendix C. The test items were recorded by a female talker who has a midwestern American accent. Clients are instructed to repeat as much of each recorded statement as possible. Performance is scored by the percentage of words repeated verbatim. These sentences allow the audiologist to estimate how well the client can recognize utterances that might occur in general telephone conversations, even when the client does not know the topic of conversation.

The final speech sample used for testing speech recognition is formulated after Erber's (1985) QUEST?AR exercise. The client speaks via telephone to a clinician stationed in another room. The client asks a list of 30 related questions to the clinician, who provides live-voice scripted answers for each. The questions are logically ordered and proceed in a conversational manner, so that the semantic context cues for recognizing the answers increase as the conversation progresses (just as would be the case in a real-world conversation). The questions and answers that we use during testing are presented in Appendix D. The clinician monitors his or her voice level with a Realistic (Model 33-2050) sound level meter while speaking, striving for an average peak intensity of 82 dBA SPL. The client's task is to write down the clinician's answer before asking the next question on the test list. The responses are scored by percentage of keywords correctly recognized. By scoring only keywords, the audiologist obtains a reflection of how well clients recognize the gist of messages. This speech sample helps to predict how well the client will perform in an interactive, live-voice conversation.

We have tested 20 Nucleus cochlear-implant users with the first test list, 19 with the second, and 18 with the third test list. Testing occurred in quiet, in the room described in Appendix 4-1.

Two lists of the SPIN test were presented, one in each of two conditions, the adapter condition and the no-adapter condition. For the adapter condition, subjects were permitted to adjust their speech processor sensitivity to a comfortable listening level. For the no-adapter condition, subjects were instructed to hold the telephone receiver no farther than $\frac{1}{2}''$ from the earpiece microphone of their cochlear implant. By comparing test scores from the two conditions, we determined whether or not the adapter provided significant benefit.

The results obtained with the SPIN test are presented in Table 4-2. A two-factor (adapter, context) repeated measures analysis of variance of percent words correct yielded significant main effects for the adapter condition ($F(1,18) = 6.5$, $p = .02$), context ($F(1,18) = 8.8$, $p = .008$), and a significant interaction ($F(1,18) = 10.7$, $p = .004$). To investigate the interaction, paired t-tests were performed. Subjects scored better for high than low context sentences when using the telephone adapter ($t = 3.4$, $df = 18$, $p = .003$). No difference between the two contexts surfaced when subjects did not use the adapter. Subjects performed better with the adapter than without it when listening to the high context sentences ($t = 3.02$, $df = 18$, $p = .007$). No advantage of using an adapter was found for the low context sentences.

These findings suggest that the TLP-102 telephone adapter is helpful when sentence context is high. We share these findings with cochlear implant users who are considering purchasing the adapter, as well as allow them to try the adapter first-hand. Similar data could be collected with adapters and amplification devices that are appropriate for hearing-aid users. On the basis of these findings, we also counsel family members to identify the topic of their utterances when talking to the cochlear-implant user in order to increase contextual cues. For example, a family member might say, "Car. I will pick up the car."

One of the most frequently asked questions that audiologists hear from cochlear-implant candidates or hearing-aid candidates is, *Will I be able to use the telephone like I did before I lost my hearing?* Results with the conversational sentences and the QUEST?AR procedure, in addition to results obtained with the SPIN test, can provide data for counseling.

All of our cochlear-implant subjects were tested using the TLP-102 telephone adapter. Subjects recognized an average of 23.3 percent of the words in the conversa-

TABLE 4-2   **Scores for the Conversational Sentences (adapted from Erber, 1985) List and the QUEST?AR Task (Erber, 1985)**

	SPEECH LIST			
	SPIN (% KEYWORDS CORRECT)			
SUBJECT	LOW CONTEXT ITEMS	HIGH CONTEXT ITEMS	SENTENCES (% WORDS CORRECT)	QUEST?AR (% KEYWORDS CORRECT)
CI1	20%	60%	45%	57%
CI2	12%	8%	DNT*	77%
CI3	4%	24%	14%	57%
CI4	48%	84%	89%	100%
CI5	4%	16%	19%	98%
CI6	12%	32%	53%	96%
CI7	8%	20%	14%	32%
CI8	0%	0%	0%	6%
CI9	0%	28%	26%	99%
CI10	20%	52%	56%	88%
CI11	0%	0%	14%	12%
CI12	8%	0%	4%	54%
CI13	4%	12%	18%	78%
CI14	0%	4%	6%	37%
CI15	0%	0%	1%	35%
CI16	0%	4%	35%	72%
CI17	0%	0%	6%	48%
CI18	4%	16%	14%	94%
CI19	0%	0%	26%	DNT*
CI20	0%	0%	3%	DNT*
M	7.2%	18.0%	23.3%	63.3%
(SD)	(11.6)	(23.4)	(23.2)	(30.4)

DNT* = Did not test

tional sentence list (SD = 23.2). For the QUEST?AR task, subjects on average comprehended 63.9 percent (SD = 31.3) of the keywords. Individual scores for the conversational sentences and the QUEST?AR task appear in Table 4-2.

Table 4-3 provides biographical and audiological data for all of the Nucleus subjects who participated in the studies reviewed in this chapter. The audiological data suggest that on average, the subjects are representative of the population who use the Nucleus cochlear implant. Their average word recognition scores are similar to those reported for other groups of cochlear-implant users (Dowell, Seligman, Blamey, & Clark, 1987; Tye-Murray & Tyler, 1989). Thus, we share the results from our telephone studies with candidates who are considering cochlear implantation. We

TABLE 4-3 **Biographical and Audiological Data for the Cochlear-Implant Subjects**

SUBJECT	AGE (YRS)	LENGTH OF COCHLEAR IMPLANT USE (MOS)	AGE AT HEARING LOSS ONSET (YRS)	DURATION OF PROFOUND DEAFNESS (YRS)	THE IOWA SENTENCE TEST AUDITON-ONLY (% WORDS CORRECT)
CI1	69	25	5	5	73%
CI2	42	39	6	5	73%
CI3	72	33	13	1	41%
CI4	32	56	27	1	95%
CI5	54	54	26	7	77%
CI6	46	33	16	10	71%
CI7	46	54	5	28	57%
CI8	64	23	14	26	0%
CI9	34	42	29	1	87%
CI10	45	30	13	29	66%
CI11	72	67	13	3	5%
CI12	57	63	8	22	30%
CI13	66	40	43	20	47%
CI14	35	74	20	8	57%
CI15	68	30	17	17	0%
CI16	58	56	47	5	76%
CI17	34	71	3	19	33%
CI18	43	42	1	40	63%
CI19	68	65	61	1	22%
CI20	56	18	21	28	52%
M	53.1	45.3	19.4	13.8	51.3%
(SD)	(13.8)	(17.4)	(15.8)	(11.9)	(28.5)

The Iowa Sentence Test (Tyler, Preece, & Tye-Murray, 1986) consists of 100 sentences spoken by a total of 20 different talkers. The sentences are presented in a sound-treated booth at a level of 73 dBA SPL (measured at the level of the cochlear implant microphone).

suggest that the average Nucleus cochlear implant user will recognize some words in conversational sentences in optimal conditions (i.e., a quiet listening environment while using the adapter recommended by the manufacturer).

By comparing the performance scores presented in Table 4-3 with those presented in Table 4-2 we can make the following generalization: Cochlear-implant users who are able to recognize some speech without the help of lipreading are usually able to comprehend some speech over the telephone. For instance, subject CI1 scored 73 percent words correct on the Iowa Sentence Test in an audition-only condition. He scored 45 percent words correct while listening to the conversational sentences presented with the telephone, and 57 percent keywords correct on the QUEST?AR task.

CONCLUSIONS

In this chapter, we have described procedures for assessing how well clients can detect telephone rings, identify telephone signals, and recognize speech. The procedures may be used with clients who use either hearing aids or cochlear implants. The scores obtained may justify the client's candidacy for particular assistive telephone devices or telephone training and practice. They may also provide necessary documentation to seek third party reimbursement.

Data from a group of Nucleus cochlear-implant users permit us to conclude the following:

1. Visual alerting devices may not be necessary when the cochlear-implant user is in the same room as the telephone.
2. Open-set recognition of telephone signals is poor.
3. Some words in conversational sentences can be recognized.
4. The recommended Cochlear Corporation TLP-102 telephone adapter is helpful when sentence context is high.

FINAL REMARKS

While objective data is important in the selection, evaluation, and fitting of assistive devices, practical considerations and subjective reports must not be overlooked. For instance, although a telephone adapter may enhance speech recognition, it might introduce new problems for some clients. Schum and Tye-Murray (1992) surveyed 45 Nucleus cochlear-implant users regarding their use of assistive listening and alerting systems. Fifty-three percent of the respondents indicated that they use a telephone adapter with their cochlear implants. When asked to rate how satisfied they were with the adapter, a mean satisfaction rating of 7.0 was obtained on a scale from 1 to 10, where

1 indicates very unsatisfied and 10 indicates very satisfied. When asked to qualify their ratings, many respondents reported that the adapter improved speech understanding over the telephone. However, they found the adapter "awkward" and "time-consuming to connect the adapter to the speech processor" when attempting to answer incoming calls. This was particularly problematic for respondents who have arthritis. Additionally, some complained that the adapter cannot be coupled to public telephones.

Whenever possible, it is desirable for clients to try an assistive device in their everyday environments. When devices are not available for loan, the audiologist might permit a month-long trial period after the client purchases a telephone assistive device. If the client is dissatisfied with its performance, he or she may return it.

Frequently, clients who converse fluently under good conditions will report speech recognition problems for long distance and public telephone communication. Thus, subjective assessments might include asking the client about how well he or she recognizes speech when conversing long distance and/or when using a public telephone in a noisy area. A client's report may indicate need for other assistive devices, for example, a TDD (Telecommunication Device for the Deaf) or a long-distance portable telephone amplifier that fits over the receiver of hearing-aid-compatible public telephones. Potential problems such as this should be considered when counseling clients about assistive devices.

Finally, when testing hearing-aid users, the objective assessment can include real-ear measures that have been obtained with a probe microphone. Fikret-Pasa and Garstecki (1993) collected real-ear measures for five different telephone amplifiers. For a stimulus, they used a speech-shaped waveform comprised of 80 pure tones. The pure tones ranged between 100 and 8,000 Hz. The authors cited two advantages of using probe microphone measures. First, they provide an objective assessment of the spectral and intensity characteristics of the signal that is received by the client. Second, the results can be compared directly (and immediately) to the client's audiometric thresholds. The real-ear response measures can complement the results from the tests described in this report, and help audiologists to recommend the optimum assistive devices for their clients.

REFERENCES

Bilger, R.C. (1984). *Manual for the clinical use of the Revised SPIN Test*. Champaign-Urbana, IL: University of Illinois Press.

Castle, D.L. (1977). Telephone training for the deaf. *The Volta Review, 79*, 373–378.

Castle, D.L. (1984). Unit 6: Using codes for telephone calls. *Telephone training for hearing-impaired persons—amplified telephones, TDDs, codes*, 2nd Edition, pp. 77–90. Rochester, NY: National Technical Institute for the Deaf.

Castle, D.L. (1988). *Telephone strategies: A technical and practical guide for hard-of-hearing people*. Bethesda, MD: Self Help for Hard of Hearing People, Inc.

Cochlear Corporation, Inc. (1989). *Clinical protocol manual for the implantation of the Nucleus 22-channel cochlear implant system in severely hearing-impaired adults.* Available from Cochlear Corporation, Inc., Englewood, CO.

Cochlear Corporation, Inc. (1991). New cochlear telephone adapter. *Communique*, Fall, p. 1.

Cohen, N.L., Waltzman, S.B., & Shapiro, W.H. (1989). Telephone speech comprehension with use of the Nucleus cochlear implant. *Annals of Otology, Rhinology, and Laryngology, 98*, 8–11.

Dorman, M.F., Dove, H., Parkin, J., Zacharchuk, S., & Dankowski, K. (1991). Telephone use by patients fitted with the Ineraid cochlear implant. *Ear and Hearing, 12*, 368–369.

Dowell, R., Seligman, P., Blamey, P., & Clark, G. (1987). Speech perception using a two formant 22-electrode cochlear prosthesis in quiet and in noise. *Acta Otolaryngologica, 104*, 439–446.

DynaMetric, Inc. (1992). *Summary of telephone logger patch characteristics*, dated February 6, Monrovia, CA. Patent number 4,446,335.

Erber, N. (1985). *Telephone communication and hearing impairment.* San Diego, CA: College Hill Press.

Fikret-Pasa, S., & Garstecki, D.C. (1993). Real-ear measures in evaluation of frequency response and volume control characteristics of telephone amplifiers. *Journal of the American Academy of Audiology, 4*, 5–12.

Kalikow, D.N., Stevens, K.N., & Elliott, L.L. (1977). Development of a test of speech intelligibility in noise using sentence materials with controlled word predictability. *Journal of the Acoustical Society of America, 61*(5), 1337–1351.

Schum, L., & Tye-Murray, N. (1992). A survey of assistive listening and alerting system use by adult cochlear implant users. Paper presented at the Assistive Devices for the Hearing Impaired: Tutorials, Applications, and Research Conference, Iowa City, IA.

Tye-Murray, N. (1994). Communication strategies training. In J. P. Gagne, & N. Tye-Murray, Eds. *Journal of rehabilitative audiology: Monograph on aural rehabilitation research.* Academy of Rehabilitative Audiology, pp. 193–208.

Tye-Murray, N., & Tyler, R. (1989). Auditory consonant and word recognition among cochlear implant users. *Ear and Hearing, 10*, 292–298.

Tyler, R., Preece, J., & Tye-Murray, N. (1986). The Iowa Phoneme and Sentence Test (Laser Videodisc). Iowa City: Department of Otolaryngology—Head and Neck Surgery, The University of Iowa.

APPENDIX 4-1: DESCRIPTION OF THE TEST SITE

The room measures 11.5′ by 19.0′, excluding an entry hallway. The room contains office furniture (four desks, two computers, one table, six chairs) and a television unit that remains stationary throughout testing. The room's concrete floor is covered with carpet. The room has a metal pane ceiling suspended by 3/4″ iron grids. The ceiling unit is covered with 3/4″ sound attenuation pads and the walls are covered with Gipson wall board. A 5.5′ by 6.5′ double-paned window is covered entirely with cotton-lined draperies. All of the studies reported in this chapter were performed in this room.

APPENDIX 4-2: DESCRIPTION OF THE COCHLEAR CORPORATION TLP-102 TELEPHONE ADAPTER

The TLP-102 telephone adapter is manufactured by DynaMetric, Inc. in Monrovia, CA (Patent No. 4,446,335). This adapter provides a full signal level analog output to a cord with a miniphone plug that inserts into the external input jack of the Nucleus Mini System (MSP) 22 speech processor and deactivates the environmental earpiece microphone. The adapter is small in size and can be semi-permanently affixed to the side of any modular telephone, even a digital telephone. The adapter plugs into the modular handset jack on the telephone base. The handset coil cord then plugs into the modular jack on the adapter (DynaMetric, Inc., 1992). A photograph of the adapter connected to the Comdial office telephone (used in the present studies) and the Nucleus MSP speech processor appears in Figure 4-4. The telephone adapter simultaneously provides an audio output from the receiver of the telephone and the electrical output which is routed to the speech processor. According to the calibration guide provided by Cochlear Corporation (1989), when the acoustic output of the telephone receiver is 82 dBA SPL (as measured with the receiver pressed gently against an MX-41/AR ear cushion attached to a 1/2″ sound level meter microphone), the electrical signal delivered to the MSP speech processor is in an appropriate range for comfortable listening. For the test materials used in the present studies, the adapter was providing a typical peak input voltage to the MSP speech processor of 0.2 volts.

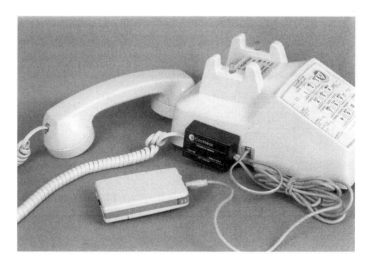

FIGURE 4-4 **Photograph of the TLP-102 adapter connected to the Comdial office telephone and the Nucleus Mini-System 22 speech processor**

APPENDIX 4-3: CONVERSATIONAL TEST ITEMS, ORGANIZED BY CONVERSATIONAL GOAL (ADAPTED FROM ERBER, 1985)

CONVERSATIONAL GOAL

1. Make arrangements
   Do you want to go shopping on Thursday?
   I'll meet you in front of the University Hospital.[1]
   Can we have lunch tomorrow?[2]
   We'll see you at the football game.*

2. Confirm arrangements
   Remember, your appointment is at 3:30.[3]
   Did you say that you would drive me to work today?[4]
   The trip to Des Moines is scheduled for November 23rd.*
   You're going to the restaurant, aren't you?*

3. Obtain information
   What time will the shuttle arrive from the Cedar Rapids airport?[5]
   Where will the family reunion be held?*
   Are you going to the church social?*
   Is Bill home?*

4. Give information
   Jane had a baby girl.[6]
   There's been a car accident in front of our house.[7]
   We won the game, but it wasn't easy.[8]
   I found that cake recipe that you asked for.[9]

5. Make social contact
   Tell me about your new grandson. (Erber, 1985, p. 70)
   How do you like your new job? (Erber, 1985, p. 70)
   Mary tells me you've been sick.*
   What did you do last weekend? (Erber, 1985, p. 70)

6. Plan future action
   Be sure to turn on the oven at 4:00.[10]
   I'll be a little late for the meeting. (Erber, 1985, p. 71)
   Please stop and buy milk at the grocery store.*
   We'll be on vacation next month.*

7. Get help
   Please send a plumber as soon as possible. (Erber, 1985, p. 71)
   My car has a flat tire! (Erber, 1985, p. 71)
   I'm not feeling well. Can you come over?[11]
   I need to run an errand. Would you watch my children?*

8. Respond to

Would you like to contribute to the Policeman's Fund?*

Is this 333-1212?*

Who is your presidential candidate of choice?*

Are you interested in our special prices on portrait packages?*

Is this the Smith residence?*

---

[1]Erber (1985, p. 70) presents this sentence as "I'll meet you in front of the Mayflower Hotel."

[2]Erber (1985, p. 70) presents this sentences as "Let's have lunch tomorrow. OK?"

[3]Erber (1985, p. 70) presents this sentence as "Remember, your interview is at 3:30."

[4]Erber (1985, p. 70) presents this sentence as "Did you say that you would drive me to the airport?"

[5]Erber (1985, p. 70) presents this sentence as "What time will the shuttle arrive from Garymede?"

[6]Erber (1985, p. 70) presents this sentence as "Jennie had a baby girl."

[7]Erber (1985, p. 70) presents this sentence as "There's been an accident in front of our house."

[8]Erber (1985, p. 70) presents this sentence as "We won, but it wasn't easy."

[9]Erber, (1985, p. 70) presents this sentence as "I found that pizza recipe you asked for."

[10]Erber (1985, p. 71) presents this sentence as "Be sure to turn on the oven at 4:30."

[11]Erber (1985, p. 71) presents this sentence as "I'm not feeling very well. Please come over."

*Locally produced test item.

APPENDIX 4-4: SCRIPT USED FOR THE QUEST?AR TASK (KEYWORDS ARE UNDERLINED) (ADAPTED FROM ERBER, 1985, P. 97)

TOPIC: The clinician's vacation in Alpine, California.

1. Client asks: Why did you go there?
Audiologist responds: To visit my in-laws.

2. Client: When did you go?
Audiologist: March 18, 1992.

3. Client: How many people went with you?
Audiologist: Two.

4. Client: Who were they (names)?
Audiologist: My husband Don and my daughter Kelsey.

5. Client: What did you take with you?
Audiologist: Too much luggage and some toys for my daughter.

6. Client: Where is the place where you went?
Audiologist: Alpine is in the mountains 30 miles east of San Diego.

7. Client: How did you get there?
Audiologist: We drove.

8. Client: What did you see on the way?
Audiologist: Beautiful scenery and lots of rain.

9. Client: Did you make any stops along the way?*
   Audiologist: <u>Yes</u>, we <u>visited</u> <u>relatives</u> in <u>Albuquerque</u>, <u>New</u> <u>Mexico</u>.

10. Client: What time did you get to Alpine?
    Audiologist: About <u>6:00</u> <u>Sunday</u> <u>evening</u>.

11. Client: What did you do first?
    Audiologist: We <u>went</u> <u>to</u> <u>Sea</u> <u>World</u>.

12. Client: What did you see?
    Audiologist: <u>Shamu</u>, the whale, <u>and</u> <u>talented</u> <u>dolphins</u> <u>and</u> <u>sea</u> <u>otters</u>.

13. Client: What happened there?[1]
    Audiologist: We <u>got</u> <u>drenched</u> with water <u>during</u> the <u>whale</u> <u>show</u>.

14. Client: What else did you do?
    Audiologist: We <u>went</u> <u>to</u> <u>Disneyland</u>, out to <u>dinner</u>, <u>shopping</u>, and <u>hiking</u>.

15. Client: What was the most interesting thing that you saw on your trip?[2]
    Audiologist: The <u>mountains</u> in <u>southern</u> <u>Utah</u>.

16. Client: What was the most interesting thing that you did?
    Audiologist: We <u>toured</u> the <u>historic</u> <u>San</u> <u>Diego</u> <u>Mission</u>.

17. Client: What souvenirs did you buy on your trip?[3]
    Audiologist: Some <u>Christmas</u> <u>ornaments</u>.

18. Client: What kind?
    Audiologist: Some <u>Victorian</u> ornaments. I <u>collect</u> ornaments <u>from</u> <u>places</u> I <u>visit</u>.

19. Client: How much did they cost?
    Audiologist: <u>$3.00</u>.

20. Client: What did you do just before you came home?
    Audiologist: We <u>rested</u> because we <u>knew</u> we <u>had</u> a <u>long</u> <u>trip</u> <u>home</u>.

21. Client: When did you leave to come home?[4]
    Audiologist: <u>Early</u> on a <u>Sunday</u> <u>morning</u>.

22. Client: Did you make any stops on the way home?[5]
    Audiologist: <u>Yes</u>, we <u>visited</u> <u>relatives</u> in <u>Colorado</u> <u>and</u> at the <u>Air</u> <u>Force</u> <u>Academy</u>.

23. Client: Did anything unusual happen on your trip home?[6]
    Audiologist: We <u>saw</u> <u>herds</u> of <u>deer</u> <u>and</u> <u>elk</u> <u>at</u> my <u>brother-in-law's</u> <u>on</u> a <u>Colorado</u> <u>mesa</u>.

24. Client: How long were you gone?
    Audiologist: For <u>16</u> <u>days</u>.

25. Client: How was the weather?*
    Audiologist: We had some <u>warm</u>, <u>sunny</u> <u>days</u> <u>and</u> some <u>cold</u>, <u>rainy</u> <u>days</u>.

26. Client: What happened on the way home?
    Audiologist: We encountered a <u>bad</u> <u>snow</u> <u>storm</u> going <u>through</u> the <u>mountains</u>.

27. Client: What time did you get home?
    Audiologist: About <u>2:30</u> on a <u>Thursday</u> <u>afternoon</u>.

28. Client: How did you feel then?
Audiologist: <u>Glad</u> to be <u>home</u> <u>again</u>.

29. Client: When are you going back?
Audiologist: <u>Probably</u> in <u>two</u> <u>years</u>.

30. Client: Do you think that I should go sometime? Why?
Audiologist: <u>Yes,</u> <u>if</u> you <u>like</u> the <u>mountains</u> and <u>southwestern</u> <u>culture</u>.

[1]Erber (1985, p. 97) presents this sentence as "What happened at the (place where you went)?"
[2]Erber (1985, p. 97) presents this sentence as "What was the most interesting thing that you saw?"
[3]Erber (1985, p. 97) presents this sentence as "What did you buy?"
[4]Erber (1985, p. 97) presents this sentence as "When did you leave?"
[5]Erber (1985, p. 97) presents this sentence as "What happened on the way home?"
[6]Erber (1985, p. 97) presents this sentence as "Did anything unusual happen? What?"
[7]Erber (1985, p. 97) presents this sentence as "How long did you stay?"
*Locally produced sentence.

► 5

Alerting and Assistive Systems

Counseling Implications for Cochlear Implant Users

LORIANNE K. SCHUM
NANCY TYE-MURRAY
The University of Iowa Hospitals

INTRODUCTION

Philosophy

While it is clear that cochlear implants can make a significant difference in the lives of persons with profound hearing loss, it is equally clear that the implants alone may not meet all of their communicative needs. In providing audiological rehabilitative services to cochlear implant recipients, we have identified that clients continue to require some listening and/or visual support assistance in communicative situations, as well as alerting assistance (Schum & Tye-Murray, 1992).

As with any hearing aid prosthesis, the listening benefit derived from cochlear implants varies among users. Cochlear implant users vary in how well they can detect

This study was supported by research grant DC00242 from the National Institutes of Health/NIDCD, grant RR59 from the General Clinical Research Centers Program, Division of Research Resources, NIH, and the Iowa Lions Sight and Hearing Foundation.

and identify environmental sounds and at what distances. For example, some cochlear implant wearers easily are able to identify the basic warning signals in their environments (telephone rings, doorbells, smoke detectors, children calling, etc.), while others are not. Alternatively, cochlear implant users sometimes identify *basic* environmental signals, but not *lifestyle-specific* signals, for instance, the clothes dryer stopping. Cochlear implant users also vary in their ability to recognize speech, both in audition-only and in audition-plus-vision conditions. Some can converse fluently over the telephone, while others experience frequent communication breakdowns in face-to-face conversations under optimal listening conditions. Regardless of the benefit derived from the cochlear implant, all clients experience events when they cannot use their devices, such as when they are sleeping, or when their hair is wet after showering. These are the times when they may not be alerted to necessary warning signals in their homes.

While the content of this chapter basically applies to adult cochlear implant users, much of the information may be applicable to children who use cochlear implants and their parents. Generally speaking, parents desire that their children grow up experiencing meaningful communication, safety, and world experiences, regardless of hearing loss. Assistive listening, visual support, and alerting systems can help children to have complete access to these inputs. While most young cochlear implant wearers use assistive listening systems in their classrooms, consideration also can be given for use of alerting, assistive listening, and visual support systems at home and in other public accommodations.

During pre-implant evaluations, audiologists, physicians, and psychologists attempt to instill realistic expectations for what listening benefit a cochlear implant will and will not provide. Clinicians may encounter different profiles with respect to assistive listening and alerting system use among new cochlear implant users, particularly: 1) clients who desire to enhance communication or enjoy music in particular situations, but are uncertain as to how they might use assistive systems with their speech processors; 2) clients who express alerting needs, but require instruction and guidance in the selection of alerting systems to best meet their needs; and 3) clients who are so excited with their newly restored hearing, especially after a prolonged period of deafness, that they disregard circumstances that continue to interfere with effective communication, or preclude detection of necessary warning signals.

When thinking of the need for alerting system use among cochlear implant users, audiologists might recall the "three psychological levels of hearing" described by Ramsdell (1978, p. 501): 1) the "symbolic (or social) level," where hearing is used for conversational purposes; 2) the "signal (or warning) level" which alerts one to events in the environment, to which one must sometimes effect changes; and 3) the "primitive (or auditory background) level" which creates the feeling that one is "part of a living world." Cochlear implants restore these three levels of communication for most users, at varying degrees. However, when the device is not worn (for instance, when sleeping), there remains the need to be *signaled* to changing events, and the need for the client to feel *connected* with his or her surroundings. In such a case, the use of visual or vibratory alerting systems may instill a psychological connection with one's surroundings and a sense of confidence that he or she will be informed of events that require a response, such as a child calling or a smoke alarm. (See also Compton, 1989.)

In summary, audiological rehabilitation for cochlear implant recipients does not end with connection and programming of the speech processor. We advocate that *the long term goal for clients is that they achieve independent communicative functioning in all communicative encounters.* Typically, this is achieved via cochlear implantation, communicative strategies training, and use of alerting, assistive listening and/or visual support systems. Leder, Spitzer, Richardson, & Murray (1988) concluded that after use of (an) assistive device(s), cochlear implant recipients reported improvements in their independence, communicative ability, and quality of life.

Terminology

In this chapter, we use the term *systems*, rather than *devices*, because it better describes all the methods clients may employ for alerting and hearing augmentation. For instance, a trained hearing ear dog, or pet dog, signalling a visitor at the door can be a reliable alerting system. For this reason, we favor the definition for *alerting systems* proposed by McCarthy, Campos, Balkany, & English (1987, p. 462), "Any device [or system] designed to act as [a] signal indicator and warning system."

We also have chosen to elaborate on the category known as "assistive listening systems." Systems that specifically enhance auditory signals (for example, an FM system), are referred to as *assistive listening systems.* Systems that visually augment auditory signals (for example, a closed-caption decoder) are referred to as *visual support systems.* Both types of systems are designed to improve speech recognition performance.

Chapter Organization

Much of this chapter is based upon what we learned from surveying adult cochlear implant users about their knowledge and experience with alerting, assistive listening, and visual support systems in January, 1992 (Schum & Tye-Murray, 1992). From trends observed in the survey data, we have identified particular counseling implications.

The remainder of this chapter is divided into four sections. The first section provides pre- and post-implant *needs assessment and counseling guidelines.* Short-term objectives are provided for approximating a goal of independent communicative functioning for cochlear implant users, through use of assistive technology, in addition to their implant devices.

In the second section, the *alerting needs* of cochlear implant users are discussed. Much of this section applies to hearing aid users with severe degrees of hearing losses, as well.

The third section cites options for hearing augmentation via *assistive listening and visual support systems* to meet the sometimes unique communicative needs of cochlear implant users (and possibly, hearing aid users with severe to profound degrees of hearing impairment). The intent here is not to provide an exhaustive list of all available devices that might be indicated for cochlear implant users. Such a list would become outdated as more devices are available over time. Instead, our intent is to differentially discuss the *types* of systems most likely to meet the communication needs of individuals with severe to profound hearing loss, especially those who wear cochlear implants.

Furthermore, rather than list all the particular communicative situations where assistive systems might be indicated, we will discuss the types of communicative encounters, for example, interactive as opposed to non-interactive communicative situations, where systems may facilitate communication. Appendix 5-1 categorizes communicative encounters as *interactive* or *non-interactive*, and warning needs as *basic* or *lifestyle-specific* (see also Compton, Chapter 12; and Compton, 1991).

The fourth section provides some final remarks regarding alerting and assistive systems counseling within an audiological rehabilitation program.

NEEDS ASSESSMENT AND COUNSELING

In order to obtain information for assessment and counseling, we surveyed the alerting, assistive listening, and visual support system use of 81 adult cochlear implant recipients in January, 1992 (Schum & Tye-Murray, 1992). The survey appears in Appendix 5-2.

Sixty-three of the survey respondents were implanted at The University of Iowa Hospital. The remaining eighteen were implanted at other cochlear implant centers, but were evaluated audiologically at The University of Iowa Hospital after thirty months of cochlear implant experience. Of the respondents, 45 wore the Melbourne/Cochlear Nucleus device (described by Patrick & Clark, 1991; Burton-Koch, Seligman, Daly, & Whitford, 1990 and Tong, Black, Clark, Forster, Millar, & O'Loughlin, 1979), 33 wore the Utah/Symbion/Richards Ineraid device (described by Eddington, 1978, 1980, 1983) two wore the House/3M device (described by House & Berliner, 1982; House & Urban, 1973), and one wore the UCSF/Storz device (described by Loeb, Byers, Rebscher, Casey, Fong, Schindler, Gray, & Merzenich, 1983; Merzenich, Rebscher, Loeb, Byers, & Schindler, 1984; Schindler, Kessler, Rebscher, Yanda, & Jackler 1986; Schindler & Kessler, 1989). The respondents ranged in age from 27–76 years old. The purposes of the survey were to determine:

1. How widely used are specific alerting, assistive listening, and visual support systems by adult cochlear implant users?
2. How informed are adult cochlear implant users about available systems?
3. Through what sources do adult cochlear implant users learn about and purchase systems?
4. How satisfied are adult cochlear implant users with currently available systems?
5. What new systems would adult cochlear implant users like to see made available?

Throughout this chapter, our strategy is to present data from particular items in the survey (Schum & Tye-Murray, 1992), and then consider their implications for assessment and counseling. Another large scale and thorough survey of sensory device use and needs by persons with severe to profound degrees of hearing losses was conducted by Harkins and Jensema (1987) using the focus-group method.

Knowledge and Purchase Sources

The Schum and Tye-Murray (1992) survey data generated surprising findings about cochlear implant users' knowledge of systems, and where they purchased systems. For example, the largest number of respondents (48 percent) learned about systems from consumer self-help group meetings and/or publications, such as Self Help for Hard of Hearing People, Inc. (SHHH). Less often, they obtained information from professional sources, such as audiologists (33 percent of the time), and general sources, such as department store catalogs and retail electronics stores (19 percent of the time).

With regard to purchases, however, the respondents indicated that they usually bought devices from general sources (39 percent of the time) rather than self-help sources, such as mail-order catalogs (33 percent of the time), or professional sources (28 percent of the time) (Schum & Tye-Murray, 1992). This finding may indicate three trends. First, the respondents may have comparison-shopped and found that chain retail electronics stores sell devices at lower costs due to higher volume sales. Second, many closed-caption decoders (the most frequently used visual support system used by the respondents) are frequently purchased from department stores. Third, the quality of devices purchased may be lower end. That is, the relatively high use of devices purchased from general sources suggests that clients may not be buying better quality devices.

The bottom line to acknowledge from this data is that cochlear implant recipients often learn about and purchase devices from sources other than audiologists. This information substantiates a need for audiologists to pursue orientation, counseling, and marketing of alerting and assistive systems more actively. As Leavitt (1989) stated, "Most hearing-impaired persons lack the breadth of training necessary to be effective self-advocates for the rehabilitation technology they need" (p. 2). For audiologists who are interested in marketing their professional consultation services to cochlear implant recipients, Palmer (1992) provides a well-thought-out model for the dispensing of assistive listening and alerting devices. Her model favors a professional consultation fee so that the actual dispensing of devices can be made at near cost to the audiologist (see also Sutherland, Chapter 13; and Compton, Chapter 12).

Preoperative Counseling

The objective of pre-operative counseling is for the audiologist to orient clients and their family members to alerting and assistive systems while imparting realistic expectations for cochlear implant use. The data described above suggests that little preoperative counseling about alerting and assistive systems occurs, since postoperatively clients reported learning about systems from sources other than their audiologists (Schum & Tye-Murray, 1992).

During preoperative discussions with clients, audiologists probably will learn that the most commonly used system prior to cochlear implantation is a visual support system: television closed-captioning. As a matter of fact, 17 percent of the survey respondents used no other visual support, assistive listening, or alerting systems during their years of profound deafness and cochlear implant use (Schum & Tye-Murray, 1992).

To facilitate preoperative counseling, audiologists might administer a brief checklist such as the one presented in Appendix 5-3. The checklist can determine clients use of, and interest in, various alerting, assistive listening, and visual support systems. It is helpful for the audiologist to personally administer the checklist during interviews with clients, rather than have them complete it on their own, since the names of certain devices may not be familiar to clients. The audiologist can administer the checklist prior to implantation, and then review it with the client and family after several months of cochlear implant experience. Although the checklist is simplistic, it determines the extent to which counseling and orientation about alerting and assistive systems will be indicated. For example, clients who require extensive preoperative counseling may indicate that they "have no need for" many alerting devices, suggesting that they may rely on family members to alert them to environmental warning signals. On the other hand, clients who require less extensive preoperative counseling may be those who check "currently use" for many alerting systems, and express that they are "interested in" some of the assistive listening options. For these clients, preoperative counseling may consist primarily of encouraging continued postoperative use of the alerting systems that are already utilized. Finally, the audiologist can assure clients that assistive listening and visual support options will be evaluated postoperatively, after a period of adjustment and trial with the cochlear implant in all listening situations.

The checklist in Appendix 5-3 can serve as a guide for imparting realistic expectations to prospective cochlear implant users, as well. The audiologist can highlight systems on the checklist and review with clients why those systems may be indicated in conjunction with a cochlear implant. It is beneficial to review the checklist in an assistive devices demonstration center, or with a display manual of available systems. For example, when audiologists counsel prospective clients for cochlear implantation that they probably will not be able to use the telephone as well as when their hearing was normal, options for enhancing telephone communication can be demonstrated (see also Slager, Chapter 3). For example, Cochlear Corporation, Inc. dispenses a telephone adapter that bypasses the telephone receiver and plugs from the telephone directly into the Mini Speech Processor (MSP) (Cochlear Corporation, Inc., 1991) (see also Tye-Murray and Schum, Chapter 4). The result is a more comprehensive and encouraging counseling discussion of realistic expectations for prospective cochlear implant users. Furthermore, from this early counseling session, clients learn how communication can be facilitated through means beyond just the cochlear implant ear-level microphone. While the audiologist does not want to overwhelm prospective cochlear implant users during preoperative evaluations, clients can be assured that the long-term goal for them will be towards independent communicative functioning in all listening and warning situations after implantation.

From the checklist or interview, the audiologist can assess clients' use of basic alerting systems. Audiologists might assume that clients with longer durations of deafness use more alerting systems. To the contrary, Figure 5-1 demonstrates that duration of deafness was not correlated with greater use of alerting systems by the survey respondents (Schum & Tye-Murray, 1992).

However, when clients are introduced to visual or vibratory alerting devices for smoke detection, telephone rings, and doorbell rings, they usually are receptive to purchasing and using such devices. Given that new cochlear implant users may be preoccupied for several months adjusting to their devices, it is advantageous to have these basic warning systems in place prior to implantation. Some lifestyle specific warning needs, for instance, alarm clock alerting, can be accommodated prior to implantation, as well.

A helpful and far more comprehensive needs assessment tool has been developed by Palmer, Garstecki, & Rauterkas (1990), in the form of a computer program entitled the "Interactive Product Locator of Assistive Devices for Hearing-Impaired Individuals" for use with a hard drive that has Hypercard™. This flexible program is designed

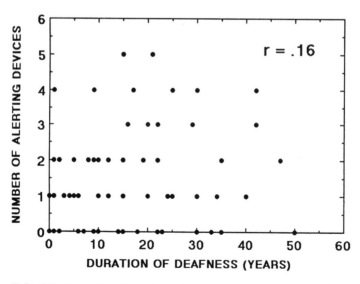

FIGURE 5-1   **Number of alerting systems used as a function of the survey respondents' durations of deafness**

to assist the audiologist in assessing and recommending assistive and alerting systems best suited to clients' individual needs.

With a lending assistive devices demonstration center, clients see how alerting systems work, and then have opportunities to borrow them and evaluate their benefits wherever needed: at home, while travelling, or in the workplace. The pre-implant period is a good time for clients to try and compare alerting systems for which they express interest. Experiencing how their communicative needs can be met, even before receiving a cochlear implant, can be motivating to clients. When possible, family members should be present for demonstration and orientation to alerting systems. Written instructions for use should be provided when clients borrow devices for home trials.

The preoperative period is also a nice time to introduce cochlear implant candidates to self-help consumer organizations such as SHHH and Cochlear Implant Club International, if they are not already members. Journals and newsletters from these organizations provide information about alerting and assistive listening systems, and their local and national meetings provide wonderful opportunities for clients to try and compare new alerting, assistive listening, and visual support technology. In fact, Table 5-1 demonstrates that members of self-help consumer organizations tended to use more assistive listening and alerting systems than did nonmembers.

Unfortunately, Table 5-2 reveals that many (55 percent) of the respondents were not members of either of the above two self-help consumer organizations, although many expressed interest in membership, as shown in Table 5-3. It would seem that clients' knowledge of assistive technology might be strengthened by encouraging membership in either or both of these organizations.

Preoperative counseling may conclude with the audiologist assuring clients that their need for assistive listening and/or visual support systems will be evaluated postoperatively, after a period of adjustment with the cochlear implant.

TABLE 5-1   **Group Mean Number of Assistive Listening and Alerting Systems Used**

SELF-HELP GROUP MEMBERS*	NONMEMBERS*	SIGNIFICANCE
4.28 systems	3.26 systems	p > .05 **

*Members (N=36); *Nonmembers (N=45)
**unpaired t-test

TABLE 5-2   **Memberships in Self-Help Organizations (N=81)**

SHHH ONLY	CICI ONLY	BOTH	NON-MEMBERS
11%	17%	17%	55%

TABLE 5-3 **Nonmembers (of either or both organizations) Interested in Joining SHHH or CICI.**

SHHH (N = 59)	CICI (N = 54)
45%	53%

Postoperative Counseling

Early Postoperative Counseling

Early postoperative visits can be tiring, and occasionally stressful, for new cochlear implant users, especially if they are participating in a research protocol. There is much data to be collected, sometimes by several different professionals. For this reason, it may not be advantageous to discuss the need for assistive listening and visual support systems during the first several months. The new cochlear implant recipient should have ample time and opportunity to participate in a variety of interactive and non-interactive communicative experiences. Ideally, the client and family will receive instruction and guided practice in communication strategies during these early months of cochlear implant use.

After new cochlear implant recipients have worn their devices for about six months, the audiologist should ascertain whether they have had opportunities to purchase and use the basic and lifestyle-specific alerting systems that were recommended during preoperative counseling. In other words, *the objective for early postoperative counseling is to ensure that clients' alerting needs are being met.* At this time, clients sometimes need reminding that although the cochlear implant has restored partial hearing, the device will not always provide necessary warning, for instance, when sleeping.

Later Postoperative Counseling

The objective for later postoperative counseling is to determine the need for assistive listening and visual support systems. Usually by nine to twelve months of cochlear implant use, clients have experienced most or all of the communicative situations that they will likely encounter in their daily routines. Review of the originally completed checklist (Appendix 5-3) can occur again at this time. The audiologist can ask clients and family members about which non-interactive and interactive communicative situations continue to present listening problems. As concerns are expressed for particular communicative situations, the audiologist can refer to the checklist and demonstrate the types of systems indicated for those situations. In some cases, clients may express that listening is not especially problematic in particular situations, but that further augmentation of the speech signal is desired. For example, some cochlear implant users desire to try assistive listening systems in conjunction with their closed-caption decoders. They are satisfied with their decoders, but simply want further sound enhancement.

Assistive listening systems require careful coupling considerations. For this reason, it is preferable to have clients try them at this later postoperative period, when they are fully adjusted to the mechanics of using their speech processors. Clients may, however, already be experimenting with some assistive devices prior to this time. For example, they may have taken the initiative to try telephone listening devices, especially telephone adapters which were dispensed with their speech processors.

Annual Follow-up Counseling

The objective for annual follow-up counseling is to ensure that clients' communicative needs are being met, as fully as possible, through regular use of their cochlear implants and assistive and alerting systems. Practice and encouragement may be indicated at this time. Communication partners can be involved in the practice sessions. Annual visits also provide an opportunity to introduce the latest technological advances in sensory systems to clients.

ALERTING SYSTEMS

Now that we have considered the preoperative and postoperative counseling sessions, let us consider specific classes of systems. First, we will discuss alerting systems.

The extent to which the cochlear implant survey respondents used alerting systems was alarmingly low. Table 5-4 indicates the percentage of respondents who used each alerting system on the checklist.

Unfortunately, the data in Table 5-4 provide testimony to the fact that alerting needs of cochlear implant users typically are not met. We suspect that many of the respondents simply were unaware of the variety of alerting systems currently avail-

TABLE 5-4   **Alerting Systems Presently Used by the Cochlear Implant Respondents (N = 81)**

ALERTING SYSTEM	PERCENT
Baby cry signaler (N = 7 clients with children age 6 years and under)	57%
Pet dog or cat	37%
Alarm clock signaler	31%
Telephone signaler	28%
Visual alert smoke alarm	22%
Doorbell signaler	21%
Trained hearing dog	2%
Door knock signaler	1%

able, since all the respondents expressed interest in learning more about alerting options. However, when discussing assistive technology needs, an audiologist's role is to inform clients of systems that may be helpful to achieve independent communicative functioning. This discussion should be conducted in a "comfortable, supportive, and nonjudgmental atmosphere" (Compton, 1991, p. 317) with complete respect for clients' opinions and decisions, especially given that their decisions may be culturally based (Compton, 1991).

Table 5-5 reveals the respondents' mean satisfaction ratings for different alerting systems, and the respondents' qualifiers for their ratings (Schum & Tye-Murray, 1992).

Table 5-5 also provides clinically useful data to consider when comparing and contrasting alerting systems with clients. The survey respondents expressed concern for the visibility of lights, reliability and costly repairs of alerting systems. Whenever visual alerting was desired, strobe lights were preferred. The reliability of devices can be assessed by repeated use in an assistive devices demonstration center and trial use in clients' homes. Clients might be encouraged to ask manufacturers about potential repair costs at the time that they consider purchase of devices.

Audiologists should avoid making assumptions about clients' use of alerting systems. For instance, as noted earlier in this chapter, duration of deafness did not influence the extent to which the survey respondents used alerting systems (see Figure 5-1). Consequently, audiologists should not assume that clients who have been deaf for 30+ years have their homes completely "rigged" with visual or tactile alerting devices. In our experience, many clients rely on family members for alerting and simply are unaware of alerting systems available for them.

Demographic findings from the survey are summarized in Table 5-6. Female cochlear implant users indicated having significantly more (p < .05) alerting systems

TABLE 5-5   **Rank Order of Alerting Systems by Satisfaction Ratings (where 1 = very unsatisfactory and 10 = very satisfactory)**

SYSTEM	RATING	LIMITING FACTORS
Trained hearing dogs	10.0	
Alarm clock signalers	9.4	Reliability of pillow vibrating devices
Pet dogs	9.2	
Telephone signalers	8.7	Light visibility Breakdowns Costly repairs
Smoke alarm signalers	8.4	Light visibility
Doorbell signalers	8.4	Reliability Breakdowns Costly repairs
Pet cats	7.3	Reliability
Baby cry signalers	6.3	Too sensitive

TABLE 5-6   **Alerting System Use as a Function of Respondent Demographics**

	GROUP MEAN NUMBER OF SYSTEMS USED	SIGNIFICANCE*
Males (N = 42)	1.19	p < .05
Females (N = 39)	1.95	
Young (N = 30) (ages 27–49 years)	1.87	p > .05
Mature (N = 51) (ages 50–76 years)	1.29	
Living alone (N = 25)	1.60	p > .05
Not living alone (N = 56)	1.52	

*unpaired t-tests

than did the male respondents. Additionally, many of the females reported having "homemade" alerting configurations, which were designed by themselves or relatives and were quite ingenious. Young cochlear implant wearers (ages 27–49 years) tended to use more alerting systems than did mature (ages 50–76 years) cochlear implant wearers, although not to a significant degree. Contrary to what might be suspected, the respondents who lived alone did not use significantly more alerting systems than those who lived with others.

Table 5-7 shows the frequency of use for particular alerting systems by the respondents who lived alone, versus those who did not live alone. A disturbing trend was revealed when tabulating that data: About one-third of the respondents who lived alone did not have any alerting systems, not even a visual alert smoke detector.

Also surprising was the fact that respondents living alone had fewer trained hearing ear dogs, pet dogs, and pet cats. Table 5-8, however, summarizes the respon-

TABLE 5-7   **Alerting Systems Used by Clients Who Live Alone versus Clients Who Do Not Live Alone**

	ALONE (N = 23)	NOT ALONE (N = 58)
Alarm clock signaler	39%	28%
Telephone signaler	35%	26%
Doorbell signaler	30%	17%
Visual alert smoke alarm	22%	22%
Pet dog or cat	22%	43%
Trained hearing dog	0%	3%
Door knock signaler	0%	2%

TABLE 5-8   **Respondents' Knowledge and Use of Trained Hearing Dogs (N = 81)**

Have <u>knowledge</u> of trained hearing dogs	89%
Have <u>no knowledge</u> of trained hearing dogs	11%
Have <u>inquired</u> about trained hearing dogs	20%
Have <u>not inquired</u> about trained hearing dogs	80%
Are <u>interested</u> in a trained hearing dog	22%
Are <u>not interested</u> in a trained hearing dog	75%
Already have hearing dogs	3%

dents' status with regard to trained hearing ear dogs. Only 3 percent of the respondents had trained hearing ear dogs. The respondents who had pet dogs or trained hearing ear dogs, rated them as superior alerting aids (see Table 5-5).

For cochlear implant users with alerting needs that currently are not being met, and who would like the companionship of pet, a trained hearing ear dog (or an intelligent pet dog) might be a foremost recommendation. Unlike hearing aid users who may have selective alerting needs, such as telephone and alarm clock alerting, cochlear implant users require alerting to most or all warning signals, especially during sleeping hours. As Compton (1991) points out, "There is a positive correlation between degree of hearing impairment and the need for alerting devices" (p. 310). For this reason, trained hearing ear dogs easily meet alerting requirements for cochlear implant users. The advantage of an official hearing ear dog, as opposed to a pet dog, is that it may accompany its owner into public accommodations. Pet cats were considered to be less reliable than dogs in their alerting ability, as evidenced in the satisfaction rating data in Table 5-3.

We receive many inquiries from cochlear implant recipients in our clinic who are interested in knowing their candidacy for owning a trained hearing ear dog. Patient libraries, with instructional materials such as videotapes and brochures produced by hearing ear dog training centers, can help to inform clients about the alerting skills of hearing ear dogs and criteria for ownership.

Another means to meet the global alerting needs of cochlear implant users, besides hearing ear dogs, are devices that respond to a choice of warning signals, for instance, smoke detectors, telephone rings, doorbells, baby cries, and alarm clocks. Typically, these programmable devices can provide alerting for four to five different signals by way of remote, frequency modulated (FM) transducers, which are all received by a central visual alerting device. Vibratory or LED wrist-worn accessories are also available. Programming of these devices reportedly is easier with some than others. This is good reason for potential users to try them in their homes before purchasing, especially if they travel frequently and want to be able to reprogram the device away from home.

Thus, in addition to trained hearing ear dogs, multi-signal warning systems can provide users with both basic and lifestyle-specific alerting. This appeals to many clients because it is less confusing, more space efficient, and portable than several different devices. Of course, individual alerting systems are available for most basic or lifestyle-specific alerting needs, as well. Some clients are not candidates for, or are not interested in, a hearing ear dog. Others do not want the sophistication and expense of a multi-signal alerting system. For detailed information about currently available alerting systems, refer to Garstecki, Chapter 10.

The same alerting needs apply to hearing aid users with severe-to-profound hearing losses and children who use cochlear implants. Naturally, parents and siblings provide necessary alerting, for example, to a smoke alarm. But, why not allow children the opportunity to learn to respond to signals independently and feel connected with their environments? When children are fully adjusted to their cochlear implants, they may enjoy having special alerting systems of their own. They will have the same basic alerting needs as adults, but perhaps fewer lifestyle-specific alerting needs. Most children will find it enjoyable to have their own visual-alert or vibratory alarm clock, for example. A strobe alerting smoke detector in a child's room is an excellent idea. Parents of preadolescent hearing-impaired children sometimes express the desire for them to overcome their dependence on family members. Bringing alerting systems into the home at early ages may foster greater independence while making it fun and special for the children.

ASSISTIVE LISTENING AND VISUAL SUPPORT SYSTEMS

While the selection of appropriate assistive listening systems for clients who use hearing aids is done only after careful consideration of all the available configurations, the issue becomes even more complex for cochlear implant users. The first question that must be addressed is whether a client's needs will best be met with an assistive listening or a visual support system. As a general guideline, if clients recognize speech in audition-only conditions, assistive listening systems alone may be suitable. However, if open-set speech recognition ability is limited, then visual support systems may be preferable, either alone or in conjunction with ALDs. This, of course, can sometimes differ from what clients desire. Cochlear implant users often want to "practice listening" as much as possible and are afraid that if they start to rely on visual text, their listening skills will not develop. Other times, cochlear implant users desire as many inputs as possible. For example, some clients want to use both an assistive listening device and a closed-caption decoder. Finally, the situational and listening demands of clients must be considered. Although clients may exhibit good audition-only speech recognition, their communication needs might necessitate the use of visual support systems in order to fully obtain spoken messages. For example, an executive who frequently meets with unfamiliar talkers at business meetings may contract with a computer note-taking service (see also Crandell and Smaldino, Chapter 7; Slager, Chapter 3; and Compton, Chapter 12).

When considering the use of any assistive listening system, audiologists and clients must heed the following precautions:

> Any desire to couple an assistive listening device to the external jack of a cochlear implant speech processor should <u>not</u> be attempted without the prior approval and specific advice of the cochlear implant manufacturer to ensure compatibility with the speech processor and safety for the cochlear implant wearer. Under <u>no</u> circumstances should any device that is powered from a wall socket be connected to a speech processor, for example, a television or a stereo system. In such a case, damage to the external speech processor and/or the implant electrode array could occur. As a rule, <u>only</u> those devices that are battery-operated should be connected to a speech processor.
>
> After following the manufacturer's coupling specifications, if the cochlear implant wearer perceives <u>any</u> unusual sound perceptions (for example, loud noises or popping sounds), use of the assistive listening device should be ceased immediately and the cochlear implant manufacturer should be contacted for troubleshooting advice.

Table 5-9 provides information regarding the extent to which assistive listening and visual support systems were used by the survey respondents. Table 5-10 also provides their satisfaction ratings for the various systems and qualifiers for their ratings. Closed-caption decoders were the most widely used system of either category, and respondents were extremely satisfied with the derived benefit (Schum & Tye-Murray, 1992).

While the data clearly suggests that assistive listening and visual support systems were not used widely by this survey population, we received many inquiries about these systems. Frequently asked questions included the purpose of particular systems (for example, oral interpreting), and how systems could be used with cochlear implants (for example, direct input to a portable personal stereo).

Perusing the respondents' satisfaction ratings and cited limitations of assistive listening and visual support systems in Table 5-10, evidences that speech clarity continues to be a concern for assistive listening systems. In general, systems with text displays (i.e., visual support systems) were more highly regarded than systems designed to enhance the speech signal.

Probably the most needed area for assistance in listening or visual support is that of the telephone. It is not uncommon for several cochlear implant recipients in a caseload to simply not use the telephone at all and rely on other family members to relay telephone messages. In keeping with our goal for clients to achieve independent communicative functioning, conversational skills over the telephone can be evaluated and practiced, as described in Chapter 4 by Tye-Murray and Schum. Many of our clients have learned to use telephone amplifiers, or telephone adapters specifically suggested for their speech processors.

TABLE 5-9   **Assistive Listening and Visual Support Systems Used by the Cochlear Implant Respondents (N = 81)**

Closed-caption decoder	73%
Telephone adapter (N = 45 Cochlear Nucleus Users)	53%
TDD relay message service (N = 44 respondents who lived in states with relay systems at the time of survey)	39%
TDD	28%
Telephone answering machine	20%
Telephone amplifier	19%
Direct audio input	16%
Sign language interpreter service	7%
Note-taking service (Computer or handwritten)	7%
Fax machine	6%
Others (Stethoscope, HA telecoil, convex rearview mirror in car)	5%
Tape recorder (for meetings, lectures, etc.)	4%
Group listening system (FM, loop, infrared, hardware)	2%

When fluent conversation cannot be achieved via a telephone listening device, then clients might be encouraged to consider a telecommunication device for the deaf (TDD). The availability of telecommunication relay systems and TDDs in public offices makes this a more desirable option for clients (see also Slager, Chapter 3).

Oftentimes, clients screen incoming calls with answering machines to determine if callers are familiar or unfamiliar, and to establish the topic of conversation. If the caller is familiar, they may pick up the telephone receiver and converse. If the caller is unfamiliar, cochlear implant users sometimes return calls explaining that they have hearing losses and would like to take the lead in conversation, or they call back via telecommunications relay systems. The use of answering machines is a prime example of how clients learn to make use of everyday technology to meet their special communication needs. Another such example, includes the popular use of facsimile (fax) machines in the workplace. Clients indicate that they use this as a visual alternative to telecommunications. Computer networking, for example, e-mail, is yet another alternative to traditional telecommunications in the work office.

Similarly, clients will discover simple everyday means to facilitate speechreading. One respondent cleverly learned that additional rearview mirrors strategically placed in the car allow her to receive lipreading cues from her passengers, while still driving safely, of course! The mirrors can be removed and placed in her friends'

TABLE 5-10 **Rank Order of Assistive Listening Systems by Satisfaction Ratings (where 1 = very unsatisfactory and 10 = very satisfactory)**

SYSTEM	RATING	LIMITING FACTORS
Fax machines	9.2	
Closed-caption decoders	8.9	Delays in captioning Misspellings Visibility Size of device
Sign language interpreters	8.3	Sign too fast
TDD relay services	7.8	Awkward Not private Often lines are busy Time-consuming
Telephone amplifiers	7.4	Speech clarity
Answering machines	7.3	Speech clarity
TDDs	7.3	Slow Expensive long distance Impersonal Breakdowns Costly repairs
Note-taking services	7.2	Expensive Reliant on note-taker's judgments
Telephone adapter	7.0	Speech clarity Cumbersome Awkward
Direct audio inputs	6.8	Cords too short Static Occasional poor connections
Group listening systems	5.6	Speech clarity
Tape recorders	5.0	Speech clarity

cars, too. This kind of ingenuity should be recognized and encouraged. As a matter of fact, it can be fun, economical, and sometimes more likely to meet clients' needs than commercially available devices.

Demographic differences in the extent to which the respondents used assistive listening and visual support systems are revealed in Table 5-11. The female respondents tended to use more assistive and visual support systems than the males, although this difference was not significant. The younger (27- to 49-year-old) respondents used significantly ($p < .05$) more systems than did the mature cochlear implant wearers (50- to 75-year-old). Young adult clients seem to request assistive devices that couple to speech processors more often than mature clients because of their interest in listening to music

TABLE 5-11   **Assistive Listening and Visual Support System Use as a Function of Respondent Demographics**

	GROUP MEAN NUMBER OF SYSTEMS USED	SIGNIFICANCE*
Males (N = 42)	2.74	p > .05
Females (N = 39)	3.23	
Young (N = 30) (ages 27–49 years)	3.81	p < .05
Mature (N = 51) (ages 50–79 years)	2.52	

* unpaired t-test

and attending movie theaters. The most frequent request that we hear is for a device that will allow clients to listen through portable personal stereos.

As stated before, cochlear implant speech processors can be coupled to most assistive listening systems and even portable personal stereos, as long as attention is paid to the specific precautions (noted earlier in this chapter) and guidelines from the cochlear implant manufacturer. Of utmost importance is the manufacturer's recommendation for the proper adapter and shielded cable for impedance matching between the speech processor and the assistive listening device. Sometimes an interfacing accessory is also necessary. For example, Cochlear Corporation, Inc. dispenses the "Audio Input Selector" for use with their Mini Speech Processor (Cochlear Corporation, Inc., 1989). With the proper connecting cables, the Audio Input Selector allows users to interface induction loops, telephones with magnetic leakage, and receive direct audio input. Again, however, any interfacing should not be attempted without technical assistance from the cochlear implant manufacturer in order to ensure the safety of the wearer and the integrity of the speech processor. The Audio Input Selector also can enhance the signal-to-noise ratio for listening, with placement at a desired external sound source, such as a television.

When evaluating the effectiveness of various assistive listening systems, the audiologist can provide clients with the manufacturers' recommended cabling configurations and two or three different systems to try at home. Thus, clients can conduct paired comparison trials in specific listening situations. Comparative trials can be conducted at conventions, such as SHHH annual conventions, where manufacturers have assistive listening devices available for trial use while listening to program sessions, as well. Attendees usually leave conventions knowing which system works best for them.

All these same opportunities for assistance in listening and visual support, of course, are available for children using cochlear implants. Closed-caption decoders provide a means to connect the child, not only with entertainment on television, but also to world happenings with, for example, a news broadcast. We all remember playing in the living room, sort of "half-listening" to the news as children. This is how we grew up knowing about the not-so-close world around us. Children, too, can grow up playing and "half-watching" visual text and films on the television news broadcast. The benefits of such systems for children are endless. Of course, portable personal stereos with the proper adapter and cable, to input children's speech processors would be an especially popular idea, once the children are skilled users of their cochlear implants. Telephone devices might be popular amongst preadolescent and adolescent age cochlear implant wearers.

As for hearing aid users with severe-to-profound hearing losses, the coupling concerns obviously are not as complex as they are for cochlear implant users. However, when severe distortional hearing loss is a concern, the audiologist might evaluate the benefits derived from visual support systems, as opposed to assistive listening systems.

FINAL REMARKS

Recommendations for assistive listening, visual support, and alerting systems are best made within the scope of a comprehensive audiological rehabilitation program with clients, as well as their family members. That is, conversational fluency is most likely to be achieved with not only appropriate assistive listening or visual support systems, but also with the use of assertive communication strategies. For instance, while the use of an auxiliary microphone in the center of a table at a restaurant certainly will facilitate conversation, occasional communication breakdowns might still occur. Clients need to be competent managers of their listening environments and skilled users of directive repair strategies (Erber & Lind, 1994; Tye-Murray, 1994; Kaplan, Bally, & Garrettson, 1985)

Most clients entering the cochlear implant process at our center have not received comprehensive audiological rehabilitation training prior to implantation. Typically, they exhibit good understanding of their hearing losses, a few report having taken "lipreading lessons," and to widely varying degrees they have been introduced to assistive and alerting systems. It has been our observation, however, that those clients and their families who become proficient in the use of appropriate communication strategies are able to derive the greatest benefit from their cochlear implants and also from the assistive listening and visual support systems that they use.

Our experience with cochlear implant users leads us to believe that most are receptive to the use of assistive and alerting systems. As a matter of fact, the findings obtained in our survey (Schum & Tye-Murray, 1992) suggest that cochlear implant users desire to know more about systems. The systems they most frequently want to know more about are listed in Table 5-12.

Not only do cochlear implant users desire to know more about systems, they also desire new systems. In the survey, respondents were asked to make a "wish list" of systems they would like. Frequently requested items appear in Table 5-13.

TABLE 5-12   **Alerting and Assistive Listening Systems that Respondents Most Frequently Wanted to Know More about**

Group listening systems (FM, induction loop, and infrared)
Direct connection audio input
Visual alert smoke alarms
Door knock signalers
TDD use with relay systems

TABLE 5-13   **Alerting, Assistive Listening, and Visual Support Systems that Respondents Most Frequently Requested as "Wish" Items**

Tornado/severe weather warning system for hearing-impaired individuals
Computer that identifies environmental sounds and speech with visual text displays
Cochlear implant suitable to wear while sleeping
Wind noise suppressor feature on the speech processor (aside from the sensitivity dial)
Telephone adapter (Ineraid users)
Induction coil to access induction loop systems (Ineraid users)
Optional headset microphone (for use when doing vigorous outdoor activities)

Audiologists may wonder why these clients appear so interested in learning more about systems, given that their mean percentages of use are somewhat low. The respondents were asked to complete the following statement: I would have more assistive listening, visual support, and alerting systems if . . . Their answers appear in Table 5-14 (Schum & Tye-Murray, 1992).

Finally, the fairly low incidence of systems used does not appear to be due to consumer dissatisfaction. Table 5-15 evidences the respondents' satisfaction ratings for a variety of consumer issues related to alerting and assistive systems (Schum & Tye-Murray, 1992).

Alerting, assistive listening, and visual support systems are necessary for cochlear implant users. They should not be viewed as extraneous. However, they do represent additional expenses that some clients cannot incur. Audiologists must continue to evaluate means for seeking reimbursement of professional consultation time spent in the selection of systems. Service organizations will sometimes assist in securing assistive and alerting systems for clients.

Too often, audiologists tend to focus on the selection and fitting of primary prosthetic devices, whether they be hearing aids or cochlear implants. However, the inherent limitations of these primary hearing devices dictate that comprehensive audiological service is not complete until full consideration is given to clients' need for assistive technology.

TABLE 5-14   **I would have more assistive listening, visual support, and alerting systems if . . . (N = 81)**

I could have home trial periods.	80%
I felt that I needed them.	48%
I were more informed of available items.	44%
I could afford them.	43%
speech were clearer through devices.	40%
I could have personal demonstration and instruction in use of devices.	26%

TABLE 5-15   **Mean Satisfaction Ratings for Consumer Issues on a Scale from 1 – 10 (N = 81)**

Cochlear Implant 1 = very unsatisfactory 10 = very satisfactory	7.7
Hearing aid for other ear (N = 12 HA users) 1 = very unsatisfactory 10 = very satisfactory	4.5
Instructions for ALDs and alerting devices 1 = very unclear and confusing 10 = very clear and understandable	7.2
Cost of ALDs and alerting devices 1 = very underpriced 10 = very overpriced	6.5
Warranties for ALDs and alerting devices 1 = very inadequate 10 = very adequate	5.8
Quality of assistive listening devices 1 = very poor 10 = very good	7.2
Quality of alerting devices 1 = very poor 10 = very good	7.0

CONCLUSIONS

The results of the survey (Schum & Tye-Murray, 1992) permit five conclusions to be made. In general, the cochlear implant respondents described in this chapter

1. did not possess alerting, assistive listening, and visual support means to fulfill all their communicative needs.

2. were not fully informed of currently available alerting, assistive listening, and visual support systems.

3. were interested in trying more systems if personal demonstration, instruction, and home trial periods are provided.

4. were satisfied with the quality, warranties, costs, and written instructions of available systems.

5. are seeking technological improvements and new alerting, assistive listening, and visual support systems.

REFERENCES

Burton-Koch, D., Seligman, P., Daly, C., & Whitford, L. (1990). A multipeak feature extraction coding strategy for a multichannel cochlear implant. *Hearing Instruments, 41,* 3:28–30.

Cochlear Corporation, Inc. (1991). New cochlear telephone adapter. *Communique,* Fall, p. 1.

Cochlear Corporation, Inc. (August, 1989). *Handbook for audio input selector.*

Compton, C.L. (1989) Assistive technology: Up close and personal. *Seminars in Hearing, 10*(1) 104–120.

Compton, C.L. (1991). Chapter 26: Clinical management of assistive technology users - Issues to consider. In G.A. Studebaker, F.H. Bess, & L.B. Beck (Eds.), *Vanderbilt Hearing Aid Report II,* pp. 301–318. Parkton, MD: York Press.

Eddington, D.K. (1978). Auditory prothesis research with multiple channel intracochlear stimulation in man. *Annals of Otology, Rhinology, and Laryngology, 87,* (Suppl. 53), 5–39.

Eddington, D.K. (1980). Speech discrimination in deaf subjects with cochlear implants. *Journal of the Acoustical Society of America, 68,* 885–891.

Eddington, D.K. (1983). Speech recognition in deaf subjects with multichannel intracochlear electrodes. *Annals of the New York Academy of Sciences, 405,* 241–258.

Erber, N.P., & Lind, C. (1994). Communication therapy: Theory and practice. In J.P. Gagne, & N. Tye-Murray (Eds.), *Research in audiological rehabilitation: Current trends and future directions. Journal of Rehabilitative Audiology,* Monograph Supplement 25.

Harkins, J.E., & Jensema, C.J. (1987, July). Focus-group discussions with deaf and severely hard of hearing people on needs for sensory devices. Technology Assessment Program, Gallaudet Research Institute.

House, W.F., & Berliner, K.I. (1982). Cochlear implants: Progress and perspectives, *Annals of Otology, Rhinology, and Laryngology,* (Suppl. 91), 1–124.

House, W.F., & Urban, J. (1973). Long-term results of electrode implantation and electronic stimulation of the cochlea in man. *Annals of Otology, Rhinology, and Laryngology, 82,* 504–517.

Kaplan, H., Bally, S.J., & Garrettson, C. (1985). *Speechreading: A way to improve understanding (second edition).* Washington, DC: Gallaudet University Press.

Leavitt, R.J. (1989). Considerations for use of rehabilitative technology by hearing-impaired persons. *Seminars in Hearing, 10,* 1–10.

Leder, S., Spitzer, J., Richardson, F., & Murray, M. (1988, January). Sensory rehabilitation of the adventitiously deafened: Use of assistive communication and alerting devices. *The Volta Review,* 19–23.

Loeb, G.E., Byers, C.L., Rebscher, S.J., Casey, D.E., Fong, M.M., Schindler, R.A., Gray, R.F.,

& Merzenich, M.M. (1983). Design and fabrication of an experimental cochlear prosthesis. *Medical and Biological Engineering and Computing, 21,* 241–254.

Mahon, W.J. (1985). Assistive devices and systems. *The Hearing Journal, 384*:7–14.

McCarthy, P.A., Campos, C.T. Balkany, T., & English, B. (1987). Chapter 13: Recent developments in rehabilitative audiology. In J.G. Alpiner, & P.A. McCarthy, (Eds.), *Rehabilitative Audiology: Children and Adults,* pp. 459–494. Baltimore, MD: Williams and Wilkins.

Merzenich, M.M., Rebscher, S.J., Loeb, G.E., Byers, C.L., & Schindler, R.A. (1984). The USCF cochlear implant project. State of development. *Advances in Audiology, 2,* 119–144.

Palmer, C.V. (1992). Assistive devices in the audiology practice. *American Journal of Audiology, March,* 37–57.

Palmer, C.V., Garstecki, D.C., & Rauterkus, M. (1990, November). An interactive product locator of assistive devices for hearing-impaired individuals. Paper presented at the Annual Convention of the American Speech-Language-Hearing Association, Seattle, WA.

Patrick, J.F., & Clark, G.M. (1991). The Nucleus 22-channel cochlear implant system. *Ear and Hearing, 12,* (Suppl. 1). 3S–9S.

Ramsdell, D.A. (1978). Chapter 19: The psychology of the hard-of-hearing and the deafened adult. In H. Davis, and S.R. Silverman (Eds.), *Hearing and Deafness (fourth edition),* pp. 499–507. New York: Holt, Rinehart, and Winston.

Schindler, R.A., Kessler, D.K., & Rebscher, S.J., Yanda, J.L., & Jackler, R.K. (1986). UCSF/Storz multichannel cochlear implant: Patient results. *Laryngoscope, 96,* 597–603.

Schindler, R.A., & Kessler, D.K. (1989). State of the art of cochlear implants: The UCSF/Storz experience. *American Journal of Otology, 8,* 79–83.

Schum, L.K., & Tye-Murray, N. (1992). Assistive and alerting systems used by cochlear implant recipients. Paper presented at the Assistive Devices for the Hearing Impaired: Tutorials, Applications, and Research Conference. The University of Iowa, Iowa City, Iowa. June 11–14.

Tong, Y.C., Black, R.C., Clark, G.M., Forster, I.C., Millar, J.B., & O'Loughlin, B.J. (1979). A preliminary report on a multiple-channel cochlear implant operation. *Journal of Laryngology and Otology. 93,* 679–695.

Tye-Murray, N. (1994). Communication strategies training. In J.P. Gagné & N. Tye-Murray (Eds.), *Research in audiological rehabilitation: current trends and future directions. Journal of Rehabilitative Audiology,* Monograph Supplement *25.*

APPENDIX 5-1

Circumstances where cochlear implant users may desire alerting, assistive listening, and visual support systems:

I. Basic Warning Signals
   A. Fire alarms
   B. Smoke detectors
   C. Doorbell/knock
   D. Telephone ring
   E. Civil sirens
   F. Intruders
   G. Vehicles

II. Lifestyle-Specific Warning Signals
   A. Emergency vehicle sirens
   B. Car horns
   C. Alarm clock
   D. Children
   E. Attention
   F. Oven/microwave timer
   G. Washer/dryer shutting off
   H. Mechanical malfunctions
   I. Security alarms
   J. Others

III. Interactive Communication
   A. Face-to-face
   B. Telephone
      1. signals
      2. conversation

C. Groups
   1. home
   2. workplace
   3. social gatherings
   4. meetings
   3. classrooms

IV. Non-interactive Communication
   A. At home
      1. television
      2. radio
      3. stereo
   B. At work
      1. announcements
   C. At public accommodations
      1. religious services
      2. movies
      3. concerts
      4. dramatic arts presentations
      5. lectures
      6. professional conferences
      7. sports events
      8. airport terminals

APPENDIX 5-2

SURVEY OF ASSISTIVE LISTENING, VISUAL SUPPORT, AND ALERTING SYSTEM USE BY ADULT COCHLEAR IMPLANT RECIPIENTS

NAME: ————————————————————————

AGE: —————————————————————————

DATE: ————————————————————————

YEARS OF PROFOUND DEAFNESS *IN BOTH EARS* BEFORE YOU
RECEIVED YOUR COCHLEAR IMPLANT: ————

COCHLEAR IMPLANT: (Circle one)

    Nucleus   Ineraid

    House   UCSF/Storz

CHECK THE STATEMENT THAT BEST DESCRIBES YOUR SITUATION:

    ———— "Most of the time, I work *outside* the home."

    ———— "Most of the time, I work *inside* my home."

    ———— "I work part-time *outside* the home, and part-time *inside* my home."

    ———— "I am retired."

    ———— "I am disabled."

FOR THE PURPOSE OF THIS SURVEY:

WHENEVER YOU SEE THE TERM *ASSISTIVE LISTENING DEVICE* **IT REFERS TO "ANY NON-HEARING AID DEVICE DESIGNED TO IMPROVE A HARD-OF-HEARING PERSON'S ABILITY TO COMMUNICATE, AND TO FUNCTION MORE FULLY DESPITE HEARING LOSS EITHER BY TRANSMITTING AMPLIFIED SOUND MORE DIRECTLY FROM ITS SOURCE TO THE LISTENER OR BY TRANSFORMING IT INTO A VISUAL OR TACTILE SIGNAL"** (Mahon, 1985, p. 7).

WHENEVER YOU SEE THE TERM *ALERTING DEVICE* **IT REFERS TO ANYTHING DESIGNED TO "ACT AS [A] SIGNAL INDICATOR AND WARNING SYSTEM"** (McCarthy et al., 1987, p. 462)

YOU MAY REFER TO THESE DEFINITIONS AS OFTEN AS NECESSARY, WHEN ANSWERING THE QUESTIONS IN THIS SURVEY.

1. INSTRUCTIONS: Place an (X) in the column that best describes your use of, interest in, or need for, each listed system.

	CURRENTLY I USE	I USED TO USE	I HAVE INTEREST IN	I DO NOT NEED
ASSISTIVE LISTENING SYSTEMS:				
Closed-Caption Decoder for TV	_____	_____	_____	_____
Telecommunication Device for the Deaf (TDD)	_____	_____	_____	_____
Direct Audio Input (to speech processor from battery-operated radio, tape-player, or portable stereo)	_____	_____	_____	_____
Telephone Adapter (for speech processor)	_____	_____	_____	_____
Telephone Amplifier (any type)	_____	_____	_____	_____
Telephone Answering Machine	_____	_____	_____	_____
TDD Relay Message Service	_____	_____	_____	_____
Group System (FM, loop, hardwire, infrared)	_____	_____	_____	_____
Fax Machine	_____	_____	_____	_____
Oral Interpreter	_____	_____	_____	_____
Sign Language Interpreter	_____	_____	_____	_____
Note-taking Service	_____	_____	_____	_____
Tape recorder (for meetings, etc.)	_____	_____	_____	_____
Other (specify): _____	_____	_____	_____	_____
ALERTING SYSTEMS:				
Telephone Signaler	_____	_____	_____	_____
Doorbell Signaler	_____	_____	_____	_____
Door Knock Signaler	_____	_____	_____	_____
Smoke Alarm Signaler	_____	_____	_____	_____

	CURRENTLY I USE	I USED TO USE	I HAVE INTEREST IN	I DO NOT NEED
Alarm Clock Signaler/ Vibrator	_____	_____	_____	_____
Baby Cry Signaler	_____	_____	_____	_____
Pet Cat or Pet Dog	_____	_____	_____	_____
Trained Hearing Ear Dog	_____	_____	_____	_____
Other (specify): _____	_____	_____	_____	_____

IF YOU MARKED ITEMS IN COLUMNS 1 0R 2 OF QUESTION 1, GO TO QUESTION 2.

IF YOU DID <u>NOT</u> MARK ITEMS IN COLUMNS 1 OR 2 OF QUESTION 1, SKIP TO QUESTION 4.

2. On a scale from 1–10, where 1 means VERY DISSATISFIED and 10 means VERY SATISFIED, indicate below how satisfied you are with *each* of your assistive listening and alerting devices and the reason for your rating. Do this for all the devices you reported *current* or *discontinued* use of from PAGE 1. (YOU DO NOT NEED TO REPORT THE BRAND NAME, JUST THE *TYPE OF DEVICE*.)

   1——2——3——4——5——6——7——8——9——10
   very   very
   dissatisfied   satisfied

   DEVICE: _____
   SATISFACTION RATING (WRITE A NUMBER): _____
   REASON FOR YOUR RATING (BE SPECIFIC): _____
   _____

IF YOU MARKED ITEMS IN COLUMN 2 OF QUESTION 1, GO TO QUESTION 3.

IF YOU DID <u>NOT</u> MARK ITEMS IN COLUMN 2 OF QUESTION 1, SKIP TO QUESTION 4.

3. Referring to QUESTION 1, if you reported discontinuance of any assistive listening and alerting devices in COLUMN 2, please list those devices and from the list below, and select your reasons for discontinued use. (WRITE THE *LETTERS* OF *ALL* STATEMENTS THAT APPLY TO YOUR REASONS)

REASONS FOR DISCONTINUED USE:

    A. I did not need it any more.
    B. The device broke down.
    C. I lost the device.
    D. The device was not compatible with my implant.
    E. I try to get by with only my cochlear implant.
    F. The device was cumbersome.
    G. The device was uncomfortable.
    H. The device was a nuisance.
    I. The device was *never beneficial*.
    J. The device was *not beneficial with my implant*.
    K. Other (specify) _____

DEVICE: _____

REASON(S) FOR DISCONTINUED USE: _____

4. Complete the following statement. "I would have more assistive listening and alerting devices if . . .": (CHECK *ALL* THAT APPLY)

____ A. I felt that I needed them.

____ B. I felt more informed of available devices.

____ C. I could afford them.

____ D. I could have home trial periods.

____ E. I thought they would be of better quality.

____ F. the written instructions were better.

____ G. I could receive personal instruction and/or demonstration of the devices.

____ H. they had longer warranty periods.

____ I. they were not so complicated or confusing.

____ J. the flashing signals would be brighter.

____ K. the volume of the signal would be more variable (i.e., louder and softer).

____ L. speech sounded clearer through the device.

____ M. closed-captioning was improved or available on more television shows.

____ N. I had someone to setup/connect the device at home.

____ O. if one was available to meet the following specific need: _____

____ P. other (please specify) _____

5. Do you have residual hearing in your non-implanted ear?

____ YES   ____ NO

IF YOUR ANSWER TO QUESTION 5 WAS "NO", SKIP AHEAD TO QUESTION 12.

6. If your answer to QUESTION 5 was YES, do you *own* a *hearing aid* for your *non*-implanted ear?

____ YES   ____ NO

IF YOUR ANSWER TO QUESTION 6 WAS "NO", SKIP AHEAD TO QUESTION 11.

7. If your answer to QUESTION 6 was YES, do you *use* that hearing aid in your *non*-implanted ear?

____ YES   ____ NO

IF YOUR ANSWER TO QUESTION 7 WAS "YES", SKIP AHEAD TO QUESTION 9.

8. If your answer to QUESTION 7 was NO, explain why you do not use that hearing aid:

_____

_____

_____

AFTER COMPLETING QUESTION 8, SKIP AHEAD TO QUESTION 11.

9. If your answer to QUESTION 7 was YES, do you use any of the following devices *with* your hearing aid? (check all that apply)

____ group listening system (FM, induction loop, or an auxiliary microphone for direct input with your hearing aid) for conferences, meetings, or social events

____ telecoil (T-switch) for telephone listening

____ TV listening system (FM, induction loop, infrared, or direct connection audio input with your hearing aid)

____ other (please specify):

_____

10. If your answer to QUESTION 7 was YES, do you use any of the following devices in that ear *without* your hearing aid? (check all that apply)

_____ one-on-one listening system (such as a personal pocket-size amplifier)

_____ group listening system at my church/synagogue

_____ group listening system (FM, infrared, or loop system with an auxiliary microphone) for conferences, meetings, or social events,

_____ special TV receiver

_____ other (please specify):

---

11. If your answer to QUESTION 6 was NO, do you use any of the following devices with that *non-implanted* ear? (check all that apply)

_____ one-on-one listening system (such as a personal pocket-size amplifier)

_____ group listening system at my church/synagogue

_____ group listening system (FM, infrared, or loop system with an auxiliary microphone) for conferences.

_____ meetings, or social events

_____ special TV receiver

_____ other (please specify):

---

12. Where 1 means VERY DISSATISFIED and 10 means VERY SATISFIED, indicate a satisfaction rating for your cochlear implant.

SATISFACTION RATING FOR COCHLEAR IMPLANT: _____

13. Using the same rating scale, where 1 means VERY DISSATISFIED and 10 means VERY SATISFIED, indicate a satisfaction rating for your hearing aid, if you *currently* **own** one for your *non-implanted* ear.

SATISFACTION RATING FOR HEARING AID: _____

Does not apply; I don't own a hearing aid anymore: _____

14. Do you live alone? _____ YES _____ NO

IF YOUR ANSWER TO QUESTION 14 WAS "NO", SKIP AHEAD TO QUESTION 16.

15. If you live alone, approximately how far do your nearest neighbor and your nearest relative live? (Give an approximate distance)

_____ approximate distance to nearest neighbor

_____ approximate distance to nearest relative

16. If your answer to QUESTION 14 was NO, list the ages and relationship to you of all other persons presently living in your home. Also indicate with an **X** the hearing status (HEARING or HEARING-IMPAIRED) of each person.

AGE	RELATIONSHIP	HEARING	HEARING-IMPAIRED
___	_____	___	___
___	_____	___	___
___	_____	___	___
___	_____	___	___
___	_____	___	___
___	_____	___	___

17. List all the pet dogs or pet cats that live *inside* your home.

DOGS	CATS
_____	_____
_____	_____
_____	_____
_____	_____

18. While sleeping *without* your cochlear implant (or hearing aid) on, check each warning signal that you would be alerted to with a *special alerting system for the hard-of-hearing*:

_____ the doorbell

_____ a door knock

_____ a smoke alarm

_____ the telephone ring

_____ your children

_____ your pet(s)

_____ the alarm clock

_____ a tornado warning (or other civil) siren

_____ other (please specify) _____

19. Referring to QUESTION 18, if you *are not alerted to some of those signals with a special alerting device for the hard-of-hearing*, are you usually alerted to them in some other way?

_____ YES   _____ NO

If YES, how?

_____

_____

20. Of all the assistive listening and alerting devices you have tried at home, what percentage *were not beneficial* and therefore *never used, but not returned for a refund or credit.*

    (specify a percentage never used and never returned) _____ %

21. Of all the assistive listening and alerting devices you have used, what percentage *were not beneficial* and so you *did return them for a refund or credit.*

    (specify a percentage returned) _____ %

22. Referring to QUESTION 21, list each device that you returned and the reason for return. (YOU DO NOT NEED TO REPORT THE BRAND NAME; JUST THE TYPE OF DEVICE)

    DEVICE: _____

    REASON: _____

23. Of the assistive listening and alerting devices you have, *how many* were: (indicate a number before each item below)

    _____ purchased at a retail electronics store

    _____ purchased through a catalog specializing in assistive and alerting devices

    _____ purchased through a catalog of different products

    _____ purchased from an audiologist

    _____ purchased from a hearing aid dispenser

    _____ purchased at a department store

    _____ purchased from someone who designed and built it him- or herself

    _____ purchased or rented from a telephone company

    _____ purchased through a newspaper or magazine advertisement

    _____ homemade by a friend or relative

    _____ borrowed or given as a gift from a friend or relative

    _____ obtained through Vocational Rehabilitation

    _____ other (please specify): _____

24. Do you receive mail order catalogs of assistive listening and alerting devices?

    _____ YES   _____ NO

25. Are you a member of the *national* SHHH (Self Help for the Hard-of-Hearing) organization? (If you are, you receive their bimonthly journal publications.)

_____ YES _____ NO

26. Do you live near a *local* SHHH chapter?

_____ YES _____ NO _____ I DON'T KNOW

IF YOUR ANSWER TO QUESTION 26 WAS "NO" OR "I DON'T KNOW", SKIP AHEAD TO QUESTION 28.

27. If your answer to QUESTION 26 was YES, do you regularly attend the local SHHH meetings?

_____ YES _____ NO

28. Are you a member of Cochlear Implant Club International (CICI)? (If you are, you receive their quarterly journal publication entitled *Contact*.)

_____ YES _____ NO

29. If your answer to QUESTION 25 or 28 was NO, have you been informed of both these organizations and their publications?

_____ YES _____ NO

30. If you are interested in membership information for either of these two organizations, please check below.

_____ I am interested in membership information for SHHH.

_____ I am interested in membership information for CICI.

31. Refer to *question 1* and list all the assistive listening and alerting devices which you have *no knowledge* of:

_____

_____

32. Do you know what a trained hearing ear dog is?

_____ YES _____ NO

33. Have you ever inquired about having a trained hearing ear dog?

_____ YES _____ NO

IF YOUR ANSWER TO QUESTION 33 WAS "NO", SKIP AHEAD TO QUESTION 35.

34. If your answer to QUESTION 32 was YES, what was the outcome? (please explain)

_____

_____

_____

35. Are you interested in knowing more about trained hearing ear dogs?

    ____ YES   ____ NO

36. Thinking of the assistive listening and alerting devices that you *have knowledge of (not only that you own)*, how were you informed of each? (In each space, write a number of how many devices you learned about from that source.)

    A. Demonstration and/or explanation by:
       ____ a retail salesperson
       ____ an audiologist
       ____ a hearing-aid dispenser
       ____ a telephone sales representative
       ____ a friend or relative who made the device
       ____ a hearing-impaired friend or relative
       ____ deaf educator
       ____ presentation at a SHHH meeting
       ____ presentation at a senior citizens' center
       ____ display at a Health Fair
       ____ a speech pathologist
       ____ a Vocational Rehabilitation counselor
       ____ other person (please specify):

       _____

    B. Description and/or picture in:
       ____ a department store catalog
       ____ a catalog from a company that specializes in assistive listening and alerting devices

_____ a catalog of assistive devices from the telephone company

_____ a catalog from an electronics store

_____ a catalog or brochure from an audiologist or hearing dispenser

_____ SHHH or CICI *Contact* magazine

_____ a textbook of assistive and alerting devices

_____ a newspaper or magazine article

_____ an audiologist's office

_____ a hearing aid dispenser's office

_____ other person (please specify):

_____.

37. On a scale from 1 to 10, where 1 means VERY UNDERPRICED and 10 means VERY OVERPRICED, rate the **price** of most assistive listening and alerting devices.

(Write a number between 1 and 10) _____

38. On a scale from 1 to 10, where 1 means VERY POOR and 10 means VERY GOOD, rate the *quality* of most assistive *listening* devices (listed on the top half of *question 1*).

(Write a number between 1 and 10) _____

39. On a scale from 1 to 10, where 1 means VERY POOR and 10 means VERY GOOD, rate the *quality* of most *alerting* devices (listed on the bottom half of *question 1*).

(Write a number between 1 and 10) _____

40. On a scale from 1 to 10, where 1 means VERY UNCLEAR AND CONFUSING and 10 means VERY CLEAR AND UNDERSTANDABLE, rate the **written instructions** provided with most assistive listening and alerting devices.

(Write a number between 1 and 10) _____

41. On a scale from 1 to 10, where 1 means VERY INADEQUATE and 10 means VERY ADEQUATE, rate the **warranties** on most assistive listening and alerting devices.

(Write a number between 1 and 10) _____

42. The specific **option** or **attachment** I would like to see made *for my cochlear implant* is a/an: (please complete the sentence) _____

_____

_____.

43. The specific *assistive listening* device I would like to see made is a/an: (please complete the sentence) _____

_____

_____ .

44. The specific *alerting* device I would like to see made is a/an: (please complete the sentence) _____

_____

_____ .

THANK YOU VERY MUCH FOR YOUR TIME!

APPENDIX 5-3

ALERTING, ASSISTIVE LISTENING, AND VISUAL SUPPORT SYSTEMS CHECKLIST

CLIENT'S NAME: _____

DATE: _____

INSTRUCTIONS TO THE CLINICIAN: Place an (X) in the column that best describes client's use of, interest in, or need for, *each* listed system.

	CURRENTLY I USE	I USED TO USE	I HAVE INTEREST IN	I DO NOT NEED
ASSISTIVE LISTENING SYSTEMS:				
Closed-Caption Decoder for TV	_____	_____	_____	_____
Telecommunication Device for the Deaf (TDD)	_____	_____	_____	_____
Direct Audio Input (to speech processor from battery-operated radio, tape-player, or portable stereo)	_____	_____	_____	_____
Telephone Adapter (for speech processor)	_____	_____	_____	_____

	CURRENTLY I USE	I USED TO USE	I HAVE INTEREST IN	I DO NOT NEED
Telephone Amplifier (any type)	_____	_____	_____	_____
Telephone Answering Machine	_____	_____	_____	_____
TDD Relay Message Service	_____	_____	_____	_____
Group System (FM, loop, hardwire, infrared)	_____	_____	_____	_____
Fax Machine	_____	_____	_____	_____
Oral Interpreter	_____	_____	_____	_____
Sign Language Interpreter	_____	_____	_____	_____
Note-taking Service	_____	_____	_____	_____
Tape recorder (for meetings, etc.)	_____	_____	_____	_____
Other (specify): _____	_____	_____	_____	_____

ALERTING SYSTEMS:

	CURRENTLY I USE	I USED TO USE	I HAVE INTEREST IN	I DO NOT NEED
Telephone Signaler	_____	_____	_____	_____
Doorbell Signaler	_____	_____	_____	_____
Door Knock Signaler	_____	_____	_____	_____
Smoke Alarm Signaler	_____	_____	_____	_____
Alarm Clock Signaler/ Vibrator	_____	_____	_____	_____
Baby Cry Signaler	_____	_____	_____	_____
Pet Cat or Pet Dog	_____	_____	_____	_____
Trained Hearing Ear Dog	_____	_____	_____	_____
Other (specify): _____	_____	_____	_____	_____

▶ 6

Television Viewing for Persons with Hearing Impairment

DONALD J. SCHUM
LYNN VANCE CRUM
The University of Iowa Hospitals

INTRODUCTION

Americans spend a significant amount of time viewing television. Television has become the principal source of news, information, and entertainment for a significant proportion of the population (U. S. Department of Commerce, 1992). It is estimated that typical American adults spend over four hours per day watching television (Television Bureau of Advertising, 1992). Persons with hearing impairment deserve equal access to broadcast media. However, the degree and nature of their hearing loss may severely restrict the amount and quality of information they actually receive. Despite these restrictions, television viewing remains a high priority among individuals who are deaf (Liss & Price, 1981). The need for useful assistive technology for television viewing has been rated as a high priority, along with the need for assistive technology for telephone use and alerting signals (Leavitt & Freeburg, 1987). In fact, listening difficulties while watching television are often the principal reason for self-referral for an audiological or hearing-aid evaluation. The person with the hearing impairment may often need the television turned up louder than required by other family members.

A variety of technologies have been developed or adapted in order to improve access to broadcast media by persons with hearing impairment. The purpose of this chapter is to review the technology and issues relevant to improving access to television programming. Included in this review will be technologies designed to augment the auditory signal (FM, infrared, etc.) and also technologies designed to substitute for the auditory signal (open and closed captioning). Further, a variety of specific patient variables that need to be considered when evaluating the usefulness of each of the available technologies will be discussed. We will attempt to foster an understanding by the reader that complete access to broadcast media can be achieved only when the assistive technology is chosen specific to patient needs.

THE PROBLEM

Television listening is difficult for persons with hearing impairment for a variety of reasons. First of all, the presence of a hearing impairment by definition is likely to lead to reduced audibility of the audio signal when played at normal volume settings. Typical conversational speech reaches the ear of the listener at an overall level of approximately 50 to 70 dB SPL (Pearsons, Bennett, & Fidell, 1977). It is logical to assume that most televisions are set to provide this sound intensity for the typical, normally hearing listener. However, at these levels, a significant portion of the auditory signal will be inaudible for persons with hearing outside of the normal region. Simply turning up the volume of the television is problematic. Normally hearing listeners may object to this increase in volume. Further, most television sets do not allow for the frequency shaping that may be useful, if not necessary, for sloping hearing losses. The use of conventional hearing aids can help to increase the audibility of the audio signal from the television.

Unfortunately, hearing aids alone do not always solve television listening problems. An additional reason why television viewing is difficult for persons with hearing impairment is that there may be significant levels of noise or other auditory competition present. Levels of noise and competing signals that may seem inconsequential for listeners with normal hearing may be extremely disruptive for listeners with hearing impairment. Noise and echo may arise in the listening environment in which television viewing is taking place or even within the audio signal from the television. A common practice in television and movie production is to mix dialogue with background speech, environmental noise, or music. Although these background sounds are intentional and assumed to add to the overall quality of the audio track, patients with hearing impairment often report that this competition disrupts their perception of the intended signal. Conventional hearing aids typically do little to improve the signal-to-noise ratio of an audio signal already consisting of speech and competition (Van Tasell, 1993).

In addition, hearing impairment is common in the elderly. Due to changes in the central nervous system that accompany the normal aging process, many elderly individuals will have difficulty extracting information from broadcasted material (Cole & Houston, 1987). Given the sometimes rapid pacing of broadcasted material, and also given that listeners do not have the opportunity to request clarification from broadcasted material, elderly viewers are at a greater risk of missing information during television viewing. The presence of hearing impairment only serves to make a difficult situation worse.

Assistive listening devices can serve to lessen the difficulties faced by persons with hearing impairment in two important ways: increasing audibility and improving the signal-to-noise ratio (Pehringer, 1989; Ross, 1991). Unfortunately, there are two situations in which assistive listening devices cannot completely solve the television listening problems of persons with hearing impairment. First, if there is significant background competition in the original broadcasted programming, the assistive device cannot improve the signal-to-noise ratio. Also, if the listener has a severe-to-profound hearing loss, even an amplified audio signal may not be useful. In either of these cases, a substituted signal presented in another modality (i.e., captioning) may be necessary.

ASSISTED LISTENING FOR TELEVISION VIEWING

As stated previously, the purpose of assistive listening devices for television viewing is to increase the overall audibility and the signal-to-noise ratio of the audio signal. This goal is accomplished by picking up the signal before it is significantly corrupted by background noise and reverberation, and delivering it directly to the listener's ear at an individually chosen listening level. Assistive devices pick up the audio portion of the broadcast either as an electrical signal before it leaves the television set or via a microphone placed adjacent to the television's loudspeaker. In either case, the level of the audio signal at the listener's ear is typically higher than the noise in the environment, producing a more favorable signal-to-noise ratio. The problems associated with reverberation also are alleviated. These assistive devices typically allow for the independent control of sound intensity. Therefore, the television can be set at a comfortable level for those listeners with normal hearing, with the assistive listening device providing the amplification needed by the listener with hearing impairment. Further, some assistive listening devices allow for control over the electroacoustical parameters such as frequency response and maximum output (similar to hearing aids). Control over such parameters allows for more precise tailoring of the device to the specific amplification needs of the listener with hearing impairment. A variety of specific approaches have been used to bring the audio signal directly to the client's ear.

Hardware Options

Hardwire

Many television sets have an earphone jack that allows the use of an earphone for television listening. This offers a relatively low expense option for television listening for persons with hearing impairment. Figure 6-1 depicts a viewer listening to the audio portion of a television broadcast via a hardwired connection. The audio signal is deliv-

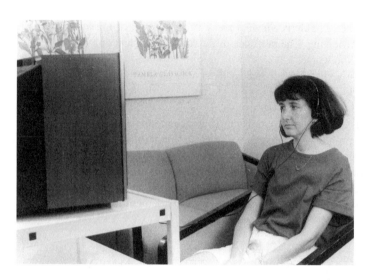

FIGURE 6-1   **A viewer receiving the audio signal from the television via a hardwire connection.**

ered directly to the listener through earphones. There are some significant limitations, however, to the widespread use of this option for assisted listening during television viewing. First of all, in many situations, when an earphone is plugged into the side of a television, the main loudspeaker is taken out of the circuit. Therefore, if other viewers in the room wish to hear the television signal, they cannot hear at the same time that an earphone is being used. Second, televisions typically do not allow for any frequency shaping of the signal. Therefore, there may be an inadequate high-frequency response through the personal earphone for a person with a significant hearing impairment. Third, many patients find the notion of being hardwired to the television inconvenient. If they sit any distance from the television, they are required to stretch a wire across the room. This trip hazard is significant and often is enough to deter a person from using such a system. However, if the listener typically views television alone, and the hearing impairment is not too severe, the use of a hardwire earphone may provide a reasonable solution for assisted listening during television viewing.

Some models of hearing aids allow for an electrical signal to be fed directly into the amplifying circuit. In such an instance, the audio signal from the television can be input directly into the hearing aid, as shown in Figure 6-2. The audio signal can then be amplified and spectrally shaped appropriately for the listener with hearing impairment. Individuals with cochlear implants are advised not to use hardwire devices that are powered from wall sockets because of potential safety hazards to their speech processors and electrode arrays (see Schum & Tye-Murray, Chapter 5).

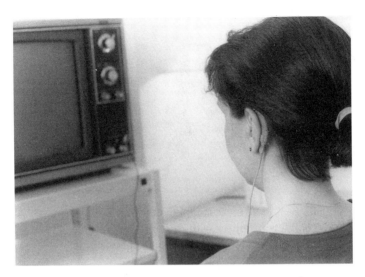

FIGURE 6-2   **A viewer receiving the audio signal via a direct electrical input into her hearing aid.**

FM Transmission

An FM transmission system consists of two basic parts, as depicted in Figure 6-3. A receiver with a microphone is placed near the source of the signal. The audio signal is converted to an FM signal and transmitted into the environment. The second part of this system consists of an FM receiver tuned to the broadcast frequency of the mate transmitter. The receiver picks up the FM signal and converts it to an audio signal that is delivered to the listener's ear via an earphone. FM transmission technology is used in a variety of products, not necessarily restricted to hearing impairment applications. For example, most popular baby cry monitors use an FM signal. Many household intercom systems also transmit via the FM modality. Crandell and Smaldino (Chapter 7) and Lewis (Chapter 8) discuss in detail the technology involved and the advantages and limitations of FM transmission technology, especially as related to use in schools and academic settings. A variety of reliable FM transmission systems have been developed for hearing-impaired students in the classroom. These systems also would work well for television viewing in the home. However, the expense and level of sophistication of these devices is generally more than is necessary for typical at-home television viewing. Therefore, less elaborate FM transmission systems have been developed for non-academic purposes. These include relatively simple FM transmitters and receivers with volume controls and at times some range of frequency response adjustment. In nearly all applications, both the transmitter and receiver are battery powered.

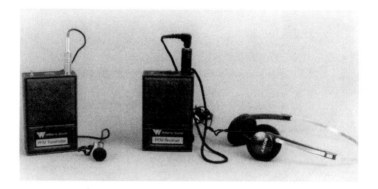

FIGURE 6-3 **The basic components of an FM system. At the left is the transmitter with its input microphone. At the right is the receiver with a set of headphones.**

Often cited limitations to FM transmission technology in hearing-impaired applications are the likelihood of electronic interference with the signal, and the potential for spill-over from one FM transmission system to another that may be operating at the same broadcast frequency. However, these limitations are not likely to be significant for most typical at-home television listening. Very few individuals have a high level of FM electronic activity within their home. Therefore, there is a small likelihood of the FM transmission being corrupted from extraneous signals. Further, it is also unlikely that a person is going to have more than one FM system operating in the same household. However, if a family is interested in having more than one FM system set up within the home, the audiologist can advise them as to how to broadcast on different frequencies. The range of FM transmission systems can be up to several hundred feet. Again, for most at-home television viewing applications, the distance over which the transmission will take place will be more in the range of 5 to 20 feet. Therefore, there should be no limitations on broadcast distance.

Although it is technically possible to pick up the signal electrically before it reaches the television loudspeaker, in most FM transmission applications in the home, it is likely that the microphone on the FM transmitter will simply be placed near the loudspeaker of the television. This arrangement should provide an acceptable signal-to-noise ratio in most listening environments. Further, this allows the television volume to be set independently for normally hearing listeners in the room. The person with hearing impairment can then adjust the volume of the FM receiver independent of the volume of the television.

In terms of transducers on the FM receiver, a variety of earphone arrangements are available, such as over-the-ear Walkman™ style headsets, or ear buds. Some personal FM systems also have neck loops available. Therefore, a person with a "T" circuit on his or her hearing aid can use it in combination with an FM system. In some cases, direct electrical input from the FM receiver to the patient's personal hearing aid is also available. FM systems can be used with cochlear implants, as long as the implant manufacturer's specific recommendations for coupling are followed.

Compared to some of the other television assistive listening systems, a personal FM system has the advantage of being fully portable. Although the client may primarily be interested in using the personal FM system for at-home television viewing, the transmitter and receiver can be used in a variety of other applications. The quality of the transmission is not limited by line of sight transmission (as is the case with infrared technology) or is not limited by the presence of an induction field (as with induction technology). Again, the reader is referred to Chapters 7 and 8 for a more complete discussion on the benefits and limitations of FM technology.

Induction

In an induction transmission system, the signal is picked up either electrically or acoustically and fed to an amplifying unit. This amplifying unit converts the original signal into an electromagnetic signal that is transmitted to a wire loop which encloses some space. The components of an induction loop system are shown in Figure 6-4. The amount of space that can be enclosed by the induction can be as small as a single chair, the size of a single room within a home, or as large as a full-sized auditorium. The amplifier typically is powered via the 110-volt household current. The person with hearing impairment who wears a hearing aid with a "T" circuit can pick up the electromagnetic signal when placed within the field generated by the loop. The listener simply needs to activate the "T" circuit within the hearing aid. For persons who do not have a hearing aid with a "T" circuit, a separate induction receiver (similar in size and shape to an FM receiver) can be used. The output signal from this induction receiver can be fed

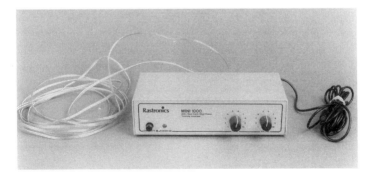

FIGURE 6-4 **The basic components of an induction system. At the right is the input microphone. In the center is the main amplifier, which sends an electromagnetic signal through the wire loop, shown on the left.**

to any one of a number of earphone arrangements. Gilmore (Chapter 9) describes in great detail the technological limitations and benefits of induction technology.

A variety of commercially available induction systems have been developed for persons with hearing impairment. These include amplifiers and loops of sufficient size and power to provide a relatively adequate signal for a complete auditorium. Personal use systems also have been developed with less powerful amplifiers and loop sizes more appropriate for a typical living or family room.

The principal advantage of induction technology for television listening is that the person who already wears a hearing aid does not have to remove the hearing aid in order to pick up the electromagnetic signal. The person simply needs to activate the "T" circuit on his or her hearing aid. There are two principal disadvantages to the induction system for television use. First of all, the person needs to be wearing a hearing aid with a "T" circuit. Therefore, if the person does not have a "T" circuit, or does not choose to wear his or her hearing aid at that time, he or she cannot pick up the electromagnetic signal. The second principal disadvantage is the lack of portability of the system. Typically, the wire loop is mounted in a semi-permanent position, for example, underneath the carpeting or behind the baseboard. It is not a simple process to pull the loop out and to re-loop another room, although it is technically possible to simply lay the loop around whatever space the listener may be in. This option would be considered impractical for most users. Again, the reader is referred to Gilmore (Chapter 9) for a more complete discussion of induction technology for persons with hearing impairment.

Television Band Radios
Another option for watching television available to persons with hearing impairment is to obtain a portable radio that is tunable to the audio portion of the television signal. The use of such a device for television listening is depicted in Figure 6-5. The person with hearing impairment can tune to the chosen television station, place the radio near, and adjust the volume to the appropriate level. Further, these radios often allow for the use of an earphone. Therefore, the person can access the audio signal of the radio directly and have it delivered to the ear via any one of the various earphone arrangements. In this setting, the volume used by the person with hearing impairment can be relatively high without disturbing other television viewers.

The use of a television band radio is a relatively low-cost option for television listening. The portable radios that are sensitive to television bands typically do not run much more in cost than traditional portable radios. There are two principal disadvantages of this system. First of all, there is a somewhat limited portability with such a system. The user needs to place the radio close to where he or she is sitting, and thus does not have the option of moving freely around the room. However, this is not a severe restriction, as most television viewing takes place with the viewer in a relatively stationary position. The second principal disadvantage of this option is that television band radios typically do not offer control over the electroacoustic response of the signal in a way similar to a hearing aid. Therefore, for a person with severe

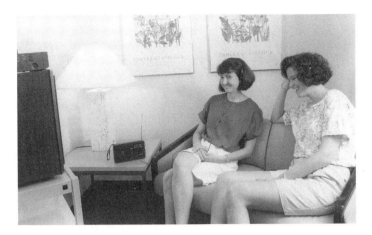

FIGURE 6-5   **The viewer on the left is receiving the audio portion of the television signal via a television band radio and an earphone. The viewer on the right is receiving the audio signal in the normal manner from the loudspeaker of the television.**

hearing loss, the television band may not provide a sufficient output, especially at higher frequencies, for adequate viewing. However, the output from such a system should be adequate for the more typical patient with a mild-to-moderate hearing loss.

Infrared
Infrared systems generally consist of two parts: the transmitter and the receiver. The transmitter is typically placed on or near the sound source (here, the television). The receiver is typically portable and worn by the listener. The use of an infrared system for television viewing is depicted in Figure 6-6. There are two ways in which the signal can be picked up by the transmitter. The audio signal can be obtained directly through a connection from an audio output or earphone jack of the sound source or through a microphone placed at the speaker of the sound source. The transmitter converts sound from the electrical input into a modulated light wave which is then transmitted to the receiver (Ankermann, 1984). Generally, the transmitter works on 110-volt house current, and the receiver is battery-operated. The receiver decodes the message coming from the transmitter and amplifies the sound. An infrared system transmits the desired speech signal directly from the source to the ears of the listener. A headset unit, for use without a hearing aid, suspends below the listener's chin, and houses the volume control. Since the signal is carried by light waves, there must be a direct line of sight between the infrared transmitter and the receiver. Therefore, personal infrared systems are used for close range hearing assistance situations. Cover-

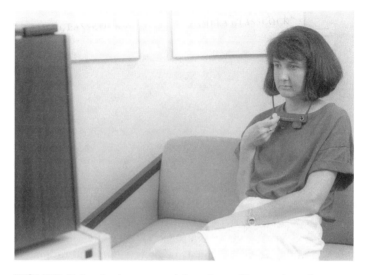

FIGURE 6-6   **A viewer receiving the audio portion of a television broadcast via an infrared system. The transmitter is located on top of the television set. The viewer wears the receiver. In this case, the viewer has control over the volume level.**

age is from 30 to 50 feet (Goldstein, 1986). For this reason personal infrared systems are ideal for television listening.

One aspect of an infrared system to be aware of is the effect of prevalence of infrared light in the immediate environment. Such sources are direct sunlight, fluorescent lights, and incandescent lamps. Depending on the intensity of the external infrared sources relative to the transmitted signal of the infrared device, the external sources could generate enough infrared energy in the listening area to drown out the signal. Due to this potential interference, the use of infrared systems generally is limited to indoors, where limited levels of direct sunlight are present (Pehringer, 1989). However, the sound quality and transmission integrity are usually excellent for indoor uses. An unlimited number of receivers can receive the signal from the single transmitter. For larger room applications (meeting rooms, theaters), a transmitter capable of generating a stronger signal will be necessary in order to ensure adequate reception in all parts of the room. Some models of receivers will allow for either direct input into a hearing aid, or for the use of a neck loop, or silhouette, in conjunction with the "T" circuit on a personal hearing aid. As with FM systems, infrared systems can be used with cochlear implants, as long as the implant manufacturer's specific recommendations for coupling are followed.

Choosing a System

Comparative Data

There is a limited amount of comparative data on the performance of the various assistive listening options. Therefore, it is difficult to turn to the literature to provide patients with clear advice in terms of which systems are more useful than others. However, there has been some work completed in this area. For example, Middleton and Ekhaml (1987) compared the use rates and the positive and negative aspects of induction loops, FM, and infrared systems. These authors found a high use rate of FM systems in different publicly accessible areas (schools, libraries, and hospitals). However, the authors found relatively high positive comments and relatively low negative comments for both infrared and FM technology. Induction loop technology was rated relatively poorly, with a variety of technical problems mentioned as negative aspects to this system. Hull (1988) provided a group of elderly hearing-impaired individuals the opportunity to use a variety of assistive listening systems, including FM and infrared technology, in a variety of listening environments. The individuals in this experimental group rated the infrared system quite highly for both ease of use and quality of transmission both at home and in publicly accessible areas.

Table 6-1 summarizes the comparative advantages and disadvantages of the various assistive listening systems available for use with television. The audiologist will often have the responsibility of recommending a specific system to a person with hearing impairment. It is incumbent upon the audiologist to evaluate a variety of lifestyle factors and personal preferences on the part of the user before recommending a specific system. Certain topics deserve further comment.

Volume Control

One of the first issues of concern is whether there will be independent control of volume on the part of the user of the assistive system as compared to other viewers of the television. If use of the assistive device eliminates the main audio signal, as in the case of some hardwired options, then the system can only be used by the person with the assistive device. This obviously places a constraint upon the use of the system. Most other options allow the user of the assistive system to set the volume independently, regardless of the chosen listening level of the other persons in the room. For example, most of the FM receivers or infrared receivers have an independent volume control. Given that persons interested in such an assistive listening system may present with a range of losses, the audiologist needs to be aware of the flexibility of such a system in terms of setting the volume. Further, some systems allow for independent settings of the volume in the right versus the left ears. This option may be necessary for a patient with a significant disparity in hearing levels between the two ears. Finally, if a person has a relatively steeply sloping hearing loss, it would be useful to be able to adjust the frequency response of the receiver. Therefore, similar to when choosing a hearing aid for a patient, the audiologist will need to know what electroacoustic parameters can be controlled on the chosen system.

TABLE 6-1   Advantages and Disadvantages of Various Assistive Listening Systems

	HARDWIRE	FM	INDUCTION	TV BAND RADIO	INFRARED
Expense	low	moderate or high	moderate	low	moderate or high
Quality of transmission	good	good, if no interference	variable	variable	good, if no interference
Electroacoustic flexibility	none	volume, perhaps tone and output	determined by hearing aid	volume, perhaps tone and output	volume, perhaps tone and output
Ease of use	poor due to trip hazard	good	acceptable	good	good
Portability	none	good	poor	good	poor
Multiple uses	none	yes	radio, stereo, stationary talker	standard radio uses	radio, stereo, stationary talker

Interference

As indicated above, some of the technologies are susceptible to interference. For example, the FM systems will be sensitive to stray radio signals in the listening environment. The infrared system will be sensitive to high levels of light in the listening environment. The induction system will be sensitive to high levels of electromagnetic energy in the listening environment. Therefore, the audiologist needs to question the patient carefully in terms of the likely presence of any of these sources of interference. If there is a chance that interference will be present, the audiologist should use that information when choosing a system.

Portability

When assessing client needs, the audiologist needs to determine whether or not the client is interested in using the system for applications other than television viewing. The person should be given examples of how some of the systems, such as the FM system, can be used in a variety of other settings other than television listening. Although the client may present to the audiologist concern only with television viewing, once other applications have been described, the client may be interested in the most portable system possible. The least portable of all the systems obviously is the hardwired system, given the direct connection to the television set. However, given the needs for direct line-of-sight transmission, the infrared system does have some limitations in terms of use. In other words, the listener needs to be in a relatively stable position. The induction loop system also has significant limitations in terms of portability, as most users would not be interested in pulling up the loop and moving it from room to room. Therefore, if the client has an interest in terms of portability, clearly the most obvious option for that patient would be a personal FM system.

Public Places

The audiologist should point out to the person with hearing impairment that the same technology that is available for at-home television viewing is often used in public entertainment venues. More specifically, due to a general concern about accessibility and specific guidelines laid out in the Americans with Disabilities Act (see Williams & Carey, Chapter 1), movie theaters and live theaters have, to a growing extent, installed a variety of assistive listening technologies. The two most popular technologies used currently are FM and infrared transmission. Typically, a central, large-room-sized transmitting unit is in place in the theater. Patrons can check out individual receivers for use during the show. Given the availability of a variety of broadcast channels, there is not a significant limitation to the use of FM technology in a facility that would have more than one theater simultaneously presenting a show. Further, given the low light levels, and the relatively stable positioning of an audience during most performances, there is not a significant technical limitation with the use of infrared technology within a movie theater. Again, in some facilities, induction neck loops are available to be used by persons who currently wear hearing aids with "T" circuits, or cochlear implants with special coupling equipment.

There is a chance that the level of expertise of the employees of theaters across the country will be low. Therefore, the audiologist should extensively train the person with hearing impairment on the function of such systems. It is likely that a person with hearing impairment will know much more about how the system within the theater works than many of the staff members of the theater. Therefore, if an individual is interested in using, for example, a neck loop in conjunction with his or her personal hearing aids, the patron may need to explain to the theater staff the specific hardware that he or she is interested in obtaining. The implementation of the Americans with Disabilities Act (ADA) is expected to increase the availability of such devices in public meeting places. Prior to the passage of the ADA, the use of assistive listening technology in public places was relatively spotty (Middleton & Ekhaml, 1987).

The person with hearing impairment who is interested in an assistive system for television viewing should also be informed that, at times, the receiver used at home will also be compatible with systems used in public meeting places. For example, if a theater has an infrared system, the personal infrared receiver that the person may use at home will also be compatible with the system used in the movie theater. Therefore, the patient does not have to go through the trouble of checking out a specific listening device when he or she goes to a theater. If the patient chooses to obtain an FM system for at-home use, the option of having tunable frequencies for the user's access should be considered. One reason for access to the tunable frequencies would be that if the person goes to a public entertainment venue that uses FM technology but is broadcasting on a different frequency, it would be handy for the user to be able to tune the receiver to the locally broadcasted frequency.

CAPTIONING

The technologies discussed so far in this chapter are designed to augment the auditory signal during television viewing. However, a significant number of persons with hearing impairment cannot successfully use even an augmented auditory signal. For these persons, a substituted visual signal, text captions, offers accessibility to television programming. Closed captions are hidden subtitles that can be seen on television sets with the use of a decoder. Until recently, a separate piece of hardware was necessary to decode the caption from the incoming television signal. A free-standing box, similar to the cable television channel selector box used in many applications, was necessary. These boxes were wired between the incoming signal (either from an antenna or cable) and the television set. These boxes typically offer the user the choice of viewing television with or without the captions present on the screen. The decoder reads a binary code from line 21 of the television signal and converts it into white characters on a black background that appear on the television screen. The size of the characters varies with the size of the television screen. On a 19" screen the characters are one-half inch high (Jensema & Compton, 1989). Since July 1, 1993, in accordance with the Television Decoder Circuitry Act, all televisions with a screen size of 13 inches or larger have been required to be manufactured with the closed caption decoder built into the television. This capability can now be implemented at a relatively low cost due to recent technical advances in microchip technology (Washington Post, 1992). Figure 6-7 depicts a viewer making use of a closed captioned broadcast. In this figure, the television signal passes through the free-standing decoder box before being fed to the television set.

Jackson and Perkins (1974) describe how closed caption television grew out of the area of captioned educational films for the hearing-impaired. They report that an obvious extension of this would be the more widespread use of captioning for televised programming. Closed caption television debuted in early 1980 with ABC, NBC, and PBS agreeing to provide approximately 20 hours per week of captioned programs (Cronin, 1980). At approximately the same time, the federal government established the National Captioning Institute as a non-profit corporation charged with the responsibility of producing and promoting closed caption television programming. A significant amount of captioning is also produced by the Caption Center of WGBH in Boston (Jensema & Compton, 1989).

Most prime time, and a significant amount of daytime, programming on the four major national networks (ABC, CBS, NBC, and PBS) is now closed captioned. A growing amount of cable programming is currently captioned, due, in part, to the fact that over half of the households in the United States now receive cable programming (U. S. Department of Commerce, 1992). The National Captioning Institute (1990) reports that, in 1990, over 200 hours per week of network television were captioned.

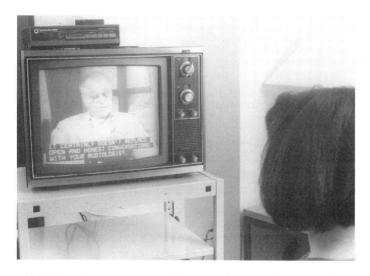

FIGURE 6-7 **A viewer making use of a closed captioned signal. The decoder is located on top of the television set.**

In addition, 170 hours per week of cable television and 85 hours per week of syndicated television were captioned.

In addition to broadcast material, there has been a push to close caption a variety of home video titles. In fact, by 1989, over 300 different movies available for home video use had been captioned (National Captioning Institute, 1990). At this time, it is relatively routine for most top-selling, new-release movies to be closed captioned by the time they are released for home video use. This captioning has greatly increased the accessibility to first run feature films by viewers with hearing impairment. Additionally, similar to the birth of the National Captioning Institute, the federal government has established the Captioned Films/Videos Service administered by Modern Talking Picture Service of St. Petersburg, Florida as a non-profit corporation. This agency loans captioned popular films on videotape to persons with hearing impairment. The service is administered through the mail at no charge to the user.

A condition where the captions are always present on the screen without the use of any type of decoding unit is referred to as open captioning. Similar to the use of subtitles for foreign language films, it is technically feasible to caption in an open form any film shown in a movie theater. However, given concern that this captioning may deter from the enjoyment of film by non-hearing-impaired viewers, there has been no push in this country to use open caption films in public facilities. Therefore, persons with hearing impairment who are interested in accessibility to feature films currently must wait until the films are released for home video use before they can view the film with the benefit of captioning.

Through the use of captioned television, the viewer who is hearing-impaired is offered the opportunity to read what he or she cannot hear. Television with the use of captioning can be an excellent educational tool, as approximately 85 percent of the more than 50 million children in the United Stated watch television every day; many for more than 32 hours each week (National Captioning Institute, 1992). Research has shown that children who are hearing impaired watch as much or more television than their hearing peers (Liss & Price, 1981). There is a paucity of specific research information of the effect captioned material will have on the understanding of the material. However, Boyd and Vader (1972) report that comprehension of a televised film was better for children with significant hearing impairments when the material was captioned. Similar results were found for adult viewers by Barras (1984).

A relatively more recent development in the area of captioning is the concept of real-time captioning. Originally, captioning was performed off line and mixed into the television signal when it was broadcast (Jensema & Compton, 1989). Since 1982, a variety of live programs have been captioned in real time (National Captioning Institute, 1992). This development has greatly increased accessibility to broadcasting, as live sports events, live entertainment events, and most importantly, live newscasts are now closed captioned in a variety of settings. Both national and local newscasts are currently closed captioned in real time. Real-time captioning is also becoming popular for live non-broadcast presentations such as lectures (Compton, 1992). However, given the technical skill necessary to create real-time captioning, this technology currently is rather expensive. This may limit its widespread use in non-broad-casted live events.

As might be expected, the accuracy of captioning varies depending on whether the captioning is done ahead of time, off line, or is done in real time. Even the best real-time captioners are still going to produce a finite number of errors in typing or transcribing. In contrast, off-line captioning offers the ability to check the accuracy and specific timing of the video and caption images. Further, real-time captioning often leads to a certain delay between the time the speech is produced, and the time that the captions are made visible on the screen. Again, given the relatively recent use of such techniques, the perceptual consequences of errors and delays in real-time captioning are simply not known at this time.

There are a variety of unresolved issues concerning the specific technical details of captioning. For example, specific data is not available on the optimal amount of time that a caption should be on the screen. It is well known that the rate at which we can read is significantly less than the rate at which we can listen. Therefore, there is concern that attempting to caption all parts of dialogue from a television program may exceed the viewers' reading capabilities. Therefore, in many situations, dialogue is often reduced when captioned to its most essential elements. This has led to situations in which the material being captioned on the screen is not tied specifically to the speech produced by the talkers. Thus, the ability for captioning to augment speechreading is somewhat limited given the lack of close simultaneous captioning and speaking. Although many hearing-impaired individuals will use both sound and captioning when viewing television, the interaction of these two effects has not yet been carefully studied.

As the audience for captioning expands, including not only individuals who are hearing impaired, but also English as a Second Language learners, young hearing children learning to read, and numerous others, the television manufacturers and caption providers are expected to pay greater attention to the needs and wishes of more special interest groups (King & LaSasso, 1992). Currently, a cooperative research project funded by the United States Office of Special Education, Gallaudet University, and The Caption Center of WGBH of Boston, has been initiated to determine which caption format features viewers with hearing impairment prefer, and which features enhance readability and comprehension of the captions (King & LaSasso, 1992).

THE ROLE OF COUNSELING

Leavitt (1985) has pointed out the relatively low level of knowledge about assistive listening devices, in general, on the part of persons with hearing impairment. Therefore, it is important for the audiologist to perform extensive counseling on the benefits and limitations of assistive technology for television viewing. The audiologist should not assume that the client is going to understand all of the subtleties of the various advantages and disadvantages of the different technology options. The audiologist should take the position that hearing aids and cochlear implants are going to have a limited benefit in certain difficult listening environments. Therefore, the need for assistive listening technology for specific applications is important.

Many clients will present to the audiologist for hearing-aid consultation due primarily to difficulties listening to the television at home. Often, either the person with the hearing impairment or a family member will comment on the relative high volume setting of the television. Although it is often the case that these patients actually do experience listening problems in a variety of other situations, it is quite possible that at-home television viewing is truly the only situation in which some sort of amplification is necessary. It is incumbent upon the audiologist to carefully question the patient to decide if a hearing aid for general listening use is truly necessary, or if the patient's primary concerns will be addressed simply by obtaining an adequate assistive listening system for the television.

Compton (Chapter 12) and Palmer (1992) provide a structured format to assess patients' needs for a variety of assistive technologies. Specifically in the area of television viewing, the audiologist should not assume that captioning is reserved only for the most severely affected patients, as all other patients can function optimally with some sort of augmented listening system. It is quite possible that persons even with mild-to-moderate hearing losses would be interested in using captioning as a supplement to assist television listening. Further, it is quite possible that patients who receive little information auditorily would still be interested in receiving whatever minimal information they can from the auditory signal. Therefore, the audiologist should at least provide the patient with the option of using both assistive listening and captioning systems during television viewing. At-home trial use of devices is an important part of the needs assessment, as clients are then able to determine the situations in which assistive listening and/or captioned material would be most useful. Hopefully, as more research is completed in the area of assistive technology for persons with hearing impairment, audiologists will be better prepared to make specific recommendations. However, given the paucity of specific research, especially in the area of television viewing, and given that the amount and quality of captioned material is increasing all the time, the audiologist should keep in mind that the clients are in the best position currently to review the benefit provided by each of the various assistive technologies.

REFERENCES

Ankermann, H.A. (1984). Infrared transmission technology. *Sound & Video Contractor, January*, 24–28.

Barras, B. (1984). Captioned TV: The third audio-visual revolution. *Hearing Instruments*, *35*(7), 16–18.

Boyd, J., & Vader, E.A. (1972). Captioned television for the deaf. *American Annals of the Deaf, February*, 34–37.

Cole, C.A., & Houston, M.J. (1987). Encoding and media effects on consumer learning deficiencies in the elderly. *Journal of Marketing Research, XXIV*, 55–63.

Compton, C.L. (1992). Assistive listening devices: Videotext displays. *American Journal of Audiology, March*, 19–20.

Cronin, B.J. (1980). Closed-caption television: Today and tomorrow. *American Annals of the Deaf, September*, 726–728.

Goldstein, W. (1986). Assistive listening devices. *Hearing Rehabilitation Quarterly, 11*(2), 4–8.

Hull, R.H. (1988). Evaluation of ALDS by older adult listeners. *Hearing Instruments, 39*(2), 10–12.

Jackson, W., & Perkins, R. (1974). Television for deaf learners: A utilization quandary. *American Annals of the Deaf, October*, 537–548.

Jensema, C.J., & Compton, C.L. (1989). Television for the hearing impaired. *Seminars in Hearing, 10*(1), 57–65.

King, C.M., & LaSasso, C.J. (1992). Your crucial role in the future of television captioning. *SHHH Journal, Sept./Oct.*, 14–16.

Leavitt, R. (1985). Counseling to encourage use of SNR enhancing systems. *Hearing Instruments, 36*(2), 8–9.

Leavitt, R.J., & Freeburg, J. (1987). Survey of ALDS interest. *Hearing Instruments, 38*(6), 28–29, 57.

Liss, M.B., & Price, D. (1981). What, when, and why deaf children watch television. *American Annals of the Deaf, August*, 493–498.

Middleton, R.A., & Ekhaml, L. (1987). The utilization of various assistive devices in schools, libraries, and hospitals. *Hearing Rehabilitation Quarterly, 12*(1), 4–11, 19.

National Captioning Institute, Inc. (1990). *National Captioning Institute Captioned Program Fact Sheet*. Falls Church, VA: Author.

National Captioning Institute, Inc. (1992). *Caption, 12*. Falls Church, VA: Author.

Palmer, C.V. (1992). Assistive devices in the audiology practice. *American Journal of Audiology, March*, 37–57.

Pearsons, K.S., Bennett, R.L., & Fidell, S. (1977). Speech levels in various noise environments. Project Report on Contract 68 01-2466. Washington, DC: Office of Health and Ecological Effects, U. S. Environmental Protection Agency.

Pehringer, J.L. (1989). Assistive devices: Technology to improve communication. *Otolaryngologic Clinics of North America, 22*(1), 143–174.

Ross, M. (1991). Listening conditions and infrared devices. *Hearing Rehabilitation Quarterly, 16*(1), 12–14.

Television Bureau of Advertising. (1992). *Trends in television*, p. 7. New York, NY: Television Bureau of Advertising, Inc.

U. S. Department of Commerce. (1992). *Statistical abstract of the United States 1992* (112th Edition), p. 551. Washington, DC: U. S. Government Printing Office.

Van Tasell, D.J. (1993). Hearing loss, speech, and hearing aids. *Journal of Speech and Hearing Research, 36*, 228–244.

Washington Post. (1992). *Financial*, p. 1 (Rep. No. 92453792). Washington, DC.

▶ 7

The Importance of Room Acoustics

CARL C. CRANDELL
University of Florida

JOSEPH J. SMALDINO
University of Northern Iowa

INTRODUCTION

The intelligibility of speech can be greatly affected by the acoustic characteristics of the room or auditorium in which it is presented. Some of the more important acoustic characteristics include reverberation time, the intensity of sound competition in comparison with the intensity of the desired message, and the distance from the speaker to the listener. Intelligibility in a room can also be influenced by linguistic and/or articulatory factors. Linguistic factors include word familiarity and/or vocabulary size of the listener, context, and the number of syllables in a word. Articulatory factors incorporate the sex of the speaker and the articulatory abilities and/or dialect of the speaker or listener. This chapter will focus on the acoustical parameters that influence speech perception in rooms. For a discussion on linguistic/articulatory variables that affect speech perception, the reader is directed to Godfrey (1984), Lehiste (1972), Sanders (1977), and Strange and Jenkins (1978).

Portions of this research were supported by a Department of Education Research Grant (Listening in Classrooms—Utah State University). The authors would like to sincerely thank Carolyn Musket and Alyssa Needleman for their assistance in the preparation of this manuscript.

REVERBERATION

Overview

In a room, speech is seldom delivered to a listener without interference from environmental distortions, such as reverberation and background noise. Reverberation is usually regarded as the most important consideration that defines the acoustical climate of a room. Reverberation refers to the persistence or prolongation of sound within an enclosure as sound waves reflect off hard surfaces (bare walls, ceilings, floors). Operationally, reverberation time (RT_{60}) refers to the amount of time it takes for a steady-state sound to decay 60 dB from its initial peak amplitude offset (Knudsen & Harris, 1978; Lochner & Burger, 1964; Nabelek & Pickett, 1974a,b; Sabine, 1964). Room reverberation increases linearly with volume and is inversely related to the amount of sound absorption in an environment. Room reverberation varies as a function of frequency and should therefore be measured at discrete frequencies. Generally, because most materials do not absorb low frequencies well, room reverberation is shorter at higher frequencies and longer in lower frequency regions. For convenience, decay time is often only reported as the mean of 500, 1000, and 2000 Hz. For a description of various measurement procedures, please see Borrild (1978), Hassall and Zaveri (1979), and/or Knudsen and Harris (1978).

Reverberation Times in Rooms

With the possible exception of anechoic chambers, all rooms exhibit some degree of reverberation. For example, audiometric booths usually exhibit reverberation times of approximately 0.1 to 0.2 seconds. Living rooms and offices often have reverberation times between 0.4 and 0.8 seconds (Knudsen & Harris, 1978; Nabelek & Nabelek, 1985). The range of reverberation for classrooms is usually reported to range from 0.4 to 1.2 seconds (Bradley, 1986; Crandell, 1991, 1992; Finitzo-Hieber, 1988; Kodaras, 1960; McCroskey & Devens, 1975; Olsen, 1988; Ross, 1978). Auditoriums, churches, and assembly halls frequently have reverberation times in excess of 3.0 seconds (Crandell, 1992; Knudsen & Harris, 1978; Nabelek & Nabelek, 1985).

Reverberation and Speech Perception in Normal-Hearing and Hearing-Impaired Listeners

Reverberation degrades speech recognition through the masking of direct sound energy by reflected energy (Bolt & MacDonald, 1949; Houtgast, 1981; Kurtovic, 1975; Lochner & Burger, 1964; Nabelek & Pickett, 1974a, b). In a reverberant environment, the reflected signals reaching the ear are temporally delayed and overlap with the direct signal, resulting in masking of speech. Vowel sounds are more intense in sound energy than consonants, therefore reverberation typically causes a prolongation of the spectral energy of the vowel phonemes, which tends to mask consonant information (particularly word final consonants). In general, speech-perception ability decreases with increases in reverberation time (Finitzo-Hieber & Tillman, 1978; Gelfand & Silman, 1979; Neuman & Hochberg, 1983; Nabelek & Pickett, 1974a, b). For example, Finitzo-Hieber and Tillman (1978) reported that while normal-hearing children obtained mean word recognition scores of 92.5 percent at a reverberation time of 0.4 seconds, recognition ability decreased to 76.5 percent at a reverberation time of 1.2 seconds.

Research has consistently demonstrated that the speech recognition of hearing-impaired listeners is more deleteriously affected by increases in reverberation than normal-hearing listeners (Finitzo-Hieber & Tillman, 1978; Neuman & Hochberg, 1983; Nabelek & Pickett, 1974a,b; Nabelek & Robinson, 1982). Additional data has indicated that several populations of "special listeners" (Nabelek & Nabelek, 1985), such as learning-disabled children and adults, listeners for whom English is a second language, young children (< 13 to 15 years), children with articulation disorders, elderly listeners, and minimally (pure-tone sensitivity from 15 to 25 dB HL) and/or unilaterally hearing-impaired listeners have greater difficulties understanding reverberated speech than normal-hearing adults (Bess, 1985; Crandell, 1991; 1992; Nabelek & Nabelek, 1985). To date, the auditory, linguistic, and/or cognitive mechanisms for these perceptual deficits are not well defined.

Recommended Criteria for Reverberation Time

Data from several studies suggest that speech perception in normal-hearing adults is not affected until reverberation times exceed approximately 1.0 seconds (Crum, 1974, Gelfand & Silman, 1979; Moncur & Dirks, 1967; Nabelek & Pickett, 1974a,b). Hearing-impaired listeners, however, need considerably shorter reverberation times for optimal speech-recognition ability. Several sources have recommended that listening environments utilized for the hearing impaired should not surpass 0.4 seconds to provide optimum communicative efficiency (Crandell & Bess, 1986; Crandell, 1991, 1992; Finitzo-Hieber, 1988; Finitzo-Hieber & Tillman, 1978; Niemoeller, 1968; Olsen, 1988). Unfortunately, a review of the literature indicates that appropriate acoustical environments for the hearing impaired are rarely achieved (Crandell, 1992; Crum & Matkin, 1976; McCroskey & Devens, 1975). Crandell and Smaldino (1994), for instance, reported that only 9 of 32 classrooms (28 percent) for the hearing impaired displayed reverberation times of 0.4 seconds or less (see Figure 7-1).

Acoustical criteria for appropriate reverberation times have not been well established for the diverse populations of special listeners previously discussed. Northern and Downs (1991) suggest that a "handicapping hearing loss in a child is any degree of hearing that reduces the intelligibility of a speech message to a degree inadequate for accurate interpretation or learning" (p. 9). Reverberation can interfere with the accuracy of speech transmission in a room, and so must also be considered potentially handicapping to many listeners. Whether the acoustics are actually interfering with

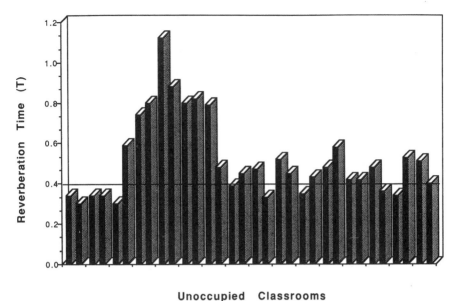

Unoccupied Classrooms

FIGURE 7-1   **The average reverberation time (500, 1000, and 2000 Hz) in 32 classrooms for the hearing impaired. The solid line indicates the recommended acoustical standard (reverberation time = 0.4 seconds)**

speech perception depends to a large degree on the integrity of the listener's auditory-linguistic system and his or her ability to use distorted cues for perception. With these considerations in mind, and until additional research is conducted, a conservative standard for reverberation times in listening environments for special listeners seems appropriate. Specifically, the reverberation time of such enclosures should follow the same acoustical recommendations utilized for hearing-impaired listeners: that is, reverberation time should not exceed 0.4 seconds.

NOISE

Overview

Noise refers to any auditory disturbance that interferes with what a listener wants to hear. Background noise diminishes speech recognition by reducing the redundant cues available in the speech signal (Cooper & Cutts, 1971; Miller, 1974; Miller & Nicely, 1955; Nabelek & Pickett, 1974a,b; Sher & Owens, 1974; Wang, Reed, & Bilger, 1978). Specifically, noise deleteriously affects speech recognition by masking less intense segments of the speech signal (primarily consonant phonemes), making them less intelligible to the listener. The masking effect of noise depends upon several parameters, including: (1) the average intensity of the noise relative to the intensity of speech; (2) the long-term acoustic spectrum of the noise; and (3) fluctuations in the intensity of the noise over time (Beranek, 1954; Knudsen & Harris, 1978; Miller, 1974; Nabelek, 1982; Nabelek & Pickett, 1974a,b). In general, low frequency noises in a listening environment are more effective maskers of speech than high frequency noises because of upward spread of masking. Upward spread of masking refers to a phenomenon in which a masking noise produces greater masking at frequencies above the frequency of the masker than at frequencies below the masker. The fact that low frequency noises have a greater effect on speech recognition than high frequency noises is important since the predominant spectra of noise found in many listening environments is low frequency. The most effective masking noises are commonly those with a spectra similar to the speech spectrum since they affect all speech frequencies to the same degree.

Sources of Ambient Noise in Rooms

Noise in a listening environment can originate from several possible sources (John & Thomas, 1957; Olsen 1977, 1981). For instance, noise from outside a building (external noise) may include local construction, traffic, and playground areas. Noise can also originate from within the building, but outside the actual room (internal noise). Rooms adjacent to high noise areas, such as the cafeteria, gymnasium, and/or busy hallways, may exhibit high ambient noise levels. A significant amount of noise originates from within the room itself (room noise). Obvious sources include talking, sliding of chairs or tables, and shuffling of hard-soled shoes on uncarpeted floors. Heating and cooling systems can also significantly contribute to room noise levels. This last form of noise (noise generated within the room) is typically the most detrimental to speech recognition since the frequency content of the message (speaker's voice) is often spectrally similar to the frequency of the noise.

Ambient Noise Levels in Rooms

A number of investigators have measured noise levels in everyday listening environments, such as homes, transportation settings, and classrooms (Bess, Sinclair, & Riggs, 1984; Blair, 1977; Crandell, 1992; Finitzo-Hieber, 1988; Markides, 1986; McCroskey & Devens, 1975; Nober & Nober, 1975; Paul, 1967; Pearsons, Bennett, & Fidell, 1977; Ross, 1978; Ross & Giolas, 1971; Sanders, 1965). Pearsons, Bennett, and Fidell (1977) reported that noise levels averaged 45 dB(A) for suburban residential settings and 55 dB(A) for urban dwellings. Mean outdoor noise levels were 2 to 10 dB more intense than indoor settings. Noise levels were measured at 54 dB(A) for department store environments and 77 dB(A) in transportation locales (train and aircraft noise). Sanders (1965) measured the noise levels in 47 occupied and unoccupied classrooms in 15 different school buildings. Mean occupied noise levels ranged from an average of 69 dB(B) in kindergarten classrooms to 52 dB(B) in classrooms for the hearing impaired. Unoccupied classroom noise levels were approximately 10 dB lower than the occupied classroom settings, ranging from 58 dB(B) for kindergarten classrooms to 42 dB(B) in classrooms utilized for the hearing-impaired. Bess, Sinclair, and Riggs (1984) measured ambient noise levels in 19 classrooms for hearing-impaired children. Median unoccupied noise levels were 41 dB(A), 50 dB(B), and 58 dB(C). When the classroom was occupied with students, ambient noise levels increased to 56 dB(A), 60 dB(B), and 63 dB(C). Crandell and Smaldino (1994) measured the ambient noise levels of 32 unoccupied classroom settings. Mean unoccupied noise levels were 51 dB(A) (range of 46–59 dB) and 67 dB(C) (range of 57–74 dB).

Speech Perception in Noise by Normal-Hearing and Hearing-Impaired Listeners

The most important consideration for speech recognition is not the absolute noise level in an environment, but rather the relationship between the level of the signal and the level of the noise at the listener's ear. This relationship, referred to as the *signal-to-noise ratio*, is commonly reported as the difference in decibels between the intensity of the signal and the intensity of the background noise. For example, if a speech signal is measured at 65 dB, and a noise is 59 dB, the signal-to-noise ratio is +6 dB. Speech-recognition scores typically achieve a plateau for favorable signal-to-noise ratios and deteriorate for less favorable signal-to-noise ratios. Crum (1974) measured word recognition in normal-hearing listeners at signal-to-noise ratios of +12 dB, +6 dB, and 0 dB. Although mean recognition scores were 95 percent at a signal-to-noise ratio of +12 dB, percent-correct scores declined to 80 percent and 46 percent at signal-to-noise ratios of +6 dB and 0 dB, respectively.

As a consequence of high ambient noise levels, relatively poor signal-to-noise ratios have been reported in many settings. Specifically, in classroom environments, the range of signal-to-noise ratios has been reported to be from +5 dB to –7 dB (e.g., Blair, 1977; Finitzo-Hieber, 1988; Markides, 1986; Paul, 1967; Sanders, 1965). Pearsons et al. (1977) reported that average signal-to-noise ratios were +9 to +14 dB in suburban and urban residential settings, respectively. In outdoor settings, signal-to-noise ratios decreased to approximately +5 to +8 dB. Additional measurements indicated that in department store settings, the average signal-to-noise ratio was +7 dB, while transportation settings yielded an average signal-to-noise ratio of –2 dB. Plomp (1978) reported that the average signal-to-noise ratio found at cocktail parties ranged from +1 dB to –2 dB.

Numerous investigations have shown that the speech-recognition performance of hearing-impaired listeners is degraded in noise when compared to normal-hearing listeners (e.g., Dubno, Dirks, & Morgan, 1984; Finitzo-Hieber & Tillman, 1978; Keith & Talis, 1972; Nabelek & Pickett, 1974 a,b; Plomp, 1978; Ross, 1978; Suter, 1985). For example, Suter (1985) reported that at a signal-to-noise ratio of –6 dB, hearing-impaired listeners obtained monosyllabic recognition scores of 27 percent correct compared to 63 percent correct for normal hearers. Moreover, research has indicated that special listeners also require higher signal-to-noise ratios than adult normal-hearing listeners to achieve equivalent recognition scores (Crandell & Bess, 1986; Crandell, 1991; Elliott, 1979; 1982; Elliott, Conners, Kille, Levin, Ball, & Katz, 1979; Finitzo-Hieber & Tillman, 1978; Nabelek & Nabelek, 1985; Nabelek & Robinson, 1982). For example, Elliott (1982) and Nabelek and Robinson (1982) reported that young children require an improvement of approximately 10 dB in signal-to-noise ratio to produce equivalent recognition scores to those of adults. It is thus reasonable to assume that commonly reported classroom listening environments have the potential of adversely affecting speech recognition in special listeners.

To support this assumption, let us examine speech-recognition data from the seminal article by Finitzo-Hieber and Tillman (1978). In this investigation, the authors evaluated monosyllabic word recognition at various signal-to-noise ratios (signal-to-noise ratio = +12 dB, +6 dB, 0 dB) and reverberation times (T = 0.0, 0.4, and 1.2 sec.). Subjects included 12 normal-hearing children and 12 hard-of-hearing children, aged 8 to 12 years. Results are presented in Table 7-1. Note that at a signal-to-noise ratio of +12 dB (a signal-to-noise ratio rarely found in a classroom), the normal-hearing children obtained mean recognition scores of 89 percent. At more commonly-reported classroom signal-to-noise ratios, recognition scores were considerably poorer. For example, at a signal-to-noise ratio of +6 dB, mean recognition scores decreased to 80 percent, while at 0 dB signal-to-noise ratio mean recognition ability decreased to an unacceptable level of 60 percent. Finally, note from this figure that hearing-impaired listeners obtained poorer recognition scores under all listening conditions.

Crandell (1993a) examined the speech recognition of children with minimal degrees of sensorineural hearing loss under commonly reported classroom signal-to-noise ratios (signal-to-noise ratios = +6, +3, 0, –3, and –6 dB). The minimally hearing-impaired children exhibited puretone averages (.5 kHz–2kHz) from 15 to 25 dB HL. Speech recognition was assessed with the Bamford-Koval-Bench (BKB) Standard Sentence test presented at a level of 65 dB SPL, while the multitalker babble from the Speech Perception in Noise (SPIN) test was used as the noise competition. Mean sentential recognition scores (in percent correct) as a function of signal-to-noise ratio are presented in Figure 7-2. Several trends from these findings are pertinent to this discussion. First, these data suggest that the children with minimal degrees of hearing impairment performed more poorly across most listening conditions.

TABLE 7-1   **Mean Speech-Recognition Scores, in Percent Correct, of Normal-Hearing and Aided Hearing-Impaired Children for Monosyllabic Words across Various Signal-to-Noise Ratios**

TEST CONDITION	NORMAL HEARING	HEARING IMPAIRED
QUIET	94.5	83.0
+12 dB	89.2	70.0
+6 dB	79.7	59.5
0 dB	60.2	39.0

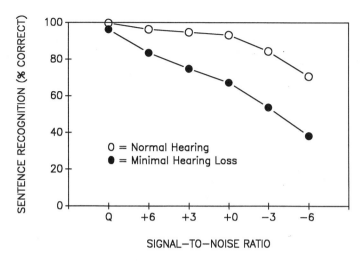

FIGURE 7-2   **Mean sentential recognition scores, in percent correct, as a function of signal-to-noise ratio for children with normal hearing sensitivity (indicated by the open circles) and minimally hearing-impaired children (indicated by the closed circles).**

Moreover, note that the performance decrement between the two groups increased as the listening environment become more adverse. For example, at a signal-to-noise ratio of +6 dB, both groups obtained recognition scores in excess of 80 percent. At a signal-to-noise ratio of –6 dB, however, the minimally hearing-impaired group were able to obtain less than 50 percent correct recognition compared to approximately 75 percent recognition ability for the normal hearers.

Criteria for Appropriate Signal-To-Noise Levels

A number of acoustical factors may influence the determination of appropriate signal-to-noise ratios in an environment. For example, the masking effect of noise depends upon the spectrum of the noise and fluctuations in the noise over time. The type of signal that is being presented (sentences, words, nonsense syllables, vowels, consonants) and/ or the power of the speaker's voice can also affect perception in noise. In general, speech perception in normal-hearing adults is not affected until the signal-to-noise ratio in the environment decreases below 0 dB (speech and noise at equal intensities). To obtain adequate communicative efficiency in noise, listeners with sensorineural hearing loss require the signal-to-noise ratio to be improved by 5 to 10 dB (Glasberg & Moore, 1989), and by an additional 3 to 6 dB in rooms with moderate levels of reverberation (Hawkins & Yacullo, 1984). Several investigators have suggested that signal-to-noise ratios in learning environments for hearing-impaired children should exceed a minimum of +15 dB (Beranek, 1954; Borrild, 1978; Crandell, 1991, 1992; Fourcin, Joy, Kennedy, Knight, Knowles, Knox, Martin, Mort, Penton, Poole, Powell, & Watson, 1980; Gengel, 1971; Finitzo-Hieber, 1988; Finitzo-Hieber & Tillman, 1978; Niemoeller, 1968; Olsen, 1988). This recommendation is based on the findings that the speech recognition of hearing-impaired children tends to remain relatively constant at signal-to-noise ratios in excess of +15 dB, but deteriorates at poorer signal-to-noise ratios. To accomplish this goal in most academic settings, unoccupied noise levels must not exceed 30–35 dB(A), or a Noise Criteria (NC) 20–25 dB curve (Borrild, 1978; Crandell, 1992; Fourcin et al., 1980; Finitzo-Hieber, 1988; Finitzo-Hieber & Tillman, 1978; Gengel, 1971; Niemoeller, 1968; Olsen, 1988). A review of prior literature indicates that these noise standards are infrequently achieved in academic settings (Crandell, 1992; Crum & Matkin, 1976; McCroskey & Devens, 1975). McCroskey and Devens (1975) demonstrated that only one of nine elementary classrooms actually met these acoustical recommendations. Crandell and Smaldino (1994) reported that none of 32 classrooms examined met recommended criteria for noise (see Figure 7-3). As with reverberation, acoustical standards for signal-to-noise ratios and ambient noise levels are not well defined for special listeners. Until such standards are clarified, we recommend that signal-to-noise ratios in learning environments should exceed +15 dB, while ambient noise levels should be no more than 30–35 dB(A).

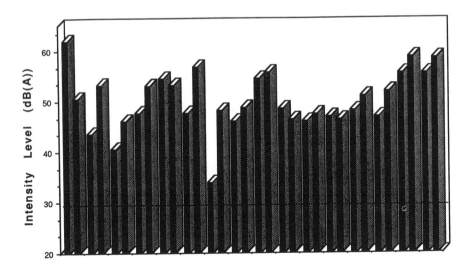

Unoccupied   Classrooms

FIGURE 7-3   **The average ambient noise levels, on the A-weighting scale, in 32 classrooms for the hearing-impaired. The solid line indicates the recommended acoustical standard (noise level = 30 dB(A)).**

NOISE AND REVERBERATION

We have discussed the singular effects of noise competition and reverberation, but these acoustic events do not occur in isolation in a room and so a discussion of their interaction is necessary. Harris, Haynes, and Myers (1960) referred to the multiplying effects of combinations of distortions to a speech signal as the *multiplicative hypotheses*. Specifically, noise and reverberation can combine in a synergistic manner to adversely affect speech recognition in a room setting (Crandell & Bess, 1986; Crum, 1974; Finitzo-Hieber & Tillman, 1978; Nabelek & Pickett, 1974a,b). That is, the interaction of the two distortions adversely affect speech recognition greater than the sum of both effects taken independently. It is reasonable to assume that the synergistic effects of noise and reverberation occur because when noise and reverberation are combined, reflections fill in the temporal gaps in the noise, making it more steady-state in nature. Recall that the most effective maskers are noises with a spectra similar to the speech spectrum. As with noise and reverberation in isolation, research indicates that hearing-impaired individuals and "special listeners" experience greater speech-recognition difficulties in noise and reverberation than adult normal hearers (Crandell & Bess, 1986, 1987; Crum, 1974; Finitzo-Hieber & Tillman, 1978; Nabelek & Nabelek, 1985).

An example of the synergetic effects of noise and reverberation on the speech perception of normal and hearing-impaired children is shown in Table 7-2. Note that even at the best signal-to-noise ratio and reverberation time (signal-to-noise ratio = +12 dB, reverberation time = 0.4 seconds) normal-hearing children do not perceive

TABLE 7-2   **Mean Speech-Recognition Scores, in Percent Correct, of Normal-Hearing and Aided Hearing-Impaired Children for Monosyllabic Words across Various Reverberation Times (RT) and Signal-to-Noise Ratios**

TEST CONDITION	NORMAL HEARING	HEARING IMPAIRED
RT = 0.0 SECONDS		
QUIET	94.5	83.0
+12 dB	89.2	70.0
+6 dB	79.7	59.5
0 dB	60.2	39.0
RT = 0.4 SECONDS		
QUIET	92.5	74.0
+12 dB	82.8	60.2
+6 dB	71.3	52.2
0 dB	47.7	27.8
RT = 1.2 SECONDS		
QUIET	76.5	45.0
+12 dB	68.8	41.2
+6 dB	54.2	27.0
0 dB	29.7	11.2

speech perfectly (83 percent) and hearing-impaired children perform poorly (60 percent). As the signal-to-noise ratio gets poorer, or as reverberation time gets longer, speech perception plummets to the worse case studied (signal-to-noise ratio = +0 dB, reverberation time = 1.2 seconds) where normal-hearing children achieve a 30 percent score and hard-of-hearing children perceive virtually none of the speech (11 percent). It should be noted that each of these listening conditions has been reported in classroom environments.

SPEAKER-LISTENER DISTANCE

Overview

In a room or auditorium, the acoustics of a speaker's voice varies as a function of the distance from the speaker to the listener. Figure 7-4 shows some of the paths of direct and indirect sound from a source to a listener in a room. At distances relatively near to the speaker, the direct sound field (indicated by the thick line) dominates the listening environment. In the direct sound field, sound waves are propagated outward in a spherical pattern and transmitted from the speaker to the listener with little to no interference

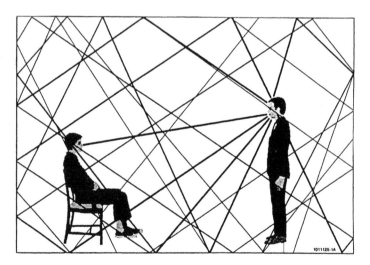

FIGURE 7-4 **Sound propagation and reflections in a room. The direct sound is indicated by the thickest line, while 1st, 2nd, 3rd, and 4th reflections are denoted by sequentially thinner lines.**

Adapted with permission of York Press from Figure 4, Chapter 17, from Wayne O. Olsen, "Classroom Acoustics for Hearing-Impaired Children," in *Hearing Impairment in Children*, edited by Fred Bess. © 1988 by York Press, Inc. Figure originally adapted from Dale, 1962.

from surfaces within the room. Direct sound pressure decreases 6 dB for every doubling of distance from the sound source; a phenomenon known as the inverse square law. For example, if the sound pressure level of the speaker's voice is 70 dB at 1 meter, sound pressure would decrease to 64 dB at 2 meters and 58 dB at 4 meters. At increased distances from the speaker, the indirect or reverberant field (indicated by the thinner lines) now predominates the listening environment. The point in a room or auditorium in which the intensity of the direct sound is equal to the intensity of the reverberant sound is referred to as the critical distance (Klein, 1971; Peutz, 1971). Operationally, critical distance can be defined by the following formula:

$$D_c = (0.20)(VQ/nT)^{-1/2}$$

where V = volume of the room in m³, Q = directivity factor of the source (the human voice is approximately 2.5), n = number of sources, and T = reverberation time of the enclosure at 1400 Hz.

Beyond the critical distance, the direct sound from the speaker arrives at the listener initially, but is followed by a number of reflected sound waves, or reverberation, which is composed of the original wave reflected off the walls, ceiling, and floor. Because there is a linear decrease in the intensity of the direct sound, and because the absorptive characteristics of structures in the room absorb some frequencies more than others, the reflected sound reaching the listener will contain a different acoustical content in the intensity, frequency, and temporal domains. Acoustic interaction of this modified spectrum with the direct sound can produce reinforcements and diminutions in the direct sound. These reinforcements and diminutions of the original signal result in an approximately equal distribution of energy beyond the critical distance of the room. It should be noted, however, that such a homogeneous distribution of sound energy may not occur in larger listening environments, particularly if the power of the sound source is limited (Klein, 1971; Nabelek & Nabelek, 1985; Peutz, 1971).

Effects of Distance on Speech Perception

Speech perception in a room depends on the distance of the listener from the source. If the listener is in the direct field (within the critical distance), reflected sound waves have minimal effects on speech perception. In the indirect field (beyond the critical distance), however, the reflections can be a problem if there is enough of a spectrum and/or intensity change in the reflected sound to interfere with the perception of the direct sound. Several investigators have reported that speech-recognition scores decrease until the critical distance of the room is reached (Crandell & Bess, 1986, Crandell, 1991; Klein, 1971; Peutz, 1971). Beyond the critical distance, recognition ability tends to remain essentially constant, particularly in small to moderately-sized enclosures. This finding suggests that speech-recognition ability can only be improved by decreasing the distance between a speaker and listener within the critical distance of the room.

In a series of investigations, Crandell and colleagues (Crandell & Bess, 1986, 1987; Crandell, 1993b) examined the effects of distance on the speech recognition of normal-hearing children in a "typical" classroom environment (signal-to-noise ratio = +6 dB; T = 0.45 seconds). Specifically, in the Crandell (1993b) investigation, PBK monosyllabic words were recorded through the KEMAR manikin at speaker-listener distances often encountered in the classroom (i.e., 6, 12, and 24 feet). The multitalker babble derived from the Speech Perception in Noise (SPIN) test was used as the noise competition (Kalikow, Stevens, & Elliott, 1977). Subjects consisted of children, 5 to 14 years of age. Results from this investigation are presented in Figure 7-5. As can be noted, there was a systematic decrease in speech-recognition ability as the speaker-listener distance increased. Specifically, mean recognition scores of 95, 71, and 67 percent were obtained at 6, 12, and 24 feet, respectively. Interestingly, even poorer recognition scores were obtained in an earlier investigation utilizing younger (5 to 7 years old) normal-hearing children (Crandell & Bess, 1986). Overall, these results suggest that normal-hearing children seated in the middle to rear of a typical classroom setting have greater difficulty understanding speech than has traditionally been suspected. Additional studies have found similar findings (Fisher, 1964; John & Thomas, 1957; Peutz, 1971; Ross & Giolas, 1971; Watson, 1964)

The effects on speech perception shown in Figure 7-5 are understandable if the results of a 1991 Leavitt and Flexer study are considered. These researchers used the Rapid Speech Transmission Index (RASTI) to estimate speech perception in a class-

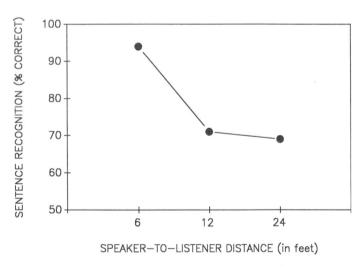

FIGURE 7-5   **Mean sentential recognition scores, in percent correct, as a function of speaker-listener distance for normal-hearing children in a "typical" classroom (signal-to-noise ratio = +6 dB; reverberation time = 0.45 seconds).**

room. RASTI is based on the assumption that noise and reverberation in a room will affect a speech-like signal in ways that can be related to speech perception. A modulation transfer function is derived as a speech-like signal that is transmitted and received in a room. Results indicated that even in a front row center seat, only 83 percent of the energy of speech was available to the listener. In the back row center, the amount of sound energy available to the listener dropped to 55 percent. Certainly, if only a fraction of the speech signal is available, poor speech perception would be expected. It should be noted that RASTI is a very simplified measure that does not fully incorporate spectrum changes that occur during speech transmission. It is clear, however, that combination effects of noise and reverberation are present in most rooms, although perhaps not adequately quantifiable at this time.

METHODS TO IMPROVE CLASSROOM ACOUSTICS

Acoustical Treatments

The speech-recognition deficits experienced by hearing-impaired individuals and special listeners highlight the need to reconsider the acoustical conditions in listening environments utilized by such populations. Certainly, stringent acoustical requirements should be employed for rooms utilized by such listeners to ensure that noise and reverberation levels are within recommended criteria. For maximum communication, signal-to-noise ratios should exceed +15 dB, unoccupied noise levels should not exceed 30–35 dB(A), while reverberation levels should not surpass 0.4 seconds (Crandell & Bess, 1986; Crandell, 1992; Crum, 1974; Finitzo-Hieber & Tillman, 1978; Niemoeller, 1968; Olsen, 1977, 1981, 1988). As noted, however, these acoustical recommendations are rarely achieved in everyday listening environments.

Noise and reverberation levels in a listening environment can be minimized in a number of ways (Finitzo-Hieber, 1988; Nabelek & Nabelek, 1985; Olsen, 1981, 1988; Ross, 1978). For example, it is imperative that rooms utilized for learning, therapy, and/ or instruction be located away from high levels of external noise, such as traffic, construction, and furnace/air conditioning unit noise. The most effective means of reducing external noise levels is through adequate planning with architects, contractors, school officials, architectural engineers, audiologists, and teachers for the hearing-impaired, prior to the design and construction of a building. Unfortunately, it appears that consultation among such disciplines prior to building construction is rare (Crandell, 1991, 1992; Elliott, 1982). Landscaping strategies such as the placement of shrubs or earthen banks, can also provide interference and absorption of exterior levels of environmental noise. An additional procedure to reduce external noise levels in the listening environment is to relocate the room and/or the noise source. If relocation of the room, or relocation of the noise source cannot be accomplished, then acoustical modifications of the room should be considered. Acoustical treatments such as thick or double concrete wall construction and double-paned windows, can help to attenuate extraneous noise sources in the room. Noise can also originate from within the building, but outside the actual room. The simplest, and often most cost-effective, procedure for reducing internal noise levels in the room is to relocate the room to a quieter area of the building. If relocation is not feasible, acoustical treatments such as double-wall construction between rooms, carpeting of hallways, and acoustically treated or well-fitting doorways can attenuate internal noise sources.

Finally, a significant amount of noise originates from within the room itself. Recall that this noise may be particularly detrimental to speech recognition since its spectrum is often similar to the frequency content of the speaker's voice. Acoustical modifications such as the installation of thick carpeting, acoustical paneling on the walls and ceiling, acoustically treated furniture, and hanging of thick curtains can reduce ambient noise generated within the classroom. In addition, the rearrangement of listeners away from high noise sources, such as fans, air conditioners or heating ducts, can also provide a more favorable listening environment. Unfortunately, a review of the literature has demonstrated that rooms often exhibit minimal degrees of acoustical modifications (Bess, Sinclair, & Riggs, 1984, Crandell, 1991, 1992). For example, Bess, Sinclair, and Riggs (1984) found that while 100 percent of classrooms had acoustical ceiling tile, only 68 percent had carpeting and 13 percent had draperies.

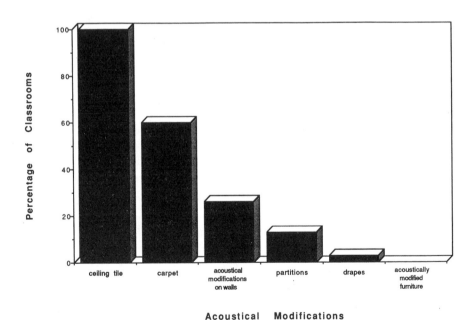

FIGURE 7-6 **Percentage of acoustical treatments for noise and reverberation in 32 classrooms for the hearing impaired.**

No classroom contained any form of acoustical furniture treatment. Recently, Crandell and Smaldino (1994) reported similar findings (see Figure 7-6). Specifically, while all of the 32 classrooms examined had acoustic ceiling tile, only 19 (59 percent) contained carpeting. Moreover, only 8 of the classrooms (25 percent) had acoustical wall modifications, 4 (12 percent) used partitions, and 1 contained drapes (4 percent). None of the rooms had acoustical furniture treatments.

Reverberation can be reduced by covering the hard, reflective surfaces in a room (i.e., bare cement walls and ceilings, glass or mirrored areas, and uncarpeted floors) with absorptive materials. Installing acoustical paneling on the walls and ceiling, carpeting on the floors, placing cork bulletin boards on the walls, curtains on the windows, and positioning mobile bulletin boards at angles other than parallel to the walls can also decrease reverberation levels in an enclosure. For a more detailed description of acoustical treatments to reduce noise and reverberation in listening environments, the reader is directed to Beranek (1954), Crandell (1991), Finitzo-Hieber (1988), Knudsen and Harris (1978), Nabelek and Nabelek (1985), Olsen (1988), and Ross (1978).

Speaker-Listener Distance

Another consideration in reducing the damaging effects of noise and reverberation is to ensure that the listener receives the speaker's voice at the most favorable speaker-listener distance possible. Specifically, the listener needs to be in a face-to-face situation and in the direct sound field, where the interaction of noise and reverberation are less detrimental to speech-recognition skills. Recall from the previous discussion that speech recognition can only be improved within the critical distance of the room. Therefore, in any learning environment, the speaker-listener distance should be as close as possible, and should not exceed the critical distance of the room. To achieve this recommendation, the restructuring of room activities must be considered. For example, small group instruction must be recommended over more traditional room settings, where the speaker instructs in front of numerous rows of listeners. Close proximity to the speaker and face-to-face contact should also aid the hearing-impaired listener in maximizing speech-reading skills. It should be noted that since the direct sound field is present only at speaker-listener distances relatively close to the speaker, the simple recommendation of preferential seating may not be adequate to ensure an appropriate listening environment for the hearing-impaired listener. The utilization of a hearing assistance device, such as a Frequency Modulation (FM) amplification system (discussed in the next section), can also decrease speaker-to-listener distance.

Hearing Assistance Technologies

If acoustic modifications are not possible due to room design or cost, improvement of the listening environment can be accomplished by using hearing assistance technologies. A summary of the most frequently used hearing assistance technologies is

TABLE 7-3   **Hearing Technologies Commonly Used to Improve Speech Perception in Rooms**

TECHNOLOGY	FEATURES
HEARING AIDS	Fit to and worn by the individual. Most beneficial in rooms with low ambient noise when desired signal is close.
Behind-the-Ear	Can incorporate tone, output, and compression controls. Some may be used with FM and inductive systems.
In-the-Ear	Can incorporate tone, output, and compression controls. Some may be used with FM and inductive systems.
ASSISTIVE LISTENING DEVICES	Improves signal-to-noise ratio and can reduce effects of reverberation.
Personal FM	Speaker wears FM transmitting microphone, listener wears FM receiver. Improves signal-to-noise ratio and virtually eliminates effects of reverberation. Can be worn alone or coupled to some hearing aids.
Soundfield FM	Speaker wears FM transmitting microphone, the receiver is connected to a small public address system. Improves signal-to-noise ratio about 10 dB and can reduce the effects of reverberation depending on speaker placement.
Hard Wired	Speaker microphone and listener earphone directly connected with wire. Can improve signal-to-noise ratio and virtually eliminate the effects of reverberation. May be coupled to some hearing aids.
Infrared	Speaker microphone transmits via light to a receiver which can be coupled to earphones, hearing aids, or small public address systems. Can improve signal-to-noise ratio and reduce the effects of reverberation. Cannot be used outdoors in daylight.
Inductance	Speaker microphone transmits via a room inductive system to a personal inductive receiver or to some hearing aids. Can improve signal-to-noise ratio and reduce the effects of reverberation.

shown in Table 7-3. Unfortunately, recent research indicates that these systems are rarely recommended for special listeners (Crandell, 1991; Davis, Elfenbein, Schum, & Bentler, 1986; Shepard, Davis, Gorga, & Stelmachowicz, 1981).

One of the most cost-effective technologies for improving listening environments is a soundfield FM system. A soundfield FM system is essentially a room public address system, in which speech is picked up via a FM wireless microphone located near the speaker's mouth, where the effects of noise and reverberation are negligible. The signal is then transmitted to an amplifier and delivered to listeners in the room via several strategically placed loudspeakers. The objectives of such a system are: (1) to improve the volume of the speaker's voice approximately 10 dB over the unamplified condition;

and (2) provide a uniform direct and/or a speech reinforcing reflected soundfield throughout the room. Several investigators have shown that if these objectives are achieved, psychoeducational and psychosocial benefits accrue for both normal-hearing and hearing-impaired listeners (Berg, 1987; Crandell & Bess, 1987; Flexer, 1989; Flexer, Millin, & Brown, 1990; Sarff, 1981; Sarff, Ray, & Bagwell, 1981; Smaldino & Flexer, 1991). For instance, Sarff (1981) utilized a soundfield amplification system in a classroom with normal-hearing children and children with minimal degrees of sensorineural hearing loss. Results indicated that both groups of children, particularly the minimally hearing-impaired children, demonstrated significant improvements in academic achievement when receiving amplified instruction. Moreover, younger children demonstrated greater academic improvements than older children.

Anderson (1991) outlined some of the benefits of classroom public address systems as follows:

(1) The system is inexpensive compared to other methods of improving classroom acoustics. It is also the most inexpensive of the electrical methods used for this purpose.
(2) It can be used with all hard-of-hearing students, and those children with speech perception/listening difficulties in noise, attention problems, and behavioral problems.
(3) Classroom public address systems can benefit children with unidentified fluctuating hearing loss, the child being medically managed that has yet to return to normal hearing, and the child with chronic conductive hearing loss. These children typically do not qualify for special help, but may have significant problems hearing, and learning, in most classrooms.
(4) The presence of the system in the classroom does not stigmatize certain children, which is often the case with auditory trainers or hearing aids. All children in the classroom are recipients of the amplified signal.
(5) The system provides some limited benefit to children while malfunctioning hearing aids or auditory trainers are repaired.
(6) Eighty-five to ninety percent of teachers readily embrace the classroom public address system and report lessened stress and vocal strain during teaching activities. This acceptance translates into careful and consistent use of the equipment.
(7) Normal-hearing students also enjoy the benefits of having classroom amplification and readily use the system for oral reports, oral reading, and when asking/answering questions.

Because of these benefits, classroom public address systems are the fastest growing component of the FM wireless market and are being placed in classrooms nationwide. There are, however, limitations of classroom public address systems which must be considered (Davis, 1992; Smaldino & Flexer, 1991):

(1) The amplification in small classrooms may be less than 10 dB because of feedback problems associated with speaker closeness and reflective surfaces. It is not clear how much benefit limited amplification can provide.

(2) Systems may not be effective in particularly noisy or reverberant classrooms. Ten dB of amplification may not be enough to overcome the effects of a high level of noise or when reverberation time approaches 1 second. Amplification of sound increases both the level of the desired direct sound and the undesired reflected sound energy.

(3) The teacher's voice may be amplified too much for some children and not enough for others, if the speaker arrangement is not appropriate for the classroom. In either case, the benefits to the student and/or teacher may be lost.

(4) Because of varying amounts of sound cancellation and distortion, it is difficult to obtain the desired uniform sound amplification throughout a classroom without careful speaker placement.

(5) Teacher and student preparation as to the benefits and use of the system is mandatory if the system is to provide maximum benefit.

The limitations are a warning that, if improperly installed or used, classroom public address systems may not produce the desired results. Audiologists aware of the complexities of the acoustic environment and the consequences of sound amplification in a classroom must be involved with the development of these systems for use in rooms.

CONCLUSIONS

The preceding discussion has highlighted some of the interactive effects of room and auditorium acoustics on the speech perception abilities of normal-hearing and hearing-impaired individuals. It was concluded that noise and reverberation levels in most listening environments are higher than would be recommended for adequate speech perception. This is particularly true in rooms used for learning where inadequate room acoustics have been shown to negatively affect the speech perception of various populations of listeners with normal-hearing sensitivity (learning-disabled children and adults, listeners for whom English is a second language, young children [< 13 to 15 years], children with articulation disorders, elderly listeners) and hearing-impaired individuals (including minimally and/or unilaterally hearing-impaired listeners). Finally, strategies were discussed to improve room acoustics, which included: (1) acoustical modifications to reduce levels of noise and reverberation; (2) minimizing the effects of speaker-listener distance; and (3) hearing assistive technologies designed to reduce the effects of inadequate room acoustics, particularly small public address systems.

REFERENCES

Anderson, K. (1991). Speech perception in children. *Educational Audiology Monograph, 1(1)*, 15–29.

Beranek, L. (1954). *Acoustics*. New York: McGraw-Hill.

Berg, F. (1987). *Facilitating Classroom Listening*. Boston: College-Hill Press, Division of Little Brown.

Bess, F. (1985). The minimally hearing-impaired child. *Ear and Hearing, 6*, 43–47.

Bess, F., Sinclair, J., & Riggs, D. (1984). Group amplification in schools for the hearing-impaired. *Ear and Hearing, 5*, 138–144.

Blair, J. (1977). Effects of amplification, speechreading, and classroom environment on reception of speech. *Volta Review, 79*, 443–449.

Bolt, R., & MacDonald, A. (1949). Theory of speech masking by reverberation. *Journal of the Acoustical Society of America, 21*, 577–580.

Borrild, K. (1978). Classroom acoustics. In M. Ross & T. Giolas (Eds.), *Auditory management of hearing impaired children*, pp. 145–179. Baltimore: University Park Press.

Bradley, J. (1986). Speech intelligibility studies in classrooms. *Journal of the Acoustical Society of America, 80(3)*, 846–854.

Cooper, J., & Cutts, B. (1971). Speech discrimination in noise. *Journal of Speech and Hearing Research, 14*, 332–337.

Crandell, C. (1991). Classroom acoustics for normal-hearing children: Implications for rehabilitation. *Educational Audiology Monograph, 2(1)*, 18–38.

Crandell, C. (1992). Classroom acoustics for hearing-impaired children. *Journal of the Acoustical Society of America, 92(4)*, 2470.

Crandell, C. (1993a). Speech recognition in noise by children with minimal hearing loss. *Ear & Hearing, 14(3)*, 210–216.

Crandell, C. (1993b). A comparison of commercially available frequency modulation sound field amplification systems. *Educational Audiology Monograph, 3*, 15–20.

Crandell, C., & Bess, F. (1986). Speech recognition of children in a typical classroom setting. *ASHA, 29*, 87.

Crandell, C., & Bess, F. (1987). Sound-field amplification in the classroom setting. *ASHA, 29*, 87.

Crandell, C., & Smaldino, J. (1994). An update of classroom acoustics for children with hearing impairment. Paper to be published in *Volta Review*.

Crum, D. (1974). The effects of noise, reverberation, and speaker-to-listener distance on speech understanding. Unpublished doctoral dissertation, Northwestern University, Evanston, IL.

Crum, D. & Matkin, N. (1976). Room acoustics: the forgotten variable. *Language, Speech, & Hearing Services in the Schools, 7*, 106–100.

Davis, D. (1992). Sound field amplification: A look more cautiously. *Educational Audiology Association Newsletter, 9(1)*.

Davis, J., Elfenbein, J., Schum, R., & Bentler, R. (1986). Effects of mild and moderate hearing impairments on language, educational, and psychosocial behavior of children. *Journal of Speech and Hearing Disorders, 51*, 53–62.

Dubno, J., Dirks, D., and Morgan, D. (1984). Effects of age and mild hearing loss on speech recognition in noise. *Journal of the Acoustical Society of America, 76*, 87–96.

Elliott, L. (1979). Performance of children aged 9 to 17 years on a test of speech intelligibility in noise using sentence material with controlled word predictability. *Journal of the Acoustical Society of America, 66*, 651–653.

Elliott, L. (1982). Effects of noise on perception of speech by children and certain handicapped individuals. *Sound and Vibration, Dec.*, 9–14.

Elliott, L., Connors, S., Kille, E., Levin, S., Ball, K., & Katz, D. (1979). Children's understanding of monosyllabic nouns in quiet and in noise. *Journal of the Acoustical Society of America, 66,* 12–21.

Finitzo-Hieber, T. & Tillman, T. (1978). Room acoustics effects on monosyllabic word discrimination ability for normal and hearing-impaired children. *Journal of Speech and Hearing Research, 21,* 440–458.

Finitzo-Hieber, T. (1988). Classroom acoustics. In R. Roeser (Ed.), *Auditory disorders in school children.* (Second Edition), pp. 221–233. New York: Thieme-Stratton.

Fisher, B. (1964). An investigation of binaural hearing aids. *Journal of Laryngology, 78,* 658–668.

Flexer, C. (1989). Turn on sound: An odyssey of sound field amplification. *Educational Audiology Association Newsletter, 5*:6–7.

Flexer, C., Millin, J., & Brown, L. (1990). Children with developmental disabilities: The effects of sound field amplification in word identification. *Language, Speech, and Hearing Services in the Schools, 21,* 177–182.

Fourcin, A., Joy, D., Kennedy, M., Knight, J., Knowles, S., Knox, E., Martin, M., Mort, J., Penton, J., Poole, D., Powell, C., & Watson, T. (1980). Design of educational facilities for deaf children. *British Journal of Audiology,* Supplement, 3.

French, N., & Steinberg, J. (1947). Factors governing the intelligibility of speech sounds. *Journal of the Acoustical Society of America, 19,* 90–119.

Gelfand, S., & Silman, S. (1979). Effects of small room reverberation upon the recognition of some consonant features. *Journal of the Acoustical Society of America, 66(1),* 22–29.

Gengel, R. (1971). Acceptable signal-to-noise ratios for aided speech discrimination by the hearing impaired. *Journal of Auditory Research, 11,* 219–222.

Glasberg, B., & Moore, B. (1989). Psychoacoustic abilities of subjects with unilateral and bilateral cochlear hearing impairment and their relationship to the ability to understand speech. *Scandinavian Audiology, Supplementum #32,* pp. 1–25. Stockholm: Almqvist & Wiksell Periodical Co.

Godfrey, J. (1984). Linguistic structure in clinical and experimental tests of speech recognition. In E. Elkins (Ed.), *ASHA report 14: Speech recognition by the hearing impaired,* pp. 52–56. Rockville, MD: ASHA.

Harris, J., Haynes, H., & Myers, C. (1960). The importance of hearing at 3Kc for the understanding of speeded speech. *Laryngoscope, 70,* 131–146.

Hassall, J., & Zaveri, K. (1979). *Acoustic noise measurements.* Naerum, Denmark: Bruel & Kjaer.

Hawkins, D., & Yacullo, W. (1984). Signal-to-noise ratio advantage of binaural hearing aids and directional microphones under different levels of reverberation. *Journal of Speech & Hearing Disorders, 49,* 278–286.

Houtgast, T. (1981). The effect of ambient noise on speech intelligibility in classrooms. *Applied Acoustics, 14,* 15–25.

John, J., & Thomas, H. (1957). Design and construction of schools for the deaf. In A. Ewing (Ed.), *Educational guidance and the deaf child.* Washington, DC: Volta Review.

Kalikow, D., Stevens, K., & Elliott, L. (1977). Development of a test of speech intelligibility in noise using sentence materials with controlled word predictability. *Journal of the Acoustical Society of America, 61,* 1337–1351.

Keith, R., & Talis, H. (1972). The effects of white noise on PB scores of normal-hearing and hearing-impaired listeners. *Audiology, 11*: 177–186.

Klein, W. (1971). Articulation loss of consonants as a criterion for speech transmission in a room. *Journal of the Audio Engineering Society, 19,* 920–922.

Knudsen, V., & Harris, C. (1978). *Acoustical designing in architecture.* Washington, DC: The American Institute of Physics for the Acoustical Society of America.

Kodaras, M. (1960). Reverberation times of typical elementary school settings. *Noise Control, 6,* 17–19.

Kurtovic, H. (1975). The influence of reflected sound upon speech intelligibility. *Acoustica, 33,* 32–39.

Leavitt, R., & Flexer, C. (1991). Speech degradation as measured by the Rapid Speech Transmission Index (RASTI). *Ear & Hearing, 12,* 115–118.

Lehiste, I. (1972). The units of speech perception. In J. Gilbert (Ed.), *Speech and cortical functioning,* pp. 187–235. New York: Academic Press.

Licklider, J., & Miller, G. (1951). The perception of speech. In S.S. Stevens (Ed.), *Handbook of experimental psychology.* New York: John Wiley.

Lochner, J., & Burger, J. (1964). The influence of reflections in auditorium acoustics. *Journal of Sound and Vibration, 4,* 426–454.

Markides, A. (1986). Speech levels and speech-to-noise ratios. *British Journal of Audiology, 20,* 115–120.

McCroskey, F., & Devens, J. (1975). Acoustic characteristics of public school classrooms constructed between 1890 and 1960. *NOISEXPO Proceedings,* 101–103.

Miller, G. (1974). Effects of noise on people. *Journal of the Acoustical Society of America, 56,* 724–764.

Miller, G., & Nicely, P. (1955). An analysis of perceptual confusions among some English consonants. *Journal of the Acoustical Society of America, 27,* 338–352.

Moncur, J., & Dirks, D. (1967). Binaural and monaural speech intelligibility in reverberation. *Journal of Speech & Hearing Research, 10,* 186–195.

Nabelek, A. (1982). Temporal distortions and noise considerations. In G. Studebaker & F. Bess (Eds.), *The Vanderbilt hearing-aid report: State of the art-research needs,* pp. 51–59. Upper Darby, PA: Monographs in Contemporary Audiology.

Nabelek, A., & Nabelek, I. (1985). Room acoustics and speech perception. In J. Katz (Ed.), *Handbook of clinical audiology,* (Third Edition). Baltimore: Williams & Wilkins.

Nabelek, A., & Pickett, J. (1974a). Monaural and binaural speech perception through hearing aids under noise and reverberation with normal and hearing-impaired listeners. *Journal of Speech and Hearing Research, 17,* 724–739.

Nabelek, A., & Pickett, J. (1974b). Reception of consonants in a classroom as affected by monaural and binaural listening, noise, reverberation, and hearing aids. *Journal of the Acoustical Society of America, 56,* 628–639.

Nabelek, A., & Robinson, P. (1982). Monaural and binaural speech perception in reverberation for listeners of various ages. *Journal of the Acoustical Society of America, 71(5),* 1242–1248.

Neuman, A., & Hochberg, I. (1983). Children's perception of speech in reverberation. *Journal of the Acoustical Society of America, 73(6),* 2145–2149.

Niemoeller, A. (1968). Acoustical design of classrooms for the deaf. *American Annals of the Deaf, 113,* 1040–1045.

Nober, L., & Nober, E. (1975). Auditory discrimination of learning disabled children in quiet and classroom noise. *Journal of Learning Disabilities, 8,* 656–773.

Northern, J. & Downs, M. (1991). *Hearing in Children* (Fourth Edition). Baltimore, MD: Williams & Wilkins.

Olsen, W. (1977). Acoustics and amplification in classrooms for the hearing impaired. In F.H.

Bess (Ed.), *Childhood deafness: Causation, assessment and management.* New York: Grune & Stratton.

Olsen, W. (1981). The effects of noise and reverberation on speech intelligibility. In F.H. Bess, B.A. Freeman, & J.S. Sinclair (Eds.), *Amplification in education.* Washington, DC: Alexander Graham Bell Association for the Deaf.

Olsen, W. (1988). Classroom acoustics for hearing-impaired children. In F.H. Bess (Ed.), *Hearing impairment in children.* Parkton, MD: York Press.

Paul, R. (1967). An investigation of the effectiveness of hearing aid amplification in regular and special classrooms under instructional conditions. Unpublished doctoral dissertation, Wayne State University.

Pearsons, K., Bennett, R., & Fidell, S. (1977). Speech levels in various noise environments. *EPA 600/1-77-025.* Washington, DC: Office of Health & Ecological Effects.

Peutz, V. (1971). Articulation loss of consonants as a criterion for speech transmission in a room. *Journal of the Audio Engineering Society, 19,* 915–919.

Plomp, R. (1978). Auditory handicap of hearing impairment and the limited benefit of hearing aids. *Journal of the Acoustical Society of America, 75,* 1253–1258.

Ross, M. (1978). Classroom acoustics and speech intelligibility. In J. Katz (Ed.), *Handbook of clinical audiology.* Baltimore: Williams and Wilkins.

Ross, M., & Giolas, T. (1971). Effects of three classroom listening conditions on speech intelligibility. *American Annals of the Deaf,* December, 580–584.

Sabine, W. (1964). *Collected papers on acoustics.* New York: Dover.

Sanders, D. (1965). Noise conditions in normal school classrooms. *Exceptional Child, 31,* 344–353.

Sanders, D. (1977). *Auditory perception of speech: An introduction to principles and problems.* Englewood Cliffs, NJ: Prentice Hall.

Sarff, L. (1981). An innovative use of free field amplification in regular classrooms. In R. Roeser & M. Downs (Eds.), *Auditory disorders in school children,* pp. 263–272. New York: Thieme-Stratton.

Sarff, L., Ray, H., & Bagwell, C. (1981). Why not amplification in every classroom? *Hearing Aid Journal, 11,* 44, 47–48, 50, 52.

Shepard, N., Davis, J., Gorga, M., & Stelmachowicz, P. (1981). Characteristics of hearing-impaired children in the public schools: Part I-Demographic data. *Journal of Speech and Hearing Disorders, 46,* 123–129.

Sher, A., & Owens, E. (1974). Consonants phonemic errors associated with hearing loss above 2000 Hz. *Journal of Speech and Hearing Research, 17,* 656–668.

Smaldino, J., & Flexer, C. (1991). Improving listening in the classroom. Paper presented at the 1991 Academy of Rehabilitative Audiology annual meeting, Breckenridge, CO.

Strange, W., & Jenkins, J. (1978). Role of linguistic experience in the perception of speech. In R. Walk & H. Pick (Eds.), *Perception and experience,* pp. 125–169. New York: Plenum Press.

Suter, A. (1985). Speech recognition in noise by individuals with mild hearing impairments. *Journal of the Acoustical Society of America, 78,* 887–900.

Wang, M., Reed, C. & Bilger, R. (1978). A comparison of the effects of filtering and sensorineural hearing loss on patterns of consonant confusions. *Journal of Speech and Hearing Research, 24,* 32–43.

Watson, T. (1964). The use of hearing aids by hearing-impaired children in ordinary schools. *Volta Review, 66,* 741–744, 787.

▶ 8

Orientation to the Use of Frequency Modulated Systems

DAWNA E. LEWIS
Boys Town National Research Hospital

FREQUENCY MODULATION DEVICES IN CLASSROOMS

The deleterious effects of noise, reverberation and distance on listeners with hearing loss has been well documented (Boney & Bess, 1984; Erber, 1971; Finitzo-Hieber & Tillman, 1978; Finitzo-Hieber, 1981; Ross & Giolas, 1971; Smith & Boothroyd, 1990). For example, Finitzo-Hieber and Tillman (1978) evaluated speech discrimination of children with normal hearing and children with hearing loss in various conditions of noise and reverberation. In all conditions the children with hearing loss performed more poorly. Even minimal hearing loss (thresholds of 15-30 dB HL) may result in poorer performance in noise and reverberation (Boney & Bess, 1984).

It has been recommended that signal-to-noise ratios in classrooms be at least +15 to +20 dB, and that reverberation times be less than 0.5 sec to provide an adequate listening environment for students with hearing loss (Gengel, 1971; Finitzo-Hieber & Tillman, 1978; Hawkins, 1988; Ross, Brackett, & Maxon, 1982). Unfortunately, few classroom environments meet these requirements (Bess, Sinclair, & Riggs, 1984; Crandell & Smaldino, 1993; Finitzo-Hieber, 1981; Ross, Brackett, & Maxon, 1982). Bess et al. (1984), for example, reported median noise levels of 41 dBA in unoccupied classrooms and 56 dBA in occupied classrooms. More recently, Crandell and Smaldino (1993) evaluated 32 unoccupied classrooms for students with hearing loss and found mean noise levels of 50.2 dBA and mean reverberation times of 0.52 sec.

A number of strategies have been recommended for reducing the effects of reverberation and noise in the classroom. One strategy is the utilization of noise reduction techniques such as carpeting, drapes, and acoustic tiles on ceilings and walls. Although these modifications may reduce the problem, Leavitt (1991) points out that use of absorptive materials in the classroom also may reduce desired energy in the speech signal, especially for frequencies above 1000 Hz. Another strategy is to reduce exposure to noise from outside sources. This can be done by situating the classroom away from high traffic areas, playgrounds, and cafeterias. Although these strategies, which depend on physical engineering, may alleviate some background noise and/or provide optimal reverberation, the child with hearing loss may still have difficulty hearing the signal of interest.

Attempts have been made to address the effects of noise on speech perception with hearing aids (Fabry, 1991a; Kuk, Tyler, & Mims, 1990; Stach, Speerschneider,

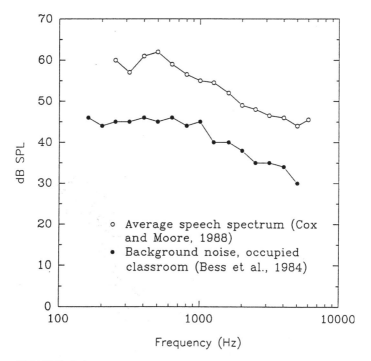

FIGURE 8-1 Long-term 1/3-octave band speech spectra from combined male/female talkers (Cox & Moore, 1988) and averaged background noise levels from 19 occupied classrooms (Bess et al., 1984).

(From Fabry 1991b. *Pediatric Amplification: Proceedings of the 1991 National Conference*: pp. 49–60. Used with permission).

& Jerger, 1987; Tyler & Kuk, 1989; Van Tasell, Larsen, & Fabry, 1988; Wolinsky, 1986). However, as Fabry (1991b) reports, a hearing aid with a single microphone cannot be expected to improve speech intelligibility in noise unless the speech and noise are spectrally different. Figure 8-1 from Fabry (1991b) illustrates the similarities between speech and noise that would be expected in a typical classroom. Note that, although the levels of the two signals are different, the shape of the curves are very similar. As Figure 8-2 (from Fabry, 1991b) shows, an adaptive high-pass filter would reduce energy below 1000 Hz for both the speech and the noise thus maintaining the same signal-to-noise ratio.

In addition, even the highest quality hearing aid cannot be expected to improve speech intelligibility if the speech signal reaching the microphone is already degraded. Leavitt and Flexer (1991) used a Rapid Speech Transmission Index (RASTI) System to measure the integrity of a speech-like signal at various locations in a classroom. With a score of 1.0 representing perfect reproduction of the transmitted signal, scores ranged from 1.0 at the reference distance of six inches from the microphone to

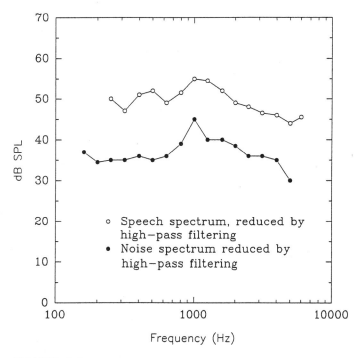

FIGURE 8-2   **As in Fig. 8-1, but with low frequencies reduced by adaptive high-pass filter processing.**

(From Fabry, 1991b. *Pediatric Amplification: Proceedings of the 1991 National Conference*: pp. 49–60. Used with permission).

0.55 at a distance of almost 11 meters (back row of the class). Even in the front row, center seat, the score was 0.83, indicating some degradation of the signal. Although these results cannot be used to predict speech perception at the various locations, they do indicate a decrease in the fidelity of a signal as it is transmitted across distance in a typical classroom. These findings have been used to demonstrate why the recommendation of preferential classroom seating alone is not a sufficient solution for the child with hearing loss.

Currently, the best means of overcoming the effects of noise, reverberation, and distance in the classroom is by placing a remote microphone 6-8 inches from the mouth of the speaker and a receiver on or near the student (Boothroyd, 1992; Fabry, 1991b; Leavitt & Flexer, 1991; Leavitt, 1991). The most common method of utilizing a remote microphone placement in the classroom environment is via a frequency-modulated (FM) amplification system. In this system the teacher wears a microphone/transmitter close to his or her mouth, and the signal is transmitted via FM radio waves to a receiver that is worn by the listener. Important characteristics which have been identified for FM-system amplification include a favorable S/N ratio, the ability to monitor one's own voice, the ability to communicate with others not wearing the FM transmitter/microphone, and binaural reception (Bess & Gravel, 1981; Ross et al., 1982; Ross, 1986). However, these goals may not be easily achieved in all situations.

The focus of this chapter is FM-system amplification for use in educational settings. First, FM transmission will be addressed briefly and then design features of current FM systems will be discussed.

FM Transmission

Until recently, educational FM transmission has been limited to 32 narrowband or 8 wideband channels in the 72-76 MHz range. Although this frequency range initially was allocated for use by educational amplification systems, there are now a number of other users occupying the band (e.g., pagers, cellular phones). These additional transmissions in the same frequency region used by FM systems pose a potential interference problem, particularly in large cities. High wattage transmissions in nearby frequency regions also may interfere with FM transmission. One principle of FM transmission is that the FM receiver responds to the strongest signal being transmitted at a particular frequency and rejects other, weaker, signals (Boothroyd, 1981; Boothroyd, 1992). Usually, this is an advantage for the FM user because the strongest signal is that sent from the FM transmitter. However, if an interfering signal is stronger than that of the FM transmitter, the user will hear the interfering rather than the intended signal.

As a result of these interference problems, the Federal Communication Commission was petitioned by Phonic Ear, Inc. for additional frequency bands to be used for FM-system transmission. In May 1992, that request was granted (FCC, 1992). Therefore, there are now 40 narrowband and 10 wideband channels available to users of FM systems. One advantage of the new bands is that users are limited to a power of one watt, reducing the potential for interference of FM-system transmission. Schools which currently use FM systems manufactured before the addition of the new channels should be able to utilize them by obtaining appropriate oscillators for the instruments.

When transmitting the FM signal to a receiver, the manufacturer may choose to utilize either wideband or narrowband channels. There are advantages and disadvantages to each. One obvious advantage of choosing narrowband transmission is that the user has a greater number of channel choices available (40 vs. 10). However, in FM transmission, the width of the channel (in Hz) is related to the level of the signal above equipment noise (Boothroyd, 1992). That is, the wider the frequency range of a particular channel, the better the signal-to-noise ratio. Therefore, narrowing the channel width from 20,000 Hz for wideband transmission to 5000 Hz for narrowband transmission may have a negative effect on the quality of the signal. Conversely, a wideband channel is equal to approximately four narrowband channels. In an area where interference from outside signals is a problem, a system using wideband transmission may be more susceptible to interference. When selecting an FM system for use in a particular setting, the audiologist and educational personnel will need to examine the environment and review the advantages and disadvantages of each type of transmission before final decisions are made. In some settings trials with different channels and bandwidths may be necessary.

Design Features

When selecting an FM system, there are also numerous design features and coupling options from which to choose. The next section will focus on design features common to most FM systems. In addition, the reader is referred to a number of excellent sources of basic information related to FM systems (Bess & Gravel, 1981; Berg, 1987; Berger & Millin, 1989; Boothroyd, 1981; Hammond, 1991; Hawkins, 1988; Logan & Bess, 1985; Madell, 1990; Ross, 1986, 1992; Ross, Brackett, & Maxon, 1982).

Transmitter/Microphone

All FM systems are composed of a microphone/transmitter and a receiver. Typically, there are three possible configurations of microphones: lavalier, lapel, and boom. In the lavalier style, the microphone and transmitter are housed in the same casing and an antenna extends downward from the unit. Alternately, a separate transmitter unit may be coupled to a lapel microphone that is clipped to the speaker's collar or to a headworn boom microphone. In these latter arrangements the microphone cord serves as the antenna. For each of these arrangements the location of the microphone relative to the speaker's mouth (6-8 inches for lapel and lavalier microphones; 1-2 inches for boom microphones) provides the improved signal-to-noise ratio. Another option, used less frequently in the classroom, is the conference microphone. In this arrangement the transmitter is plugged into a tabletop microphone that is designed to direct sounds from around the table into microphone ports in a cone-shaped base. Because the microphone will not be as close to the speaker's mouth when a conference microphone is used, the signal-to-noise ratio improvement would not be as great as that expected with the other transmitter/microphone options.

In addition to the transmitter style, the audiologist may select a directional or omnidirectional microphone. Typically, lavalier and boom microphones are directional. Lapel microphones may be either directional or omnidirectional. The purpose of a directional microphone is to amplify the speaker's voice more than sounds reaching the microphone from other directions. Theoretically, this feature should help to improve the signal-to-noise ratio (Hawkins & Schum, 1985). However, use of a directional microphone may result in fluctuations in the speaker's voice with head movement toward or away from the microphone, or from improper placement of the microphone (Lewis, 1993b; Thibodeau, 1992). Although an omnidirectional microphone will amplify sounds regardless of direction, it generally is assumed that the speaker's voice will be louder than background noise due to the proximity of the microphone to the mouth. This may not be the case in a very noisy environment. These problems could be alleviated by using a boom microphone that is closer to the speaker's mouth and will move as his or her head moves. However, some individuals find a boom microphone and its associated headband uncomfortable. In some instances, teachers may wear the headband around their necks. This permits changes in the distance between the microphone and the speaker's mouth as the head is moved, causing fluctuations in the transmitted signal. When using a headworn microphone, care also must be taken to ensure that the microphone does not obstruct the view of the lips, which would impede speechreading.

Advantages and disadvantages of each type of transmitter/microphone are summarized in Table 8-1. Discussion with the individual who will be wearing the transmitter prior to final selection may help to alleviate acceptance problems based on physical factors.

Many FM transmitters are equipped with an input Automatic Gain Control (AGC) circuit. The purpose of the AGC circuit is to reduce amplitude variations in the input signal as the speaker varies vocal effort or moves his or her head. The level at which the AGC is activated varies across manufacturers; however, in most cases this level is fixed. At least one manufacturer utilizes a variable AGC control in the transmitter. Although the AGC circuit would appear desirable, it may have some negative effects on the output signal (Boothroyd, 1992; Hawkins & Schum, 1985; Lewis, 1993b). For example, Figure 8-3 illustrates the effects of input AGC for two FM systems. The left panel presents an input/output function for a Telex TDR-7AA/TW-4 with the *mic gain* control on the transmitter set to three different settings. The right panel presents an input/output function for a Phonic Ear 471 set so that the AGC circuit is activated at 75 dB SPL (level set by manufacturer) and 90 dB SPL (adjusted level). When either system is set to maximum compression, there is very little change in output for inputs above 70-75 dB SPL. Compression of the signal may reduce amplitude variations in the speech signal that would be important for some hearing-impaired individuals (Boothroyd, 1986). Boothroyd (1992) has also pointed out "if it [the knee point for activation of the AGC circuit] is set too low, then, when the teacher

TABLE 8-1 **FM Microphone/Transmitters**

MICROPHONE STYLE	FEATURES	ADVANTAGES	DISADVANTAGES
Lavalier	• Microphone and transmitter in one case • Antenna extends from case • Microphone usually directional • Worn around the neck	• Single case may simplify use • No need for waistband or belt to attach transmitter	• Weight of device around the neck may be uncomfortable for some users • Single case for all components may complicate troubleshooting • Poor placement or head movement may affect signal
Lapel	• Microphone and transmitter are separate • Antenna in cord of lapel microphone • Microphone clips to lapel or may hang around neck • Transmitter usually clips to belt or waistband • Microphone may be directional or omnidirectional	• Lightweight microphone comfortable • May be easier to troubleshoot because of separate components • Microphone options increase flexibility	• Need for waistband or belt to hold transmitter • Poor placement or head movement may affect signal with directional microphone
Boom	• Microphone and transmitter separate • Antenna in microphone cord • Worn on headband or glasses • Microphone usually directional	• Headworn microphone improves S/N ratio • May be easier to troubleshoot because of separate components	• Poor placement or head movement may affect signal with directional microphone • Fit may be uncomfortable • Some of benefit may be lost if worn differently than recommended
Conference	• Microphone and transmitter separate • Antenna in base of microphone • Microphone placed in single location (usually tabletop) • Microphone is omnidirectional	• No need to pass microphone • Able to pick up numerous speakers from single microphone location	• May amplify other, unwanted sounds in the room • Distance of microphone from mouth of speaker greater, reducing S/N ratio advantage

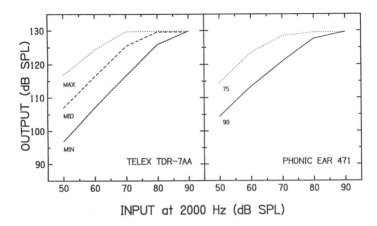

INPUT at 2000 Hz (dB SPL)

FIGURE 8-3   **Output (dB SPL) as a function of input (dB SPL) using a 2000 Hz pure tone for Telex TDR-7AA (left panel) and Phonic Ear 471 (right panel) FM systems at different input AGC settings at the FM transmitter.**

(From Lewis, 1994. *American Journal of Audiology, 3*, 70–83. Used with permission).

is not talking, noise in the room may be amplified to levels that interfere with the student's reception of his or her own speech, thus eliminating one of the intended benefits of an FM system" (pp. 14-15).

Receiver
FM-system receivers vary in the number of features they include. One important feature found on all receivers is a volume control wheel. A few FM systems have separate volume-control wheels for both the FM and environmental microphones. This option is desirable because it allows greater flexibility when setting output levels of the FM and environmental microphone modes of operation. However, most commercially available systems utilize a single volume-control wheel for both modes of transmission, limiting flexibility of the system. In addition, there may be variability in the linearity of this control in the FM and environmental microphone modes of operation (Hawkins & Schum, 1985; Lewis, Feigin, Karasek, & Stelmachowicz, 1991).

The location of the environmental microphone varies across FM receivers, depending upon how the unit is worn. Options for environmental microphone location include ear level, chest level, and/or waist level. Microphone location may have an effect on the spectral characteristics of the input signal at the microphone. Medwetsky and Boothroyd (1991) found considerable variability in the level of the short-term spectrum of speech sounds when measured at five microphone locations that would be representative of FM microphones (to the side of the speaker's mouth, on the speaker's chest) and environmental microphones (over the speaker's ear, on the speaker's chest, at the speaker's waist). These were compared to the spectrum at 5 feet in front of speaker's mouth. Considerable variability was found across microphone locations, with greatest energy loss occurring in the high frequencies when the microphones were located off-axis (i.e., not in front) in relation to the speaker's mouth.

Users of FM systems have a choice between self-contained or personal FM receivers, and among numerous coupling options for each (Figure 8-4). Self-contained FM receivers usually are used in place of personal hearing aids and must be set accordingly. An important design feature of self-contained FM receivers is the presence of internal controls. These controls may vary from one system to another but usually include at least a tone control and a maximum output control. In addition, many systems utilize a control designed to adjust the relationship between the FM and environmental microphone signals when the system is operated in the FM plus environmental microphone mode. The purpose of the FM level control is to maintain the FM signal at a level above the environmental microphone signal, maintaining the FM advantage. However, audibility of environmental signals also is important for the monitoring of one's own speech and for person-to-person communication. One decision that must be made, therefore, is how to set the relationship between the two signals and still meet the listening/communication needs of the user. For example,

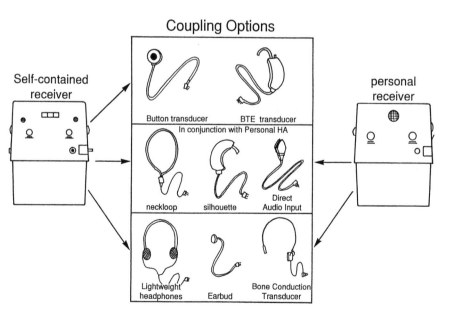

FIGURE 8-4   **Coupling options for a self-contained FM receiver and a personal FM receiver.**

(From Lewis, 1994. *American Journal of Audiology, 3*, 70–83. Used with permission.)

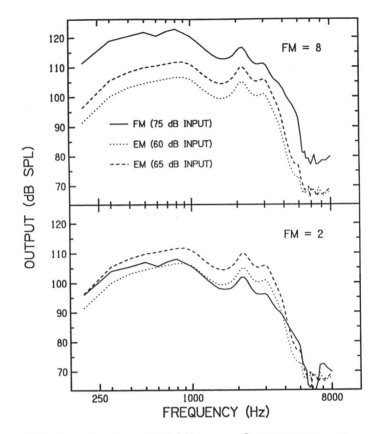

FIGURE 8-5   **Output (dB SPL) across frequency as a function of input level (dB SPL) to the FM microphone and EM at FM control settings of 8 (upper panel) and 2 (lower panel).**

(From Lewis, 1994. *American Journal of Audiology, 3*, 70–83. Used with permission).

Figure 8-5 illustrates output of an FM system for three different input signals when the FM-level control is set to maximum (upper panel) and close to minimum (lower panel). The 75 dB SPL input represents input to the FM microphone, the 65 dB SPL signal represents the user's own voice at an ear-level environmental microphone and the 60 dB SPL signal represents other voices reaching the environmental microphone (see Lewis et al., 1991 for a discussion of the rationale for use of these input levels). It is assumed that the noise level in the environment is similar at all three measurement points. Thus, the speech signal at the FM microphone likely is at a much more advantageous signal-to-noise ratio. However, as this figure illustrates, adjustment of the FM-level control may affect the FM advantage that is realized. Although output in the FM mode is 10-18 dB higher than in the environmental microphone mode at an FM-level control of 8 (upper panel), the advantage of the FM signal drops significantly when the FM-level control is set to 2 (lower panel).

When selecting an FM system for a given individual, it is important to maintain as much of an advantage as possible for the FM signal while ensuring that the environmental microphone signal will be audible to the user. This concept is illustrated in Figure 8-6 for a mild (left panel) and a severe (right panel) hearing loss. In both panels the FM system has been set so that the output in the FM mode of operation matches the desired amplified long term speech spectrum (solid line). Output in the environmental microphone mode would usually be set to some level below that in the FM mode in order to maintain a positive signal-to-noise ratio advantage for the FM signal. The dashed lines represent levels 5, 10 and 15 dB below the FM signal. For the mild hearing loss, audibility of speech in the environmental microphone mode would be maintained at any of the lower levels. However, if the hearing loss is severe, audibility of speech through the environmental microphone is compromised as the level of the amplified environmental signal is reduced.

Self-contained FM receiver units allow a choice of ear-level (behind-the-ear) and button transducers. The choice of one transducer over another impacts both the environ-

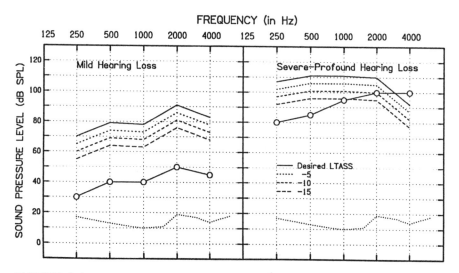

FIGURE 8-6   **Amplified long-term average speech spectrum (LTASS) as a function of frequency for a mild hearing loss (left panel) and a severe hearing loss (right panel). Solid line represents desired amplified LTASS (dB SPL). Dashed lines represent the amplified LTASS at 5, 10, and 15 dB below the desired level.**

(From Lewis, 1994. *American Journal of Audiology, 3,* 70–83. Used with permission).

mental *microphone-only* and *FM plus environmental microphone* modes of operation. If ear-level transducers are utilized, the user receives environmental signals at ear level and, if worn in a binaural arrangement, experiences binaural reception. However, feedback may be a problem when fitting individuals with severe hearing loss. Although button transducers will reduce feedback by allowing greater separation of the environmental microphone and transducer, environmental signals will be received at chest or waist level rather than at ear level, thus reducing or eliminating binaural cues. Placement of the environmental microphone at waist level introduces its own problems, because of the increased distance from the speaker's mouth to the microphone for monitoring of his or her own voice and resulting changes in the frequency-gain characteristics of the signal (Medwetsky & Boothroyd, 1991). In addition, the signal often will need to travel under clothing, desks, or books to reach the microphone.

Personal FM systems differ from self-contained systems in that they are designed to be worn in conjunction with an individual's personal hearing aid. Personal systems usually have a volume control but do not have internal controls to adjust the frequency-gain characteristics of the signal. Frequency-shaping and maximum output are accomplished by the hearing aid(s).

The choice of when to use and how to couple any FM system to a hearing aid will vary depending upon such factors as the hearing loss, hearing aids, personal/behavioral characteristics of the user and the educational environment (Lewis, 1991). Coupling options include neckloops, silhouettes, and direct audio input. A neckloop coupling may be appropriate for a student concerned about the cosmetic aspects of using an FM system, as well as for a student who is distracted by the presence of cords necessary for direct audio input coupling. In both cases, the neckloop can be placed out of sight under clothing without affecting the signal; however, use of a neckloop may have deleterious effects on the transmitted signal in the presence of other devices that emit electromagnetic energy (e.g., video display terminals, electrical wiring, fluorescent lights). In addition, the loss of low-frequency energy when hearing aids are operated in the telecoil mode (Rodriguez, Holmes, & Gerhardt, 1985; Thibodeau, McCaffrey, & Abrahamson, 1988) may preclude use of neckloop coupling for individuals whose degree of hearing loss requires significant amplification in the low frequencies. Figure 8-7 illustrates the differences that may occur when comparing the frequency response of a hearing aid alone to that same hearing aid coupled to an FM system via an inductive neckloop. The dashed line represents the output of the hearing aid alone (60 dB SPL swept puretone input). The solid line represents output of the hearing aid, in telecoil mode, coupled to a personal FM system via an inductive neckloop (75 dB SPL swept puretone input). Note that although the outputs were matched for the frequencies 1000 Hz and above, output in the low frequencies was significantly less for the FM coupling.

An inductive silhouette may be an option if the telecoil of the hearing aid is not strong enough to couple it to an FM system via a neckloop. Because the silhouette is worn next to the hearing aid, a stronger signal can reach the telecoil. However, signal variability may be a problem when using a silhouette. Figure 8-8, from Lewis et al.

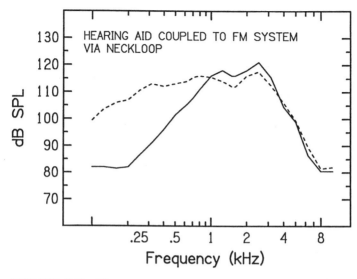

FIGURE 8-7   **Illustrates attempt to match the frequency response of an FM system coupled to a personal hearing aid via a neckloop (solid line) to that of the personal hearing aid alone (dashed line).**

(From Lewis, 1991. *Pediatric Amplification: Proceedings of the 1991 National Conference*, pp. 115–138. Used with permission).

(1991) illustrates the effect of movement of an inductive silhouette on FM output. The dashed line represents output of a hearing aid with a 60 dB SPL input. The solid line represents output of the FM system with a 75 dB SPL input. In the top panel an attempt has been made to match the two outputs. Although an acceptable match is achieved, the bottom panel illustrates how slight movement of the silhouette can result in large changes in the FM response.

Direct audio input coupling may be an appropriate option for some students. However, the cord and audio boots used to couple most hearing aids may be too fragile for active and curious preschoolers or even early elementary students, resulting in frequent breakdowns and repairs. In addition, if many students in one class use direct audio input, the necessity of maintaining a stock of appropriate cords and audio input boots for a variety of hearing aid/FM combinations in one class may impact negatively on the classroom teacher's acceptance of the FM system.

Regardless of the option chosen, it is important to remember that the response of the hearing aid coupled to the FM system may vary from that of the hearing aid alone (Friedman & Harford, 1982; Gravel & Konkle, 1982; Hawkins & Schum, 1985; Hawkins & Van Tasell, 1982; Lewis et al., 1991; Thibodeau, 1990; Van Tasell & Landin, 1980). For example, Van Tasell and Landin (1980) compared frequency-gain

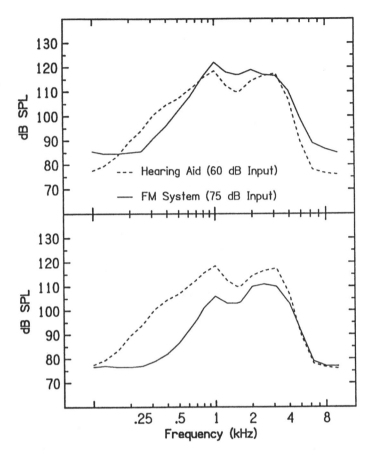

FIGURE 8-8   **Examples of the impact on FM output caused by movement of inductive silhouette. 2 cm³ coupler values (dB SPL) are displayed as a function of frequency for an optimal hearing fitting (dashed line) and FM system coupled via a silhouette to a hearing aid operating in the telecoil mode (solid line). The top panel displays a close match between the output of the hearing aid and the FM system. The bottom panel shows a decrease in FM output due to slight movement of the silhouette.**

(From Lewis et al., 1991. *Ear and Hearing*, pp. 260–280. Used with permission).

characteristics of five personal hearing aids to the responses measured with the hearing aids coupled to an FM system via a neckloop. They found differences in frequency response between the two modes of operation for all hearing aids tested. Thibodeau (1990) also reported variability in the hearing aid alone condition versus the hearing aid coupled to two different FM systems via direct audio input.

Thibodeau and Saucedo (1991) evaluated 30 same-model FM systems to examine variability across receivers, lapel microphones, and neckloops. They found numerous differences across systems, including volume-control settings in both FM and environmental microphone modes of operation, lapel microphones, and neckloops. As these findings suggest, it is important to evaluate the effect of specific coupling options on the desired response of an FM system on an individual basis.

Self-contained receivers also may be coupled to an individual's personal hearing aids via direct audio input, a neckloop, or a silhouette. In these instances, coupling concerns would be the same as discussed for personal FM systems. In addition, when coupling to personal hearing aids, care must be taken that the internal control settings of the FM receiver do not interact adversely with the internal control settings of the hearing aid. It may helpful to start with the internal controls of the FM receiver set wide open and the volume at a low level to allow the hearing aid to do the frequency shaping and output limiting. Changes in FM receiver controls then can be made as needed to obtain the appropriate response. Alternately, the FM system could be set with the output controls at minimum, initially, to ensure that it does not overdrive the hearing aid. The most appropriate settings for the FM system will vary across hearing aids, coupling options, and FM systems.

Other coupling options for FM systems include lightweight headphones or earbuds for unilateral, conductive, or minimal hearing losses, and bone conduction vibrators for conductive losses such as those involving atresia or chronic ear drainage. Whenever an a child who has normal hearing or minimal hearing loss is fitted with an FM system, it is critical to determine the maximum output of the system to avoid damage to residual hearing. Kopun (1991) reported peak 2 cm^3 coupler outputs as high as 139.5 dB SPL for FM systems coupled to nonoccluding headphones. Also, it is important that the ear remain unoccluded so that environmental sounds may be received naturally.

Recent Additions

Recent additions to FM technology in the classroom have increased the options available for students needing additional amplification in educational settings. Soundfield FM amplification systems have been recommended for students with fluctuating hearing loss, recurrent middle ear problems, unilateral hearing loss, minimal hearing loss, and for students with normal hearing whose additional handicapping conditions suggest the need for amplification of auditory signals (Benafield, Keiser, Weatherton, Eaton, & Thompson, 1992; Blair, Myrup, & Viehweg, 1989; Flexer, 1992; Flexer, Millin, & Brown, 1990; Jones, Berg, & Viehweg, 1989; Neuss, Blair, & Viehweg, 1991; Sarff, 1981). These systems consist of an FM microphone/transmitter, an amplifier, and loudspeakers placed in various locations in the classroom. The goal is to provide a uniform amplified signal that is approximately 10-15 dB above background noise.

Reported benefits of soundfield systems include an improved auditory signal for all students in the class and absence of additional receiver units for providing the amplified signal. The latter may increase acceptance by students, who will not feel they are being singled out, and by teachers, who will not be responsible for trouble-shooting individual FM units and placing them on students. The cost of soundfield amplification systems also makes them an attractive option for many schools. Al-though a soundfield system may cost more than an individual FM system, it provides amplification for the entire class, including those with unidentified or fluctuating hearing loss related to middle ear problems.

There are some limitations to soundfield amplification systems. One limitation relates to installation. Because all classrooms are not the same, the number and loca-tion of loudspeakers needed to amplify a particular room varies. If the system is not installed properly, the result may not be an improved signal (Davis, 1991; Flexer, 1992; Leavitt, 1991). Currently, there are no standards for system characteristics and few guidelines to assist schools in making installation decisions.

Soundfield systems may not be the most appropriate option for students with severe hearing loss, even when used in conjunction with personal hearing aids. Blair, Myrup, and Viehweg (1989) evaluated speech recognition ability of 10 students with mild-moderate hearing loss using personal hearing aids, personal hearing aids plus a soundfield FM system, and a personal FM system coupled to hearing aids via a neckloop. In all but one case, both hearing aids plus the soundfield system and hear-ing aids plus a personal FM system resulted in higher scores compared to hearing aids alone. In all but two cases, however, scores were best when the hearing aids were coupled to the personal FM system. The authors reported that the soundfield system provided a slightly poorer signal-to-noise ratio than would be expected with the per-sonal FM and that the system could not be used for individualized instruction.

Finally, soundfield amplification systems also are limited by their lack of port-ability. Unlike personal and self-contained FM systems, they cannot be transported easily from one class to the next and would not be available for activities such as field trips or outdoor play.

Another recent addition to FM system amplification is an ear-level FM receiver/hearing aid combination developed by AVR Sonovation, Inc. Placement of the FM receiver at ear level eliminates the need for an additional receiver unit and coupling. In addition, the receiver operates on a standard 675-size hearing-aid battery, rather than the larger batteries used in traditional FM systems. The system provides the user with FM-only, FM plus environmental microphone, and environmental microphone-only modes of operation.

The ear-level FM system is an excellent option for older students who need the improved signal-to-noise ratio of an FM system but refuse to wear traditional models due to cosmetic concerns. The transmission range of the system is significantly less (approximately 100 feet outdoors) than that of traditional FM systems (approximately 300 feet outdoors), which may limit its use in situations where distance is a factor (e.g., on the playground, in a large auditorium). The limited range, however, may be beneficial in settings where numerous classrooms are using FM systems simulta-neously by reducing the possibility of interference among systems when more than one class is transmitting on the same channel.

This particular FM system places several of its FM controls on the transmitter unit. As a result, flexibility may be limited in classes for students with hearing impairment or in classes where more than one student is wearing the FM system because the same transmitter settings would have to be used for everyone, regardless of hearing loss. Because of its recent introduction, further research will be necessary to examine benefits and limitations of the ear-level FM system.

SUMMARY

FM systems, when set and used properly, are able to overcome many of the deleterious effects of noise, distance, and reverberation. A thorough understanding of the design features and coupling options that are available must be combined with knowledge of the educational environment and the individual's specific needs. Together, this information will allow the audiologist to select the system that will be most appropriate for a given individual.

REFERENCES

Benafield, N., Keiser, H., Weatherton, M., Eaton, B., & Thompson, C. (1992). Sound field amplification in a preschool language group. Presented at American Speech-Language-Hearing Association Convention, San Antonio, TX.

Berg, F. (1987). FM equipment. In *Facilitating Classroom Listening: A Handbook for Teachers of Normal and Hard of Hearing Students*, pp. 155–190. Boston: College-Hill Press.

Berger, K., & Millin, J. (1989). Amplification/assistive devices for the hearing impaired. In R. Schow & M. Nerbonne (Eds.), *Introduction to aural rehabilitation*, pp. 31–80. Austin, Texas: Pro-Ed.

Bess, F., & Gravel, J. (1981). Recent trends in educational amplification. *Hearing Instruments*, *32*, 34–29.

Bess, F., Sinclair, J.S., & Riggs, D. (1984). Group amplification in schools for the hearing impaired. *Ear and Hearing*, *5*, 138–144.

Blair, J., Myrup, C., & Viehweg, S. (1989). Comparison of the listening effectiveness of hard-of hearing children using three types of amplification. *Educational Audiology Monograph*, *1*, 48–55.

Boney, S., & Bess, F. (1984). Noise and reverberation effects in minimal bilateral sensorineural hearing loss. Presented at American Speech-Language-Hearing Association convention, San Francisco.

Boothroyd, A. (1981). Group hearing aids. In F. Bess, B. Freeman, & J.S. Sinclair (Eds.), *Amplification in education*, pp. 123–138. Washington, DC: Alexander Graham Bell Association.

Boothroyd, A. (1986). Compression-limited amplification for the profoundly deaf. Presented at the RESNA Rehabilitation Technology 9th Annual Conference, Minneapolis, MN.

Boothroyd, A. (1992). The FM wireless link: An invisible microphone cable. In M. Ross (Ed.),

FM auditory training systems: Characteristics, selection, and use, pp. 1–19. Timonium, MD: York Press Inc.

Cox, R., & Moore, J. (1988). Composite speech spectrum for hearing aid gain prescriptions. *Journal of Speech and Hearing Research, 31*, 102–107.

Crandell, C., & Smaldino, J. (1993). A current analysis of classroom acoustics for hearing-impaired children. *American Journal of Audiology*, in press.

Davis, D. (1991) Utilizing amplification devices in the regular classroom. *Hearing Instruments, 42*, 18–22.

Erber, N. (1971). Auditory and audiovisual reception of words in low-frequency noise by children with normal hearing and by children with impaired hearing. *Journal of Speech and Hearing Research, 14*, 496–512.

Fabry, D. (1991a). Programmable and automatic noise reduction in existing hearing aids. In G. Studebaker, F. Bess, & L. Beck (Eds.), *Second Vanderbilt Hearing Aid Conference Proceedings*, pp. 65–78. Parkton, MD: York Press.

Fabry, D. (1991b). Signal processing hearing aids with the pediatric population. In J. Feigin & P. Stelmachowicz (Eds.), *Pediatric amplification: Proceedings of the 1991 national conference*, pp. 49–60. Omaha, NE: Boys Town National Research Hospital.

Federal Communications Commission. (1992). Amendment of Part 15. (92-163), ET Docket No. 91-150. *Additional frequencies for auditory assistance devices for the hearing impaired*, April 7, 1992.

Finitzo-Hieber, T. (1981). Classroom acoustics. In R. Roeser & M. Downs (Eds.), *Auditory disorders in school children: The law, identification, remediation*, pp. 250–262. New York: Thieme-Stratton.

Finitzo-Hieber, T., & Tillman, T. (1978). Room acoustics effects on monosyllabic word discrimination ability for normal and hearing-impaired children. *Journal of Speech-Language-Hearing Research, 21*, 440–458.

Flexer, C. (1992). FM classroom public address systems. In M. Ross (Ed.), *FM auditory training systems: Characteristics, selection and use*, pp. 189–210. Timonium, MD: York Press.

Flexer, C., Millin, J., & Brown, L. (1990). Children with developmental disabilities: The effect of sound field amplification on word identification. *Language, Speech and Hearing Services in Schools, 21*, 177–182.

Friedman, B., & Harford, E. (1982). A clinical evaluation of FM mini-loop auditory trainers. Presented at American Speech-Language-Hearing Association Convention, Toronto, Canada.

Gengel, R. (1971). Acceptable signal-to-noise ratios for aided speech discrimination by the hearing impaired. *Journal of Auditory Research, 11*, 219–222.

Gravel, J., & Konkle, D. (1982). Electroacoustic hearing-aid performance with neck-loop inductive coupling. Presented at American Speech-Language-Hearing Association Convention, Toronto, Canada.

Hammond, L.B. (1991). *FM auditory trainers: A winning choice for students, teachers and parents*. Minneapolis, MN: Gopher State Litho Corp.

Hawkins, D. (1988). Options in classroom amplification. In F. Bess (Ed.), *Hearing impairment in children*, pp. 253–265. Parkton, MD: York Press, Inc.

Hawkins, D., & Schum, D. (1985). Some effects of FM-system coupling on hearing aid characteristics. *Journal of Speech and Hearing Disorders, 50*, 132–141.

Hawkins, D., & Van Tasell, D. (1982). Electroacoustic characteristics of personal FM systems. *Journal of Speech and Hearing Disorders, 47*, 355–362.

Jones, J., Berg, F., & Viehweg, S. (1989). Close, distant and sound field overhead listening in kindergarten classrooms. *Educational Audiology Monograph*, *1*, 56–65.

Kopun, J. (1991). Amplification options for children with minimal and unilateral hearing loss. In J.A. Feigin & P.G. Stelmachowicz (Eds.), *Pediatric amplification: Proceedings of the 1991 national conference*, pp. 115–138. Omaha, NE: Boys Town National Research Hospital.

Kuk, F., Tyler, R., & Mims, L. (1990). Subjective ratings of noise-reduction hearing aids. *Scandinavian Audiology*, *19*, 237–244.

Leavitt, R. (1991). Group amplification systems for students with hearing impairment. *Seminars in Hearing*, *12*, 380–387.

Leavitt, R., & Flexer, C. (1991). Speech degradation as measured by the rapid speech transmission index (RASTI). *Ear and Hearing*, *12*, 115–118.

Lewis, D. (1991). FM systems and assistive devices: Selection and evaluation. In J. Feigin & P. Stelmachowicz (Eds.), *Pediatric amplification: Proceedings of the 1991 national conference*, pp. 115–138. Omaha, NE: Boys Town National Research Hospital.

Lewis, D. (1994). Assistive devices for classroom listening: FM systems. *American Journal of Audiology*, *3*, 70–83.

Lewis, D., Feigin, J., Karasek, A., & Stelmachowicz, P. (1991). Evaluation and assessment of FM systems. *Ear and Hearing*, *12*, 268–280.

Logan, S., & Bess, F. (1985). Amplification for school-age hearing-impaired children. *Seminars in Hearing*, *6(3)*, 309–321.

Madell, J. (1990). Managing classroom amplification. In M. Ross (Ed.), *Hearing-impaired children in the mainstream*, pp. 95–118. Parkton, MD: York Press, Inc.

Medwetsky, L., & Boothroyd, A., (1991). Effect of microphone placement on the spectral distribution of speech. Presented at the American Speech-Language-Hearing Association Convention, Atlanta, Georgia.

Neuss, D., Blair, J., & Viehweg, S. (1991). Sound field amplification: Does it improve word recognition in a background of noise for students with minimal hearing impairments? *Educational Audiology Monograph*, *2*, 43–52.

Rodriguez, G., Holmes, A., & Gerhardt, K. (1985). Microphone vs. telecoil performance characteristics. *Hearing Instruments*, *36(9)*, 22–24, 57.

Ross, M. (1986). Classroom amplification. In W. Hodgson (Ed.), *Hearing aid assessment and use in audiologic habilitation*, pp. 231–265. Baltimore, MD: Williams & Wilkins.

Ross, M. (Ed.). (1992). *FM auditory training systems: Characteristics, selection, and use.* Timonium, MD: York Press, Inc.

Ross, M., Brackett, D., & Maxon, A. (1982). Remediation. In M. Ross (Ed.), with D. Brackett, & A. Maxon, *Hard of hearing children in regular schools*, pp. 121–232. Englewood, NJ: Prentice-Hall, Inc.

Ross, M., & Giolas, T. (1971). The effects of three classroom listening conditions on speech intelligibility. *American Annals of the Deaf*, *116*, 580–584.

Sarff, L. (1981). An innovative use of free field amplification in regular classrooms. In R. Roeser & M. Downs (Eds.), *Auditory disorders in school children*, pp. 263–272. New York, Thieme-Stratton, Inc.

Smith L., & Boothroyd, A. (1990). Perception in noise by hearing impaired children. Presented at ASHA, Seattle, WA.

Stach, B., Speerschneider, J., & Jerger, J. (1987). Evaluating the efficacy of automatic signal processing hearing aids. *The Hearing Journal*, Mar., 15–19.

Thibodeau, L. (1990). Electroacoustic performance of direct-input hearing aids with FM amplification systems. *Language, Speech and Hearing Services in Schools, 21*, 49–56.

Thibodeau, L. (1992). Physical components and features of FM transmission systems. In M. Ross (Ed.), *FM auditory training systems: Characteristics, selection, and use*, pp. 45–73. Timonium, MD: York Press, Inc.

Thibodeau, L., McCaffrey, H., & Abrahamson, J. (1988). Effects of coupling hearing aids to FM systems via neck loops. *Journal of the American Rehabilitation Association, 21*, 49–56.

Thibodeau, L., & Saucedo, K. (1991). Consistency of electroacoustic characteristics across components of FM systems. *Journal of Speech and Hearing Research, 34*, 628–635.

Tyler, R., & Kuk, F. (1989). Consonant recognition evaluation of "noise suppression" hearing aids in speech babble and low frequency noise. *Ear and Hearing, 10*, 243–249.

Van Tasell, D., & Landin, D. (1980). Frequency response characteristics of FM mini-loop auditory trainers. *Journal of Speech and Hearing Disorders, 45*, 247–258.

Van Tasell, D., Larsen, S., & Fabry, D. (1988). Effects of an adaptive filter hearing aid on speech recognition in noise by hearing impaired subjects. *Ear and Hearing, 9*, 15–21.

Wolinsky, S. (1986). Clinical assessment of a self-adaptive noise filtering system. *The Hearing Journal, Oct.*, 29–32.

▶ 9

Orientation to the Use of Induction Loop Systems

ROBERT A. GILMORE
American Loop Systems

The induction loop system is the oldest form of wireless assistive listening technology in use today—it was developed over forty-five years ago. The use of induction-based assistive listening technology is experiencing renewed interest and popularity in the United States in large measure because of federal legislation, such as the Telephone Compatibility Act of 1988, which requires that essentially all telephones transmit to telecoil-equipped hearing aids; by the Americans with Disabilities Act of 1990, which mandates communication accessibility for hearing-impaired people; and by the many new advances in hearing-aid telecoil, audio, and assistive listening technology.

HOW CONVENTIONAL LOOP SYSTEMS WORK

The conventional large-area induction loop assistive listening system is made up of a "loop" wire (which may consist of one or more turns of cable) that is placed around the listening area, a special loop amplifier, and one or more hardwired and/or wireless (FM and/or VHF) microphones in close proximity to the speaker or speakers. The loop system may also receive input from a public address (P.A.) system via a microphone or line level output feed. Speech or other audio signals are amplified and circulated through the loop wire. The resulting electromagnetic energy radiating from the loop wire is picked up and amplified by the "telecoil" (activated by the "T"-switch or Telephone switch) found in many hearing aids, vibrotactile devices, cochlear implant processors, or by wearable induction receivers with earphones. In effect, current flow through one coil of wire (the loop), causes current to flow in a nearby coil of wire (the telecoil circuit inside the hearing aid). This process is called "induction"—hence, the term "induction loop system." The end result is an amplified faithful reproduction of the original audio signal. The signal is sent directly to the hearing-impaired listener without any physical or electrical connection to the loop wire or loop amplifier: A wireless audio link is formed between the desired sound source and the hearing-impaired listener or listeners (Figures 9-1 and 9-2). Background room noises are greatly reduced, while intelligibility is greatly increased. Induction loop systems may be used in any size area, from a single individual neck loop, to a small conference table, to a large auditorium (Figures 9-3 and 9-4).

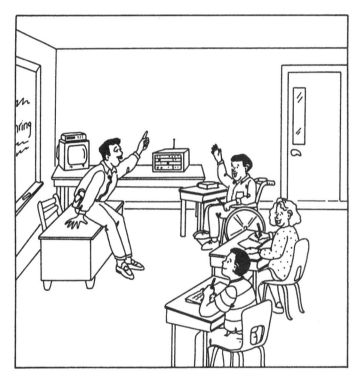

FIGURE 9-1   **In the classroom equipped with the 3-D Loop, the teacher's voice is sent from his wireless microphone to the 3-D Loop processor box on the table. The processor sends it to the special under-carpet mat, which transmits the voice signal to the student's telecoil-equipped hearing aids. Reception is unaffected by the orientation of the telecoil, and adjacent classrooms can be effectively looped without signal spillover.**

(Courtesy American Loop Systems)

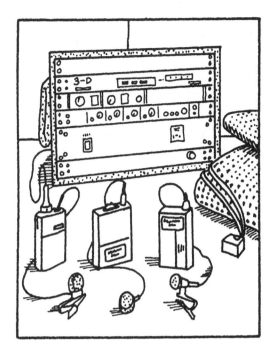

FIGURE 9-2 **Components of the 3-D Loop system include a wireless microphone, a loop processor box, a special under-carpet mat and the hearing-impaired person's own telecoil-equipped hearing aid.**

(Courtesy American Loop Systems)

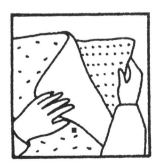

FIGURE 9-3 **A complex configuration of wiring elements enable the 3-D mat to transmit an audio signal clearly regardless of the orientation of the telecoil and with minimal signal spillover.**

(Courtesy American Loop Systems)

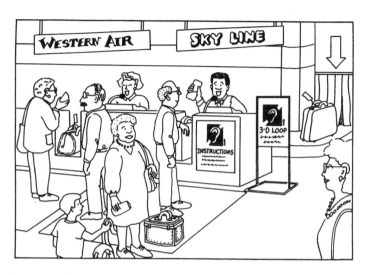

FIGURE 9-4 **With the 3-D Loop system installed, the hearing-impaired passenger can converse comfortably with the ticket agent despite the ticket counter hubbub. The audio signal from the ticket agent's microphone is sent through the 3-D Loop processor box (not shown) to the special under-carpet mat. The hearing-impaired passenger's hearing aid, switched to the "T" or "MT" position, picks up the agent's voice signal transmitted from the mat.**

(Courtesy American Loop Systems)

Induction loop systems may be designed to be permanently installed or portable. Features making loop systems portable include: use of easy-to-lay and easy-to-wind loop wire which is placed on the floor where needed and then removed later, and the "permanent" installation of loop wire in commonly used rooms then moving the loop amplifier from room to room, plugging into the loop wire in each room as needed. Alternately, the loop wire may be installed under flooring, beneath carpeting, along baseboards, around walls, and in ceilings (generally not more than 12 feet high). Some loop wires are terminated in connectors that fit together. This feature facilitates unwinding and encircling the loop wire around the area of use—the listening area. In most loop systems a loop lead-in wire is extended from the loop wire to the special loop amplifier. This feature allows the looped area to exist some distance from the loop amplifier, which may then be interfaced with a public address system or other sound source.

The use of multiple loop systems may be required to provide equal communication accessibility to all parts of a large space (e.g., a theater, house of worship, or auditorium). For example, if the perimeter measurement of the auditorium you want to make accessible is 400 feet, it would require two 200-foot loop wire systems to accommodate the entire space. A single 400-foot loop wire system would probably lack the power needed to adequately reach hearing-impaired telecoil users seated in the middle of the auditorium. The magnetic field strength within the looped area is directly proportional to the current that flows through the loop. The induction signal originates from the loop wire. The middle of the looped area is most distant from the signal source and is thus the weakest point. For this reason, the International Electroacoustical Commission (IEC) standard for loop systems is based on measurements taken in the center of the looped area. If the center of the loop system measures at IEC standard, then you can assume that the entire space is receiving adequate signal strength.

People who use classrooms, theaters, and other meeting rooms depend on effective and timely communications. However, these listening environments can have a lot of background noise; the distance from the person speaking or the public address system loudspeakers to the listeners is often great; and the hard smooth surfaces found in most of these public spaces creates a high level of reverberation. These factors combine to create very challenging listening environments, especially for hard-of-hearing people. The signal-to-noise ratio is very unfavorable. These noisy environments actually make an individual's hearing loss more of a handicap than it is under quieter conditions.

In order to comprehend speech, the hearing-impaired individual requires that sound be presented at a higher intensity than does a person with normal hearing. The usual approach to this situation is to utilize personal amplification in the form of hearing aids. The hearing aid increases the sound intensity to the level required by the listener. The hearing aid may also provide additional signal processing in which the frequency response is tailored to better suit the configuration of an individual's particular hearing loss.

Unfortunately, hearing aids amplify the *unwanted* sound along with the desired sound, being unable to differentiate between ambient room noises and the speech signals of interest. Unwanted sounds can be defined to include any acoustic signals other than those which the listener is attempting to hear at that time. In this way, any sound or speech signal may be either desirable or unwanted depending on the context of the listening event and the communication needs and desires of the listener. This interference and resulting deterioration of the intelligibility of the desired signal affects comprehension, resulting in a barrier being placed between the hearing-impaired person and equal access to educational, employment, and recreational opportunities.

New digital sound processing technology is being developed to improve the capacity of hearing aids to differentiate between noise and the desired sound. It is expected that in the next decade advanced signal processing techniques will result in a "smart" hearing aid. Nonetheless, it is unclear whether the advanced hearing aid will "know" that it is supposed to be "listening" to the person speaking over the public address system, rather than the two people chatting nearby.

In the meantime, this issue is being addressed through the use of assistive listening device technology. Conventional and 3-D loop assistive listening systems serve to essentially bridge the gap between the hearing-impaired listener and the desired sound source while attenuating the undesired competing noise (Figures 9-5 and 9-6).

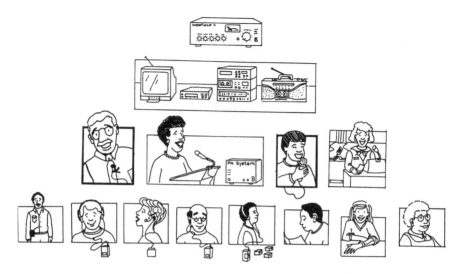

FIGURE 9-5   **Starting from the top: the loop amplifier (level one), which receives its signal from a variety of audio signal sources (level two), or from a variety of speakers using any of the many types of hardwired or wireless microphones (level three). The signal is then sent out of the loop wire to hearing-impaired people utilizing a variety of induction receivers including hearing aids, vibrotactile devices, cochlear implant systems, and induction loop receivers with headphones.**

(Courtesy American Loop Systems)

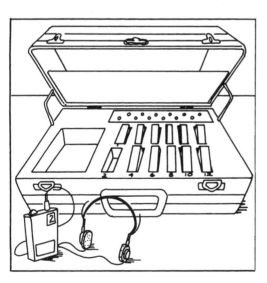

FIGURE 9-6   **Induction loop receivers with headphones are available as rechargeable units complete with recharger/ storage cases.**

(Courtesy American Loop Systems)

TELECOIL-EQUIPPED INDUCTION RECEIVERS

To access loop systems, hearing-impaired listeners only need to enter the designated "listening area"—which can be as small or as large an area as needed—and adjust their aids to the "T" (Telecoil) or "MT" (Microphone/Telecoil) position. In addition to hearing aids, vibrotactile devices, cochlear implant systems, and personal assistive listening devices such as induction receivers with headphones can all serve as the signal receiver. The listener will then receive a clear speech transmission or any other audio signal (e.g., television, VCR, stereo, or tape player) directed through the loop system.

Induction-based assistive listening systems may also be used by hearing people for language translation. Audio induction loops have also been used by visually disabled people for descriptive video and audio description services. In each of these

TABLE 9-1 **A Consumer's Guide to Telecoils**

Sensitivity:	*Request the most sensitive telecoil circuit possible*, considering the size of the hearing aid.
Type of Telecoil:	*Request a telecoil circuit with a dedicated pre-amplifier*, an active telecoil. Active telecoils are size-for-size more powerful than passive telecoils.
Telecoil Position:	*Request that the telecoil be mounted in a near-vertical position relative to the worn position.* Although a horizontal position relative to the worn position generally yields a slightly stronger (approx. 5 dB) signal when coupled normally to a hearing aid compatible telephone, this telecoil orientation severely limits the telecoil's effectiveness when used with induction loops.
MT Switch:	*Request an "MT" (Microphone/Telecoil) combination switch.* In the "MT" mode, the user has simultaneous access to both the acoustic signal, via the "M" (microphone) and the induction signal (from such devices as hearing-aid-compatible telephones and audio induction-based devices such as loops, neck loops, and silhouette inductors) via the "T" (telecoil).
Remote Control:	*Investigate a hearing-aid remote control option.* The remote control feature allows the user to switch from "O" (Off), "M" (Microphone), "T" (Telecoil), and/or "MT" (Microphone/Telecoil). In addition, such features as volume and tone control may also be adjusted. Remote control is a handy feature for people who adjust their hearing aid controls frequently or have difficulty manipulating small switch controls.
User Tested:	*Users should request a listening test using the telecoil-equipped hearing aid and a hearing-aid-compatible telephone at time of fitting.*
Clinician Tested:	*Users should also request that the hearing-aid dispenser evaluate the hearing aid's telecoil circuit using electroacoustic hearing-aid test equipment. Users should ask the hearing-aid dispenser if the make/model of hearing aid has manufacturer specifications for the telecoil.* If so, compare the electroacoustic test results of your hearing aid with the manufacturer's telecoil specifications.

cases, the listener is provided with an induction loop receiver with earphones with which to access the loop signal.

Not all telecoils are equal. Recognizing that in-the-ear and in-the-canal type hearing aids have certain space constraints, there are some telecoil features that can significantly improve the quality and usefulness of the telecoil.

When a hearing health care provider orders a telecoil-equipped hearing aid, every effort should be made to include an active telecoil circuit (i.e., one with a dedicated pre-amplifier). This type of telecoil circuit will dramatically improve the performance of the hearing aid when switched to "T". Hearing aids switched to "T" do not permit the wearers to hear their own voices or the voices of those around them. Switching to "MT" restores that capability, although in some listening environments it may add unwanted room noise back into the amplified signal. The best solution is the use of hearing aids with an "MT" combination switch position. In the "MT" mode, the hearing aid's internal microphone is not disabled when the aid is switched to "T", thereby maintaining the user's acoustic "connection" with the world around him or her. Whenever possible and practical an "MT" switch should be included in hearing aid fittings. The alternative solution of positioning additional microphones around the listening area to feed back ambient room noise to the assistive listening system would not adequately resolve this problem. Most people would be too far from a microphone and each microphone represents a "new" source of potential noise and interference.

ADVANTAGES AND LIMITATIONS OF CONVENTIONAL LOOP SYSTEMS

The major advantage of induction loop systems is that no special receivers are required by people whose aids are equipped with telecoils. Special receivers are always required by assistive listening systems using infrared light or radio frequency transmission (FM behind-the-ear hearing aids are available but are a special receiver.). This feature, unique to induction systems, results in decreased need for management of the system and increased acceptance and motivation to use the system on the part of the hearing-impaired end user.

The exact number of hearing aids currently equipped with telecoils is unknown. Best estimates put the number of hearing aids in the United States with telecoils between 20 and 35 percent of all hearing aids with the greatest number being in behind-the-ear and body-worn hearing aids. At least one state has proposed legislation requiring anyone purchasing a hearing aid in that state to be notified of telecoil technology by the dispenser. In January 1993, an organization called Friends of Telecoils was formed to further promote the use and availability of quality telecoils in devices for hearing-impaired people.

Induction loop systems can be easily installed by lay people and are comparatively inexpensive. Personal-sized (i.e., those servicing areas of 625 square feet/100 foot perimeter or less) basic induction loop systems cost about $300 or less. Loop systems can service an unlimited number of hearing-impaired people within a looped listening area. No physical connections are made to the hearing aid or hearing-impaired user of the loop. The users of the system are free to move about within the listening area. Induction loop systems may be used by people with hearing losses ranging in degree from mild to profound.

Two limitations have remained associated with the conventional induction loop system. The conventional approach to looping a room consists of encircling the area with the loop wire and providing input power from a special audio amplifier. The vertical and horizontal components of the radiated field extend in all directions, passing through nonmetallic walls and floors. The result is that adjacent rooms cannot be successfully looped and used simultaneously due to crosstalk (i.e., signal spillover). In fact, depending on the loop size and power of the system, considerable distances between two looped areas must be maintained to avoid interference. Spillover distances of 50 to 100 feet are not uncommon for large-area (i.e., 200-foot perimeter) loop systems. Shielding is theoretically possible, but present techniques and materials make it cost prohibitive and logistically impractical. It should also be noted that use of other forms of technology such as infrared and FM in conjunction with neck loops in rooms adjacent to "looped" rooms may also result in signal interference. As soon as the neck-looped FM or infrared user switches to "T", he or she is potentially open to receive the loop signal originating next door.

However, signal spillover is not always a limitation. For example, signal spillover may be used to service a larger area then can be effectively "looped" by the loop wire. In this case the signal spillover can be used to accommodate additional people seated a certain distance outside of the actual "looped" or loop wire encircled area. The usable spillover distance will vary. As always, measurements with a field strength meter and induction loop receiver should be made to determine the specific spillover distance. Another example of the creative beneficial use of signal spillover is the installation of the loop wire in the ceiling of one room to service both the room itself and the one above. This is particularly practical in places where both spaces are not used simultaneously, such as houses of worship.

The second limitation of conventional loop systems is lack of magnetic field uniformity. This can be a particular problem for young children or multi-disabled persons with limited head control. Conventional single plane approaches to looping a room result in a strong vertical field (i.e., the signal produced by the loop wire is transmitted in such a way that telecoils mounted in the near-vertical position relative to the worn position receive the optimum signal) and varying signal strengths as received by the hearing-aid telecoil when the user's head moves in the field. The system user experiences drop-outs and fading of the signal when the telecoil is moved out of the near-vertical position relative to the worn position. The extent to which this occurs can be reduced by minimizing the vertical orientation of the installed loop wire. Ideally, the loop wire should be installed at a uniformly horizontal level (relative to the floor) around the space to be made accessible. Avoid installing the loop wire vertically around doors, windows, and other structures as this tends to orient the signal in a less than optimum direction. Another concern is to avoid running the loop wire continuously on or behind ferrous metals which act as a magnetism sink and/or shield. Placing of the loop wire(s) should be done with the consideration that a narrow signal "dead spot" will occur directly over the loop wire. This region of diminished signal strength directly over the loop wire is generally less than two inches wide when measured at ear level for a seated adult. In general, do not exceed an installation height of greater than 12 feet. The loop wire may be installed under floors. In some installations the loop wire can be installed in the ceiling of the room below and effectively service both spaces. The loop wire signal passes through walls, ceilings, and floors. The degree to which this occurs is determined in part by the construction of the walls, ceilings, and floors. Basically, the greater the ferrous metal content the less the resulting signal spillover.

3-D LOOP SYSTEMS

In contrast to conventional induction loop systems, 3-D Loop assistive listening systems eliminate and/or minimize these problems so that adjacent areas can be successfully looped, and problems associated with telecoil orientation are eliminated. This

TABLE 9-2   **Attenuation of Signals**

Horizontal Attenuation of Signal*

Distance from Loop:	3 ft.	6 ft.	8 ft.	12 ft.
Conventional Induction Loop	−9 dB	−11 dB	−12 dB	−15 dB
3-D Loop with 12 ft. × 12 ft. 3-D Mat	−30 dB	−32 dB	−36 dB	≥ −40 dB
3-D Loop with 9 ft. × 9 ft. 3-D Mat	−30 dB	≥ −40 dB	≥ −40 dB	≥ −40 dB
3-D Loop with 5 ft. × 5 ft. 3-D Mat	−32 dB	≥ −40 dB	≥ −40 dB	≥ −40 dB

Vertical Inter-Room Attenuation of Signal**

Conventional Induction Loop	−20 dB
3-D Loop with 12 ft. × 12 ft. 3-D Mat	≥ −40 dB
3-D Loop with 9 ft. × 9 ft. 3-D Mat	≥ −40 dB
3-D Loop with 5 ft. × 5 ft. 3-D Mat	≥ −40 dB

*NOTE: Measurements in dB relative to center of induction assistive listening system where 0 dB = 100 mA/m at a vertical distance of 39 inches and telecoil in vertical position. Target attenuation value = ≥-40 dB.

**NOTE: Measurements in dB relative to center of induction assistive listening system in room directly below where 0 dB = 100 mA/m. The conventional induction loop system loop wire and 3-D Loop Mat were installed on the floor of the upstairs room and designed to service the entire space. Measurements were made at a height of 39 inches off the downstairs room floor with telecoil in the vertical position. The ceiling height was 9 feet. Target attenuation value = ≥-40 dB.

new design assistive listening technology has been termed "three-dimensional" (3-D) as a result of one of its operational characteristics. The 3-D Loop presents a very uniform signal to the user's telecoil-equipped hearing aid or any other induction receiver, regardless of its physical orientation in the signal field.

The 3-D Loop system is completely prefabricated, consisting of a control electronics "black box" and one or more special 3-D floor mats. The lightweight and flexible 3-D mat contains a complex configuration of wiring elements that transmit a highly controlled and extremely uniform signal irrespective of telecoil (i.e., hearing aid) position. The 3-D mat's physical design is similar to standard carpet matting (flexible mesh material) and is intended to be placed under floor covering (e.g., carpeting, wood or rubber flooring, or concrete poured floors). The necessity to have the 3-D mat covered by some form of floor covering may present an installation problem in some places.

Uneven field uniformity and crosstalk (i.e., signal spillover) to adjacent areas, characteristics that have long been associated with the conventional induction loop approach, have been resolved and/or minimized with the 3-D Loop system. The 3-D Loop system exhibits minimized signal spillover (see Table 9-2 above). The 3-D Loop system demonstrates absolute signal uniformity regardless of telecoil orientation. The 3-D Loop system is designed to be set up and operated by nontechnical people with a minimum of effort.

LOOP SYSTEM STANDARDS

The international standard for induction loop assistive listening systems is International Electrotechnical Commission Standard 118-4 (1981), in which the primary specification states that the magnetic field shall be 100 milliamperes/meter ± 3 dB with 70 mA/m as a minimum and 140 mA/m as a maximum, as measured at the center of the loop at a height of 1.2 meters above the floor. Allowing for 12 dB peaks occurring in speech, peak field strength may reach 400 mA/m. The frequency response shall be 100 Hz–5000 Hz ± 3 dB. This specified field strength ensures that telecoil users will receive an adequate signal, obviating the need to make substantial adjustments in volume control settings upon switching from "M" (microphone) to "T" (telecoil) or "MT" (microphone/telecoil). To verify the loop system calibration a field strength meter should be used. There are several commercially available field strength meters on the market. They range in price from under one hundred dollars to several hundred dollars, depending on the features. Regrettably, not all conventional loop systems are designed and built with the IEC standard in mind, and as a result, not all loop systems are created equal.

Over forty-five years after their first appearance, induction loop assistive listening systems remain a popular, cost-effective, user and management friendly choice of hearing-assistance technology.

RECOMMENDED READING

Gilmore, R. (1992a). Assistive listening systems: How ASHA members fit in. *Asha, 34*(6/7), 44–45.

Gilmore, R. (1992b). Creating communication accessibility: ASHA, loop systems and the ADA. *The Hearing Journal, 45*(6), 29–32.

Gilmore, R., & Lederman, N. (1988). The missing link: Large area listening systems. *The Voice, 4*(5), 14–-8.

Gilmore, R., & Lederman, N. (1989). Induction loop assistive listening systems: Back to the future? *Hearing Instruments, 40*(3), 14–20.

Lederman, N., & Gilmore, R. (1990). Loop technology—a viable solution. *Sound & Video Contractor*, 70–73.

Monte, D., & Gilmore, R. (1992). Classroom amplification goes 3-D. *Advance for Speech-Language Pathologists & Audiologists, 2*(14), 10–11.

▶ 10

Alerting Devices for the Hearing-Impaired

DEAN C. GARSTECKI
Northwestern University

Alerting devices for hearing-impaired individuals are electro-mechanical systems comprised of sensing, transmitting, and warning mechanisms (Compton, 1991). Traditionally, alerting devices have been used primarily by deaf individuals and by those suffering sudden, severe hearing loss. In more recent times, others with less severe and/or long-standing hearing loss have discovered the benefits of their use. For many, alerting devices serve as guideposts for navigating through life's everyday happenings . . . lights flash signaling incoming telephone calls . . . buzzers hum indicating callers at the door . . . wristbands shake calling attention to nearby problems. While many hearing-impaired individuals use alerting devices at the present time, many more will first become acquainted with them through implementation of the Americans with Disabilities Act (ADA).

With enactment of the ADA, environmental monitoring through use of assistive technology became a federally mandated option for hearing-disabled individuals. Title III (Public Accommodations) of the ADA ensures nondiscrimination toward individuals with hearing disability in the enjoyment of goods, services, facilities, privileges, advantages and accommodations of any public entity (DOJ, 1991). Accordingly, auxiliary aids, including alerting devices, must be provided for those with impaired hearing, unless undue burden would result for service providers or facility proprietors. Hearing professionals involved in implementation of Title III regulations will need to consider the role that alerting devices play in ensuring personal safety in:

1. places of lodging (e.g., inns, motels, hotels);
2. establishments serving food or drink (e.g., restaurants, bars);

3. places of exhibition or entertainment (e.g., theaters, concert halls, arenas);
4. places of public gathering (e.g., auditoriums, convention centers, lecture halls);
5. sales or rental establishments (e.g., bakeries, grocery stores, clothing stores, hardware stores, shopping centers);
6. service establishments (e.g., laundromats, dry cleaners, banks, barber shops, beauty shops, travel services, shoe repair services, funeral parlors, gas stations, offices of accountants or lawyers, pharmacies, insurance offices, professional offices of health care providers, hospitals);
7. stations used for public transportation (e.g., terminals, depots);
8. places of public display or collection (e.g., museums, libraries, galleries);
9. places of recreation (e.g., parks, zoos, amusement parks);
10. places of education (e.g., nursery, elementary, secondary, undergraduate, and post-graduate public and private schools);
11. social service center establishments (e.g., day care centers, senior citizen centers, homeless shelters, food banks, adoption agencies; and,
12. places of exercise or recreation (e.g., gymnasiums, health spas, bowling alleys, golf courses).

Title III also specifies that in places of lodging, at least one of every 25 sleeping rooms must be equipped with a visual alarm such as a door knock warning device, smoke alarm, and telephone alerting light. With a greater number of lodging rooms, a similar proportion must be equipped to accommodate the needs of hearing-impaired individuals, approximately 2 percent of the total rooms available in a lodging facility. Visual alarms must be located and oriented so that they spread light and reflection throughout a given space or raise overall light level sharply.

It is clear that with implementation of the ADA, use of alerting devices will become commonplace. In this chapter, the reader is acquainted with basic principles underlying the function of sensing, transmitting, and alerting components of available devices. Advantages and limitations of current technologies will be presented, along with examples of commercially available products.

THE SENSING STAGE

Alerting devices may be activated by acoustic, electronic, or inductive sensing mechanisms (Compton, 1991). In an acoustic sensing system, a microphone having variable sensitivity captures acoustic energy and transforms that energy into an electrical signal. The electrical signal, in turn, triggers a switching mechanism within the device that activates the alerting mechanism. It is in this way, for example, that the blare of a smoke detector will activate a signaling device that causes a warning light to flash.

The microphone of an acoustic sensing system can be placed near any potential sound source, making such a system highly versatile. One disadvantage is that the microphone may be sensitive to any acoustic signal in a given area, appearing to be indiscriminate in its alerting function. Problems relating to indiscriminate perfor-mance may be minimized by placing the sensor microphone in close proximity to the targeted signal. In addition, the pick-up sensitivity of some sensors may be varied so that the device does not respond to low-level or ambient noise, but only to sound that exceeds usual noise levels. There are other features that might be considered. For example, some devices are designed to be more sensitive to low rather than high frequency stimuli or to signals of long rather than short duration. In any case, it is wise to consider all available features and options during the device selection process, and to match device capabilities carefully with the nature of the signal to be monitored.

An example of a commercially available acoustic sensing system is the Sonic Alert (USS360) Universal Sound Monitor which is distributed by HITEC Group International, Inc. (Figure 10-1). The device contains a built-in sensor microphone and an electrical receptacle for use with a lamp or fan warning appliance. The device is powered by standard 110-volt household current. It can be used for wake-up pur-poses, monitoring young children, signaling activation of a smoke detector, or to indicate a telephone ring. The system is highly portable.

One alternative to an acoustic sensing system is an electronic system. An electronic sensing system usually generates the signal of interest and transmits it directly to the alerting appliance by means of a direct, hardwire connection. This eliminates the need for a sensing microphone. For example, a clock radio alarm may activate a triggering mechanism by the flow of electrical current through the system. The triggering mecha-nism allows electrical current to flow to an attached alerting appliance. Through electri-

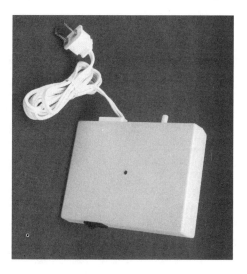

FIGURE 10-1 **Sonic Alert (USS360)**
Universal Sound Monitor

(Courtesy HITEC Group International, Inc.)

cal connections, then, a clock radio can activate an alerting lamp. One advantage of an electronic sensing system is that it is dedicated to input from a single source. It cannot indiscriminately respond to other acoustic stimuli. However, in the same vein, the hardwired connection limits range of use. Portability and user mobility are sacrificed. In addition, an electronic sensing system is likely to demonstrate limited versatility. A separate system may be required for monitoring separate sound sources.

One example of an electronic sensing system is the Sonic Alert (TR50) Telephone Signaler distributed by HITEC Group International, Inc. (Figure 10-2). Through use of a duplex plug attached to the line input jack on the telephone base, a Telephone Signaler may be attached to a warning fan or lamp.

Inductive sensing system technology provides a third option. An inductive sensing system captures electromagnetic energy generated by a signal source, such as a doorbell or telephone. This energy, as with other systems, activates an electronic switching mechanism to send current to an attached alerting appliance. One advantage of this system is that, like the electronic sensing system, it is dedicated to monitoring a designated signal source. Alternately, it also does not respond to extraneous signals or environmental noise, only to doorbells or telephones having electromagnetic ringers. Suction cup connectors tend to require some exploration in placement and they may frequently become detached. One example of an inductive sensing system is the Watchman Signaling System Sound Master (UT-WMSTR) which is distributed by HITEC Group International, Inc. (Figure 10-3). This system monitors sound from a single source. Its sound-signal control is adjustable to allow variable

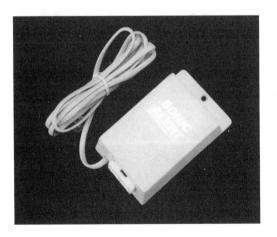

FIGURE 10-2   **Sonic Alert (TR50)
Telephone Signaler**

(Courtesy HITEC Group International, Inc.)

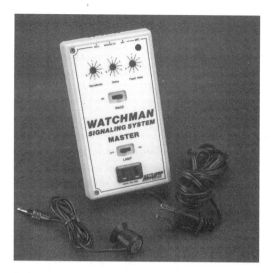

FIGURE 10-3   **Watchman Signaling System Sound Master (UT-WMSTR)**

(Courtesy HITEC Group International, Inc.)

sensitivity of the pick-up microphone. It also has an adjustable signal lamp flashing rate which may help in distinguishing signals from multiple pick-up locations.

THE TRANSMITTING STAGE

Two types of signal transmission technologies are commonly employed in alerting devices: hardwired and wireless. Hardwired signal transmission incorporates a direct connection from sensing to alerting mechanisms. Direct linkage minimizes electrical interference. Installation, operation, and maintenance of hardwired systems is straight-forward and relatively easy to manage. When troubleshooting or repairs are required, equipment malfunctions are relatively easy to isolate and remedy. Alternately, direct wired systems are typically dedicated to a single purpose, limiting their versatility in comparison with other systems.

Wireless systems depend on acoustic, inductive, or radio frequency signal trans-mission technology. In an acoustic transmission system, an open field exists between the sound source and the sensor microphone. Advantages to open-field transmission relate to increased versatility and user mobility. Such a system can be self-contained and used anywhere. One disadvantage is that, as indicated above, the sensor microphone is not selective. All sound arrives at the sensor microphone with the same level of importance.

In a wireless inductive system, signals are transduced electromagnetically from the primary source to the alerting device. The advantage is that inductive technology is relatively simple. Problems with this system are easy to troubleshoot and resolve. Inductive coupling is easy to manage. Major disadvantages to inductive signal transmission relate to vulnerability to electrical interference and variability in transmitted signal strength. In addition, while electromagnetic couplers are easy to attach to a host, sound-generating appliance, the user may need to explore optimal placement locations and be mindful that these couplers tend to be easily displaced (Compton, 1991).

Wireless radio frequency systems transmit sound energy from a sensor/transmitter unit to a receiver unit. Transmitters send FM carrier signals throughout an electrical system to receiver modules powered by standard 110-volt wall-socket current. Alerting appliances plugged into receiver modules react to activation of the transmitter unit. For example, the Ultratec Phone Module plugs directly into a telephone jack. When activated by a telephone ring, this system sends an FM carrier wave through an area's electrical system to lamp modules which are plugged into electrical wall sockets. Attached to each lamp module is an alerting appliance. The advantage to using this system is that there is no direct connection between the transmitter and receiver unit. This helps to maximize the distance between the sound source and the alerting appliance. Another advantage is that radio frequency technology is not susceptible to electrical or thunderstorm interference. On the negative side, such a system requires use of ancillary appliances and these systems tend to be more costly than systems employing alternate technologies.

THE ALERTING STAGE

Alerting devices attract their users by acoustic, vibratory, or light stimulation. In systems employing acoustic stimulation, the intent is to provide an enhanced or tailored signal that can be perceived by most individuals, regardless of hearing ability. For example, under Title III of the ADA, specific reference is made to public areas equipped with audible emergency alarms. In these areas, acoustic alarm signals are required to exceed prevailing sound levels by 15 dBA SPL or to exceed the maximum sound level typically occurring in an area by 5 dBA SPL. In addition, acoustic alarms must be presented for a minimum duration of 60 seconds. It is further specified that audible alarms must have a periodic element to their signal such as repetitive single stroke bells, signals sweeping from high to low in frequency signals, or fast 'whooping' signals as these are easier to detect than continuous signal alarms. One advantage to using an acoustic alerting system is that it does not require any unusual vigilance on the part of the user to be effective. In addition, in many acoustic alerting systems, signal frequency, intensity, duration, and presentation pattern can be tailored to provide the most effective signal possible within a given environment. One major disadvantage is that a point of diminishing returns is reached as the hearing capability of a device-user decreases. That is, an acoustic alerting system is of questionable benefit to those with severe-to-profound hearing loss. In addition, an acoustic alerting system can be obtrusive to anyone with relatively normal hearing.

In order to optimize an individual's ability to use an acoustic alerting device, it would be helpful to use strategic locations for sound-generating equipment. For example, consider use of remotely placed bells for telephone alerting needs. It may be possible to place telephone bell devices in unused phone jacks in rooms throughout a home or office area. Consider use of variable gain and variable frequency devices such as the Ringmax (WS-TEL008) device distributed by HITEC Group International, Inc. (Figure 10-4). This device is equipped with four frequency selections, four ring pattern variations, and a volume control.

Some alerting systems use vibrating receivers to alert their users. In these systems, for example, sound may be captured by the sensing microphone and serve to trigger sending of an FM carrier wave that is transmitted to a receiver unit by means of the electrical wiring system of a given household. When the receiver is activated in

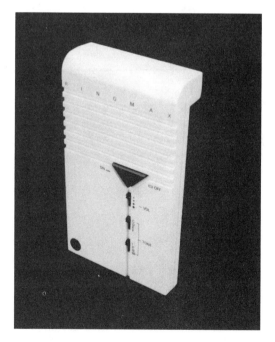

FIGURE 10-4   **Ringmax (WS-TEL008)
telephone signaler**

(Courtesy HITEC Group International, Inc.)

this way, it vibrates to signal its user. This form of alerting device may be most useful to those with combined hearing and vision problems. It also may be useful to individuals who want to be alerted to events outside of their direct line of vision. Another advantage is that some systems will accommodate up to fifteen different transmitter units, enabling their users to monitor a variety of sound sources simultaneously. Limitations relate to restrictions in effective transmission range.

One example is the Silent Call Personal Alert system. This system includes a doorbell sensor, a telephone bell sensor, a smoke detector, a general sound monitor, a personal pager, and a sleep alert system. When receivers are activated, they vibrate to alert the user. Another example is the Knock Alert (HT-K/ALERT) distributed by HITEC Group International, Inc. (Figure 10-5). The Knock Alert is a battery-operated device that alerts its users to door knockers by detecting vibrations which trigger a switch to flash a strobe light. A final example is the LilBen (GA-LILBEN) bed vibrator that is distributed by HITEC Group International, Inc. (Figure 10-6). This device is placed between mattresses or under a pillow when in use. It is constructed of shockproof plastic and it has an automatic thermal cutoff to prevent overheating.

Finally, there are devices that use light as the alerting medium. In these devices, the sound source triggers a mechanism in the device to activate an alerting light. Light signals need to be at the 100 candela level or above in order to be effective for alerting

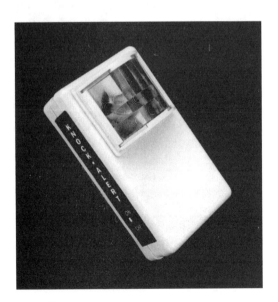

FIGURE 10-5 **Knock Alert (HT-K/ ALERT) door signaler**

(Courtesy HITEC Group International, Inc.)

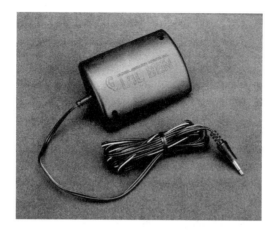

FIGURE 10-6 **LilBen (GA-LILBEN) bed vibrator**

(Courtesy HITEC Group International, Inc.)

purposes (Nober, Well, & Moss, 1990). It is best if alerting lights are positioned to reflect off walls and in a way that they may be seen in several rooms simultaneously or over a wide area. Some light systems can be coded so that signal sources can be identified by number of flashes presented. If a visual system is used for wake-up purposes, consideration should be given to use of a strobe light. Visual alarms typically are not the most effective devices for waking sleepers. A flashing light seven times brighter than that required to alert awake individuals in normal daylight is required to wake a sleeper. While strobe lights may meet signal strength requirements, they generally cannot be used with systems that code signals to differentiate between alternate sound sources.

SUMMARY

Use of alerting devices is likely to become commonplace among those with hearing disability with implementation of the ADA. Alerting device selection requires some knowledge of the benefits and limitations of various types of sensing technology.

When portability is a primary concern, preference should be given to acoustic or inductive systems with acoustic systems demonstrating greatest versatility. When emphasis is on signal transmission, direct transmission systems minimize the possible effects of electrical interference. Alternately, wireless systems maximize the potential for monitoring multiple sound sources simultaneously.

Acoustic, vibratory, and light signals are used as alerting stimuli. This enables the user to capitalize on the most effective personal means of monitoring sound sources. This also provides device options for those with progressive hearing loss and/or an inability to benefit from all the technology that is available.

In closing, this chapter highlights differences in alerting device sensing, transmitting, and alerting mechanisms. The information presented has direct application to clinical selection of alerting devices. It is recommended that these decisions be considered in the context of a comprehensive program of rehabilitative management. In this way, related factors such as personal preference, ability to use a particular device independently, and ability to maintain operation and use also are considered (Garstecki, 1988).

REFERENCES

Compton, C.L. (1991). Chapter 26. Clinical management of assistive technology users: Issues to consider. In G.A. Studebaker, F. Bess, & L.B. Beck (Eds.), *The Vanderbilt hearing-aid report II*, pp. 301–318. Parkton, MD: York Press, Inc.

Department of Justice (DOJ) (1991). 28 CFR Part 36. Nondiscrimination on the basis of disability by public accommodations and in commercial facilities: Final rule. *Federal Register, 56*, 144, July 26, 35544–35604.

Garstecki, D.C. (1988). Considerations for use of assistive devices by hearing-impaired adults. *Journal of the Academy of Rehabilitative Audiology, 21*, 153–157.

Nober, E.H., Well, A.D., & Moss, S. (1990). Does light work as well as sound? Smoke alarms for the hearing-impaired. *Fire Journal, January/February*, 27–30.

Acknowledgment
Appreciation is extended to HITEC Group International, Inc.for providing photographs of devices incorporated in this chapter.

▶ 11

Integrating Assistive Devices into the Hospital Setting

HELENE FRYE-OSIER
William S. Middleton Memorial Veterans Affairs Hospital

DONALD J. SCHUM
The University of Iowa Hospitals

INTRODUCTION

Countless opportunities exist within the medical center/hospital complex to make a positive impact on the quality of life of the patients with hearing impairment that we serve daily. Our challenge as audiologists is to evaluate all listening environments throughout the medical center, to improve those environments to minimize the need for assistive technology whenever possible, to identify the remaining barriers to successful communication, and to implement a program that provides the required assistive device and services. However, a comprehensive accessibility program in a hospital setting includes not only the appropriate assistive devices and services. An appropriate continuing education program for hospital staff members is also vital. Without the appropriate understanding of the impact of hearing loss, the role of assistive devices, and the specific understanding of how to access and use equipment and services within the hospital, there is no guarantee that even the most technically sophisticated assistive devices will be utilized appropriately. Comprehensive accessibility programs for hospitals have been described for both a generic setting (Self Help for Hard of Hearing People, Inc., 1991) and for specific settings (Jensen, Anderson, Bergquist, Boyd, Hermanson, Khal, Schum, Searls, Summerwill, Tyler, & Wolfe,

1992). These described programs highlight the need to view accessibility as more than just providing available assistive devices. Accessibility can only be insured if there is the proper understanding throughout all levels of staff within the hospital setting as to the nature of hearing impairment.

It is our hope that the information contained within this chapter will help you arrive at an approach that offers a balance between what is the ideal and what is practical. We will introduce issues for your consideration to assist you in integrating assistive devices and services in your hospital setting, highlighting aspects of patient concern and administrative support.

There are a variety of reasons why a hospital setting is a good choice for establishing a model accessibility program. First of all, most medium-to-large hospitals have an audiologist on staff. Therefore, there is a well-qualified professional on board to direct such a program. Secondly, the prevalence of hearing loss among hospital patients is probably higher than in the general population. This higher prevalence is due to the number of patients directly being seen for ear and hearing complaints, the large number of elderly patients seen in a hospital for other health problems, and the large number of patients with other related disorders such as diabetes and neurological problems. A further reason why accessibility for hearing-impaired patients is important in a hospital setting is that most communication that takes place within the hospital setting is vital. Patients are attempting to communicate with doctors, nurses, and other staff members. The content of this communication is usually quite important to both the patient and medical personnel. Further, patients may be under stress, given concern over their medical conditions. This stress may further complicate communication, as the listener may not be able to fully concentrate on the incoming message. There is very little room for error and misinterpretation of information transmitted from the medical staff to the patient. Finally, it would seem that the awareness and the willingness to learn about hearing impairment would be higher among a hospital staff, given their professional dedication to patient care.

NEEDS ASSESSMENT

The first step in an accessibility program is to review the devices and services necessary in various locations throughout the hospital. Table 11-1 provides a listing of device and service needs at various points throughout a facility. Although an audiologist may take the devices and services on this list for granted, other professionals involved in the accessibility program may not have a complete appreciation for the range of communicative needs on the part of patients and guests with hearing impairment. For example, some inpatients may prefer to watch television with an enhanced audio signal whereas others prefer closed captioning. Additionally, the Americans with Disabilities Act provides specific guidelines on the accessibility needs of public meeting areas (Williams & Carey, Chapter 1).

The next step is to review what services and devices are currently available. In

TABLE 11-1 **Hospital Location and Accessibility Needs**

AREA	NEEDED DEVICES AND SERVICES
Registration/Discharge Public waiting areas	Telecommunication access One-to-one communication Interpreter service, signage, visual message service General information displays
Emergency Treatment and Poison Control Center	Telecommunication access One-to-one communication Interpreter service
Cashier and Business Office	Telecommunication access One-to-one communication Interpreter service
Public meeting rooms	Interpreter services General information displays Large room assistive listening system
Outpatient clinics	Telecommunication access One-to-one communication Interpreter services
Inpatient rooms	Telecommunication access One-to-one communication Interpreter services Broadcast media enhancement

some cases no devices or services will be in place, and therefore the accessibility program needs to be built from the ground up. However, in other cases, it is quite possible that certain programs have been put in place by a variety of departments in the hospital that can help improve accessibility for hearing-impaired patients. It is possible that certain devices and services are available yet not widely known about. For example, does the social service or a pastoral service in the hospital have access to sign language interpreters? Does the telecommunications department within the hospital have access to a text telephone or amplified telephones? Has the maintenance or housekeeping division performed any modifications on televisions in order to provide better amplification of a signal for inpatients with hearing impairment? It is possible that specific departments have made adjustments in devices or services in response to individual inquiries at some point in the past.

An important aspect of the needs assessment within the hospital is to identify which personnel would be best suited to be involved in an accessibility program. Obviously, the audiologists are best suited to provide leadership in the area of hearing accessibility (Palmer, 1992). However, other professionals can lend invaluable input. For example, are the pastoral, social service, or patient representative personnel interested in participating in an accessibility program? Does the volunteer service group want to be involved in perhaps distributing and collecting assistive devices to inpatients in the hospital? It is wise to consider the establishment of a multidisciplinary accessibility team for a variety of reasons. First, each individual chosen from a variety of disciplines can bring expertise and talents to the team. Secondly, the use of a team as opposed to one individual person allows for the distribution of responsibility, and therefore the likelihood of continued success of the program is perhaps enhanced. It is unfortunate if an accessibility program dies out because one individual becomes overworked and disinterested in the program.

SERVICES AND EQUIPMENT

Our charge is to deliver quality assistive device services to patients and visitors via technology that is appropriate yet not overwhelming, technology that is easily recognized and whose purpose is understood by hospital support staff.

Patient Identification

Ideally, the patient's need for an assistive device was known prior to his or her arrival at your facility. A number of mechanisms can be proposed to improve the probability of that event. Many outpatient and inpatient medical facilities provide preappointment notification. The patient's preappointment letter should introduce your medical center's special needs program and a request that the patient notify the medical center's patient services representative or other designated personnel to report the need for a specific category of assistive technology. Figure 11-1 provides an example of a preappointment letter from the University of Iowa Hospital. Information concerning assistive devices is included along with other routine preappointment information. Request that your patient contact the representative prior to the scheduled appointment to allow the representative to conduct a written or telephone survey of the patient's specific need and familiarity with the facilities program options.

Promotional material at your facility should be highly visible; it is of invaluable benefit to introduce your assistive device program to potential users and their caregivers. Despite longstanding hearing loss, many patients may not fully realize the role and advantages of assistive devices (Parmiter-Jacobs, Kraemer, & Jared, 1988; Leavitt & Freeburg, 1987). Your medical media, library service, voluntary service, medical administration, and local professional associations may be of assistance in preparing and providing promotional information. In-house literature and signage is a must. Also, announcements in local print and broadcast media will further the popularity of the program. In the age of health care competition, your hospital administration may look quite favorably on such publicity.

Closed-circuit cable television capabilities or interactive video information sta-

May 14, 1993

Mr. John Smith
229 Melrose Ct.
Iowa City, IA 52246

Dear Mr. Smith:

An appointment has been scheduled for you in the

**Department of Ophthalmology—General Clinic on
June 23, 1993, at 2:00 P.M. with Dr. Jones**

**Please bring a list of all medications you are now taking, any eye drops you may be
using, glasses you prefer, and older glasses if you use them also. In addition, it would be
helpful to have a written family history of eye problems with you at the time of your
visit.** The examination will likely require dilating your pupils, so you may prefer to have a
driver with you and to bring sunglasses. Since we have to wait for the pupils to dilate, the
complete examination may be an hour or longer.

If you cannot accept this appointment, please write the Department of Ophthalmology or
call (xxx) xxx-xxxx.

Please complete the enclosed **PATIENT REGISTRATION FORM** and return in the
"Send-N-Return" envelope. Also, **please stop at the MAIN ENTRANCE Registration
area with your health insurance information 20 minutes before your appointment.**

A variety of devices are available to assist patients and visitors with hearing impairment.
If you needs such a device, please call (xxx) xxx-xxxx.

If you need interpreter services, you may call (xxx) xxx-xxxx. Hearing impaired patients
who have a Telecommunications Device for the Deaf (TDD) should call (xxx) xxx-xxxx.

Parking is available at University Hospitals as shown on the diagram on the reverse side
of this letter.

If you need help or additional information, staff at the **Information Desk inside the
Main Entrance** will be pleased to be of assistance. We look forward to serving you.

Sincerely,

June Doe
Scheduling Supervisor

FIGURE 11-1   **Preappointment Letter**

tions are available in some medical centers and hospitals. They are used for general
patient education and may serve as an efficient source of education for your inpatients
and outpatients interested in learning about the ADA, their rights, and your efforts to
meet their assistive device needs.

Brief videotaped educational programs running in key clinic waiting room areas, hospital lobbies, and gathering places will help target potential users of the benefits of the assistive loaner program at your facility; specify clearly in all material the patient services representative, his or her address, telephone, and TDD access.

Pamphlets available in all outpatient clinic areas should describe the range of services available and the methods to obtain the service. Encourage the patient to reserve the device well in advance of his or her appointment. Marquees in the outpatient clinic areas, at elevator locations, and in high-traffic areas should be used to introduce your ADA-compatible program, and to encourage all patients to express their special needs to their caregivers prior to their scheduled appointments so that at your facility, needs expressed will be needs met.

When reviewing facility needs relating to the impact of hearing impairment, the audiologist should focus on both individual and group listening needs. In other words, if the hospital has public meeting rooms, those rooms will need to be fully accessible. Therefore, group FM, loop, or infrared systems may be appropriate. Further, a complete accessibility program will make the facility accessible for not just hospital patients, but also visitors. Whatever programs are set up, there must be an understanding that visitors to the hospital will be informed about available services and devices and be encouraged to make use of the program.

Ideally, at the beginning of each patient appointment the patient should be asked if he or she requires an assistive device before the appointment proceeds. And in that utopian world of clinical possibilities, at the closure of each medical appointment, each patient should be asked if they wish to reserve an assistive device prior to their follow-up appointment. However, the patient shares in the responsibility of arranging for the appropriate device at the appropriate time. No matter how publicized the program may be, patient-initiated requests are a vital link in insuring that the program is used to its fullest potential. However, the hospital can do as much as possible to publicize the program and to encourage patient requests.

Increasing the visibility of your facilities and assistive device program will undoubtedly result in the identification of potential users. The next steps involve procuring the devices and management of the program's devices.

Procurement and Management

The logistics of how to provide assistive devices will be dictated, in part, by the type of device needed by the patient. For example, small self-contained portable hardwired patient communicators are high-use devices at most medical facilities. They often reside permanently at core locations within the medical center such as: urgent care, emergency rooms, geriatric evaluation units, radiology departments, otolaryngology clinics, medical and surgical intensive care units, recovery rooms, and with the clergy. However, even if the devices are located at different locations within the hospital setting, it is of utmost importance that some sort of centralization of equipment management be put in place. One particular office needs to have the responsibility for tracking the location of devices. Weekly or monthly checks on the location of individual units is essential in order to ensure that the devices are where they should be and are in proper working order.

Requesting use rate data from the clinic locations will assist you in placing devices. Inventory management can involve personal computer inventories or simple card files. An adhesive label attached to the loaner device allows you to track the use rate of a specific device. Collect and replace the adhesive labels monthly, and you have data on that device's use rate.

When assigning devices to core clinic locations it is imperative to assign responsibility for that device to a specific hospital employee. Establish a clear policy as to who is financially responsible if a device is not returned (patient? staff member? clinical department?). Simple, reliable devices whose function is obvious will gain favor with patients and caregivers alike. The same style patient communicator should be used throughout the medical facility whenever possible to increase visibility of the device and familiarity with function. When staff is familiar with a product's function they are more likely to cooperate in the device's successful use. Inevitably, familiarity will expand to knowledge and basic troubleshooting strategies will be more easily integrated.

Other categories of assistive devices require very little management once installed. Telephone handset amplifiers will likely be a common device in use at most medical centers. Clear signage directing users to locations where amplified handsets are available should be included at each non-amplified public telephone location. The location of amplified handset should be highly visible, and clear written instructions for use of the amplifier should be available at each telephone location. Each public telephone location should contain clear directions to the location of the nearest text telephone. Telephone relay information access numbers must become part of standard telephone signage.

Closed captioned decoders and signal-to-noise ratio enhancing television assistive technology such as infrared and FM television units represent a category of device within the medical center that requires centralized management. They may be dispensed by your building management or housekeeping or biomedical personnel. Installation policies should be cleared with your hospital safety personnel. A clear infectious disease policy should be available for the cleaning of each assistive device prior to initiating your program. That policy should describe the method of cleaning required before the device is returned to loaner stock, the documentation necessary to track the device's use, and the device's cleaning record. Your local infectious disease control officer can assist you with this segment of your program, and methods exist at all medical facilities to address these issues.

Long-term inpatients are often the greatest users of television enhancement technologies (closed caption, infrared and frequency modulated [FM] transmission). Introducing TV enhancement technologies as part of that patient's initial orientation to the hospital environment can be done through the closed circuit cable capabilities at your facility.

Systematic Internal Reviews and Outcome Measures

In addition to understanding the use rate of the devices in your accessibility program, you will benefit from the outcome statements provided by your patients. Require simple outcome statements from the users of your program. Provide self-addressed response envelopes and explain that their thoughts will help you improve your program to assist patients with special needs. Let them know that you sincerely value their input about the positive aspects of your program and any negative comments as well. Ask specifically how you might provide them with better service. Be sure to inform your users of the opportunity to purchase assistive devices through your hearing loss management program for their personal use when they are not at your facility.

The specific policies must be established ahead of time to determine when charges are appropriate to patients for professional services. The hospital facility should be completely accessible to the patient with a hearing loss at no additional charge. However, an effective accessibility program will likely lead to professional consultation with audiologists on a patient-to-patient basis concerning the impact of hearing impairment and the need for specific intervention. If a patient is referred to the audiology division for hearing-aid consultation, hearing-aid repairs, or other intervention techniques, these need to be viewed as normally chargeable procedures. The implementation of an accessibility program within the hospital should not be used as an excuse for the provision of free audiological services to individual patients.

STAFF TRAINING

A comprehensive accessibility program needs to include a training component in order to ensure success. Even the best assistive and alerting devices will not be used to their fullest extent if the hospital staff is not aware of their existence or their role. Such a staff training program needs to go beyond a simple technical orientation to the workings of such devices. In order for hospital employees to understand the need for such devices and the appropriate use of such devices, a general orientation to the impact of hearing loss will be necessary. It has been well established that many related professionals have an incomplete understanding of hearing loss (Woodford, 1987; Gibson, 1985; Johnson, Stein, & Lass, 1992; Lass, Tecca, & Woodford, 1987; Lass, Woodford, Pannbacker, Carlin, Saniga, Schmitt, & Everly-Myers, 1989; Scherz, Kallail, & Edwards, 1991). However, specific attempts at training can improve the understanding of the effects of hearing loss (Strong & Shaver, 1991). A variety of useful written material for increasing the understanding of hearing loss by related professionals has been developed (e.g., Weinstein, 1989). Table 11-2 provides an outline of a useful inservice training program for hospital staff. This material should be adapted to the needs of each specific group.

TABLE 11-2   **Outline of a Hospital Staff In-Service Program on Hearing Impairment**

I.   Overview of accessibility program (including ADA requirements)

II. Prevalence of hearing impairment
- general prevalence
- increased prevalence in hospitals (elderly, other medical conditions)
- common etiologies (adapted to group's specific clinical assignments)
- under-reporting of hearing loss
- behavioral signs of hearing difficulties

III. Impact of hearing impairment
- communication in hospital vital
- effects on speech understanding (inaudible speech, misunderstood speech)
- problem of background noise and loss of visual cues
- limitations of hearing aids
- informed consent

IV. Devices and services
- what devices/services are available
- matching to patient need
- how to access devices/services

V.   Communication strategies
- noise reduction
- visual cues
- distance between talker and listener
- communication strategies
- clear speech
- verification of transmitted information

VI. Conclusion: hospital staff has obligation to strive towards accessibility

Goals of Staff Training Programs

The goals of the staff training program can be broken down into the following four areas.

WHO Can Be Expected to Have Hearing Impairment

The hospital staff should be made aware of the overall prevalence of hearing impairment. Further, they should be oriented to the fact that the expected prevalence within a hospital setting is higher, given the large number of elderly patients within the hospital and the large number of other related medical disorders. The hospital staff should be informed that hearing impairment is often a very under-reported condition on the part of patients (Giolas, 1982; Matthews, Lee, Mills, & Schum, 1990; Schow, Smedley, & Longhurst, 1990), and that is in many respects an "invisible" condition. Therefore, the staff should be made aware of the fact that many hearing-impaired patients will not report their hearing impairment. The staff needs to be aware of the subtle signs of the presence of hearing impairment, such as apparent misunderstandings on the part of patients, request for repetition of information, or the inordinate reliance on visual cues. The medical staff should be made aware that they have a responsibility to know the patient's health history and to be able to quickly identify related medical disorders that may predict a higher likelihood of the presence of hearing impairment. Armed with this knowledge, the medical staff should have a heightened awareness of the potential presence of hearing impairment in specific subpopulations within the hospital setting.

WHY It Is Important to Identify Hearing Impairment
The hospital staff should be provided with specific examples of how misunderstanding on the part of a patient may impact the health care provision process. Further, the inherent limitations to amplification should be discussed. It should be pointed out that, at times, an assistive device may serve as an alternative to hearing aids (Pruitt, 1990). For example, a patient with limited dexterity may find a one-to-one communicator easier to use. Staff should be reminded that most communication between hospital staff and the patient is of utmost importance. A complete, accurate history cannot be obtained from a patient unless the patient can understand the specific questions being asked by the health care provider. If the medical staff is unaware of a hearing impairment, a patient may not fully understand specific instructions regarding when to take medications, when to return for follow-up visits, or when to contact the physician if symptoms do not improve. The legal and ethical concerns about informed consent should be outlined to the medical staff. The doctrine of informed consent indicates that medical personnel have certain responsibilities to ensure that a patient fully understands the full range of impact that specific medical decisions will have. They should be made aware of their responsibility in ensuring that patients understand the information provided as to alternate forms of treatments, success likelihood, potential risks of certain medical and surgical procedures. It should be impressed upon the medical staff that if they are generally aware of the potential presence of hearing impairment and if specific steps are taken to lessen the impact of such impairment, their patients will be better informed.

WHAT Devices and Services Are Available
The hospital staff should be given an overview of the sort of devices and services available within the hospital. The hospital staff should be informed that accessibility goes beyond simply having devices available. The accessibility program also relies on the full use of such devices and also on the use of associated services such as interpreter services and telecommunication relay services. The hospital staff should be informed as to which patient populations may have particular needs for such services and devices. For example, certain patients may absolutely require a closed caption decoder for television listening, whereas others may prefer to use a signal-to-noise ratio enhancing listening system. Further, it should be pointed out that whereas many severe-to-profound hearing-impaired patients may need the text telephone

placed in their room, many more patients (based on known prevalence data) may be better served by the provision of amplified handsets within their rooms.

At this point in training, the hospital staff should also be informed of what appropriate steps they can take in order to improve communication with patients. Topics such as appropriate speaking behaviors, noise reduction, and proper use of visual cues should be discussed. The staff should understand their responsibilities related to using proper communication techniques. The staff should be given as many concrete examples of appropriate communication techniques as is possible in order to expand their understanding. For example, the staff should be given the scenario of a hearing-impaired patient in a room with several visitors present engaging in unrelated conversation and the television playing in the background. The staff should be informed that the most appropriate environment for effective communication with a hearing-impaired patient would require that the visitors be asked to decrease the intensity of their speech or to move the conversation out into the hallway, and that the television be turned off before the medical personnel attempt to communicate with the patient. Additionally, the hospital staff could be informed of just how difficult it is for a hearing-impaired patient to understand what is being said by an individual attempting to communicate with a medical chart in front of his or her face, or when his or her back is turned to the patient.

HOW Devices and Services Are Accessed

The hospital staff needs to be given instructions about the most effective ways to access the available devices and services. Simple written instructions are the most useful at this point in time. Table 11-3 provides an example of an information sheet that can be distributed to hospital staff and placed at key locations such as nursing stations and registration desks. The hospital staff should be informed about what devices and services are available and who should be called in order to access such services. They should also be informed of the typical time delay expected in obtaining such devices and services. If an interpreter will not be available for typically an hour or so after being contacted, appropriate arrangements may need to be made for the short term.

Staff training should be viewed as an ongoing process. In other words, at the initiation of an accessibility program within a hospital, there may be a burst of inservices provided to various departments in order to make the appropriate staff members aware of available devices and services. However, as staff turns over and as memories grow dim, it will be important to repeat such training at appropriate intervals. Many of the people within a hospital may have continuing education requirements concerning the accessibility program: nurses, physicians, and other professional groups. The staff training component of the accessibility program may be included on an ongoing (such as annual) basis to fulfill one aspect of the continuing education needs.

When looking across the various individuals employed by a hospital, it is clear that certain groups may have a higher need for training in the accessibility program than others. Physicians, nurses, chaplains, or social workers will be in constant contact

TABLE 11-3 **Example of Information Sheet for Distribution to Hospital Employees**

SERVICES AND RESOURCES AVAILABLE TO HEARING-IMPAIRED PATIENTS

Portable Teletext Device for the Deaf

- Allows deaf patient to communicate over the telephone using a typewriter-like device.
- Available through Telecommunications (xxx-xxxx) at no cost to patient.
- Can be placed in any inpatient room.
- A teletext is also available 24 hours a day in the Telecommunications office for staff members to use to contact TDD users outside of the hospital.

Amplified Telephone

- Allows hearing-impaired patient to receive amplified sound through the telephone. These telephones also have a flashing light to alert the patient when the telephone is ringing.
- Available through Telecommunications (xxx-xxxx) at no cost to the patient.
- Can be placed in any inpatient room.
- Someone from unit needs to bring regular telephone from patient's room to Telecommunications center to swap for amplified telephone.

Sign Language Interpreter

- Allows deaf patients who use sign language to communicate with medical staff.
- Administered through Social Services (xxx-xxxx) at no cost to the patient.
- An interpreter can usually be available within a few hours. If at all possible, the services of the interpreter should be scheduled ahead of time, especially for outpatient visits.

Television Closed Captioning Devices

- Provides a written transcription of dialogue at the bottom of the television screen. Most major networks (CBS, ABC, NBC, Public Television) caption many shows.
- Available through Housekeeping (xxx-xxxx) at no charge to the patient.
- Can be placed in any inpatient room.
- Once housekeeping is called, a unit will be placed in the room within a few hours.

Personal Amplifiers

- These handle devices provide an amplified signal to the listener in order to ease communication between the patient and staff/visitors.
- Available through Otolaryngology/Speech and Hearing (xxx-xxxx) at no cost to the patient.
- Available for any inpatient or for any outpatient during a clinic visit.
- Available typically within 1–2 hours.

Hearing Aid Checks, Hearing Aid Cleanings, and Batteries

- Routine maintenance for patients who use hearing aids.
- Available through Otolaryngology/Speech and Hearing (xxx-xxxx).

TABLE 11-3 *Continued*

- Costs vary, typically $25–$100.
- Service in an inpatient unit or in the Speech and Hearing Clinic is typically available the same day.

Hearing Testing, Hearing Aid Consults, and Assistive Listening Devices Consults

- Full-range Audiological service available for patients who know or suspect that they have hearing loss.
- Available through Otolaryngology/Speech and Hearing (xxx-xxxx).
- Costs vary, depending on service. Costs are typically $50–$100. Health insurance will usually pay for many of these services, if ordered by a physician.
- These services are typically provided in the Speech and Hearing Clinic, but can be provided in an inpatient unit if warranted.
- These services should be provided in conjunction with an examination by an Otolaryngologist (xxx-xxxx).

with patients, and therefore their need for understanding the impact of hearing impairment is quite high. Other services, such as housekeeping, dietary, and medical records, may not have as high a level of interaction with patients, or the importance of their interactions may not be as crucial; their training requirements in accessibility for hearing impairment may not be as great. Even within groups of physicians and nurses, the specific need for understanding hearing impairment may vary. Physicians and nurses assigned to units such as geriatric care, otolaryngology, or oncology, may have a greater likelihood of interacting with patients with hearing impairment, so their specific training needs in the area of hearing impairment will be much higher. Physicians and nurses on units such as radiology, orthopedics, or urology, may not be in contact with hearing-impaired patients as much as other units, and their ongoing training needs may not be as great. Figure 11-2 provides a list of disciplines that may have particular inservice needs due to a high likelihood of interaction with patients with hearing impairment. Given the range of needs in the area of education about hearing impairment, a two-tiered training program may be useful. A brief orientation to the impact of hearing impairment and to the accessibility program within the hospital may be required for all new hospital employees. This sort of brief exposure may take place during new staff orientation. Then, depending on the specific assignment of the individual, more complete and detailed information can be provided on a unit-to-unit basis. The amount of information provided to a new staff member in the area of hearing impairment can be tailored to the needs of their job assignment.

When providing training to a group of hospital employees, it is important to focus a specific program to the needs of a group. When dealing with a group of physicians or nurses on a pediatric unit, prevalence information should be provided specific to likely pediatric etiologies. When providing training to a group of professionals assigned to a neurologic unit, the audiologist may want to discuss the difficulty in differentially diag-

Cardiology
Chaplaincy
Emergency medicine
Endocrinology
Family practice
Geriatrics
Oncology
Otolaryngology
Patient and guest relations
Pediatrics
Poison control
Registration/information
Social work
Telecommunications

FIGURE 11-2 **Disciplines that should be specifically targeted for in-service training.**

nosing the presence of hearing impairment from other neurologic problems that an elderly patient may possess. When speaking to a group of professionals from an oncology service, the specific ototoxic effects of certain cancer-treating medications should be discussed, and the appropriate program of audiological monitoring should be described. Hospital employees are probably going to be much more interested in the sort of information the audiologist can provide, if that information is tailored to those employees' specific needs and experiences.

The audiologist providing training in the area of hearing impairment should keep in mind that hospital employees are probably most interested in the most basic and practical information available. Therefore, the audiologist should confine his or her educational program to the most pertinent and basic information necessary. For most groups of hospital employees, it is probably not necessary to launch into a detailed discussion of the physiology of hearing. However, it is important to stick to such topics as how to communicate best with a hearing-impaired patient, or how to identify a hearing-impaired patient. Again, an educational program for staff members will have a greater impact if those staff members recognize that the audiologist is speaking directly to the needs and experiences of each individual employee.

ADMINISTRATION

The accessibility program at the hospital needs to be viewed by the central hospital administration as an ongoing budgeted program. In other words, an outlay of funds for the procurement of devices at the beginning of the establishment of the program is absolutely necessary in order to obtain the appropriate devices. However, a long-term budgetary commitment is also necessary for two important reasons. First, the equipment can only be expected to last for a certain period of time. As with all equipment within the hospital, at some point replacement items are going to be necessary. Secondly, as time goes on, better devices will become available and will at times need to be included in the accessibility program. Outdated technology will need to be updated with new devices. Thirdly, as devices become available within the hospital, their popularity may very well increase. A successful publicity program both within and outside the hospital is expected to lead to greater demand for such devices. On a year-to-year basis the number and range of devices available will likely need to be increased. Budgeting for such program increases should be undertaken as part of the hospital administration's long-range plan.

There are several ways in which the budget impact on the hospital can be lessened. The widespread purchase of free-standing closed caption decoders is not necessary for a new program, as more and more televisions are being manufactured with the decoder built into the device. The implementation of closed caption decoders within the hospital can be achieved by specifying that all new televisions purchased for patients' rooms include internal closed caption decoders. The financial burden of providing a full range of accessible telecommunication devices may be shared with the local telephone company. The hospital should enter into negotiations with its local provider as to the relative responsibility for providing text telephones in public and private areas within the hospital, amplified handsets, and lighted ring displays for inpatient telephones. The audiologist should encourage the local telephone company to meet and go beyond its statutory requirements for accessibility within the hospital setting.

Finally, the cost of obtaining many of the necessary devices for the accessibility program may perhaps be supported by local volunteer organizations. The internal volunteer program within the hospital or other local service agencies may be interested in providing financial help in obtaining appropriate devices for the hospital. A high level of publicity both within and outside the hospital concerning the accessibility program will help to engender interest on the part of service organizations in participating in the program.

A comprehensive accessibility program must have the complete support of the central hospital administration. It cannot be a program that is conceived, structured, and carried out entirely by one division within the hospital, such as audiology. The audiologist may need to promote the need for such a program to the administration in order to convince the appropriate authorities of the importance of hearing accessibility. The audiologist should be willing to cite the specifics of the Americans with Disabilities Act. However, the audiologist has the responsibility of encouraging the hospital administration to go beyond the statutory requirements of the Americans with Disabilities Act. An appropriate accessibility program needs to be tailored to the specific needs of the hospital, as opposed to simply meeting the minimum requirements of the ADA. The audiologist can also rely on both legal and ethical concerns when justifying the need for a hearing accessibility program. For example, a strong argument can be made that a patient cannot be fully informed of his or her rights as a patient if he or she has a hearing impairment, and if no measures are taken to lessen the impact of that hearing impairment when communication takes place between the patient and physician. If hearing impairment is a barrier to informed consent, the hospital has both a legal and ethical responsibility to attempt to lessen this barrier.

It should be pointed out that if the audiologist is not an employee of the hospital, he or she needs to be willing to charge appropriate fees for professional consultation. Payment for professional service is also required if outside consultants such as telephone or audio engineers are required.

The central hospital administration may respond quite favorably to the public relations advantages of having an accessibility program. In the age of competitive health care providers, programs such as hearing impairment accessibility may be quite appealing to patients in the community. The audiologist should highlight the potential public relations benefits of such a program when attempting to obtain cooperation and funding.

CONCLUSION

The success of an accessibility program within a hospital can only be insured if there is long-term cooperation and commitment on the part of the various professionals involved in such a program. Although the audiologist is the most logical choice to head such a program, the long-term success of a program is dependent on the appropriate support from a variety of other agents within the hospital. The purchase and distribution of a handful of one-to-one communicators is not enough to guarantee long-term accessibility within a facility. There must be an understanding and commitment on the part of all relevant professionals in order to ensure complete long-term success of such a program.

The central administration of the hospital should also be reminded that an effective accessibility program with the appropriate promotion should help to increase use of the audiology services within the hospital. Another expected fallout from an effective accessibility program would be increased use of audiological consultation on the part of patients, increased dispensing of assistive listening and alerting systems to be taken home by patients, and increased hearing aid dispensing.

In the chapter that follows you will learn how to select what is best for the individual, including how to conduct need assessment protocols; how to perform a similar assessment of your facilities; how to identify shortfalls in current devices, services, and training needs; and how to develop a comprehensive accessibility program to alleviate such shortfalls.

REFERENCES

Fox-Grimm, M.E. (1991). Americans with Disabilities Act (PL 101–336). *American Speech-Hearing-Language Association, June/July*, 41–46.

Gibson, G.C. (1985). The role of the family physician—a front line view. *Ear and Hearing*, *6*(1), 59–60.

Giolas, T.G. (1982). *Hearing-Handicapped Adults*. Englewood Cliffs, NJ: Prentice-Hall, Inc.

Jensen, G., Anderson, C., Bergquist, L., Boyd, M., Hermanson, C., Khal, G., Schum, D., Searls, L., Summerwill, J., Tyler, R.S., & Wolfe, S. (1992). *Report and Recommendations of the Task Force Regarding Accessibility for Persons with Hearing Impairments*. The University of Iowa Hospitals and Clinics, Iowa City, IA.

Johnson, C.E., Stein, R.L., & Lass, N.J. (1992). Public school nurses' preparedness for a hearing aid monitoring program. *Language, Speech, and Hearing Services in Schools*, *23*, 141–144.

Lass, N.J., Tecca, J.E., & Woodford, C.M. (1987). Teachers' knowledge of, exposure to, and attitudes toward hearing aids and hearing aid wearers. *Language, Speech, and Hearing Services in Schools*, *18*, 86–93.

Lass, N.J., Woodford, C.M., Pannbacker, M.D., Carlin, M.F., Saniga, R.D., Schmitt, J.F., & Everly-Myers, D.S. (1989). Speech-language pathologists' knowledge of, exposure to, and attitudes toward hearing aids and hearing aid wearers. *Language, Speech, and Hearing Services in Schools*, *20*, 115–131.

Leavitt, R.J., & Freeburg, J. (1987). Survey of ALDS interest. *Hearing Instruments*, *38*(6), 28–29, 57.

Matthews, L.J., Lee, F.S., Mills, J.H., & Schum, D.J. (1990). Audiometric and subjective assessment of hearing handicap. *Archives of Otolaryngology—Head and Neck Surgery*, *116*, 1325–1330.

Palmer, C.V. (1992). Assistive devices in the audiology practice. *American Journal of Audiology*, *March*, 37–57.

Parmiter-Jacobs, L., Kraemer, K.B., & Jared, C. (1988). When a hearing instrument is not enough: An ALD center. *Hearing Instruments*, *39*(6), 22–24.

Pruitt, J.B. (1990). Assistive listening device versus conventional hearing aid in an elderly patient: Case report. *Journal of the American Academy of Audiology*, *1*(1), 41–43.

Scherz, J.W., Kallail, K.J., & Edwards, H.T. (1991). Attitudes of family practice residents about speech-language-hearing referrals. *Family Practice Research Journal*, *11*(2), 217–223.

Schow, R.L., Smedley, T.C., & Longhurst, T.M. (1990). Self-assessment and impairment in adult/elderly hearing screening—recent data and new perspectives. *Ear and Hearing*, *11*(5), 17S–27S.

Self Help for Hard of Hearing People, Inc. (1991). *SHHH 4-Point Program for Hospitals*. Bethesda, MD.

Strong, C.J., & Shaver, J.P. (1991). Modifying attitudes toward persons with hearing impairments. A comprehensive review of the research. *American Annals of the Deaf*, *136*(3), 252–260.

Weinstein, B.E. (1989). Geriatric hearing loss: Myths, realities, resources for physicians. *Geriatrics*, *44*(4), 42–60.

Williams, J. (1992). What do you know? What do you need to know? *American Speech-Hearing-Language Association*, *June/July*, 54–61.

Woodford, C.M. (1987). Speech-language pathologists' knowledge and skills regarding hearing aids. *Language, Speech, and Hearing Services in School*, *18*, 312–321.

▶ 12

Selecting What's Best for the Individual

CYNTHIA L. COMPTON
Gallaudet University

The objective of this chapter is to provide the reader with a practical framework for quickly identifying the potential assistive device user and his or her specific equipment needs. A good working knowledge of the technology, coupled with meticulous evaluation of each client's receptive communication needs, is required before specific technologies can be recommended.[1]

All people, whether they have a normal auditory system or not, have receptive communication needs in four basic areas: (1) Face-to-face communication, (2) the enjoyment of broadcast and other electronic media, (3) telephone communication, and (4) communication of the occurrence of alerting signals and situations. It is helpful to group assistive technologies into four categories corresponding to these needs, although products can be used to meet more than one need. For example, some FM, infrared, and hardwired systems can be used to enhance not only face-to-face communication and media reception, but also can be connected to the telephone to provide monotic or diotic listening.

Assistive devices are not only for deaf or hard of hearing people. For example, normal-hearing people working in noisy factories may need visual alarms to alert them to smoke detectors. They also may benefit from visual signaling systems at home when working in the shop or when listening to the stereo precludes the reception of the doorbell ring or other auditory signals. A normal-hearing person with a central auditory processing problem may require an FM system to assist in face-to-face communication at a meeting and may need a telephone amplifier to enhance a poor connection.

---

[1]For a more detailed, generously illustrated review of these technologies, see Compton (1991) and Harkins (1991).

Most of the people we will work with, however, will have some degree of peripheral hearing loss. Most of the time we will fit these people with hearing aids; however, the personal hearing aid cannot always meet a person's communication needs. For example, it is common for a hearing-aid user to experience difficulty understanding speech in noise, from a distance, and on the telephone. A person with even a mild-to-moderate hearing impairment might be functionally deaf to a smoke alarm located down the hall and behind a closed door if she is in a deep sleep and has removed her hearing aids. She also may miss the doorbell if she is listening to the television in a room some distance from the doorbell chime—despite the fact that she is wearing her hearing aids.

Numerous auditory and nonauditory assistive devices are available to meet these communication needs. As important as the personal hearing aid, these devices may be used in addition to or in place of the personal hearing aid, cochlear implant, or tactile device. As professionals, we must be prepared not only to fit and recommend personal amplification systems and assistive devices appropriately, but also to evaluate their place within the larger framework of maximizing the communication skills of the hearing impaired person in *all* aspects of daily life. Accordingly, we also need to provide the ongoing training and counseling necessary to assure successful use of the technology.

Audiologic assessment and the selection of appropriate technology must occur within context of a comprehensive, individualized, reality-based communication needs assessment that looks at a person's lifestyle, hearing level, speech recognition, and numerous other factors before determining which type or types of technologies are best.

The needs assessment/selection process for assistive technology begins with a thorough audiologic and communication needs assessment (Figure 12-1).

CONTINUUM OF AUDIOLOGIC CARE

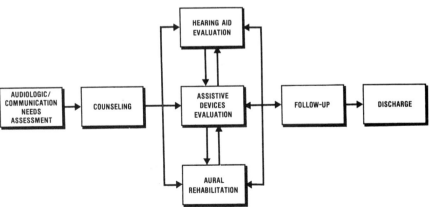

FIGURE 12-1   **The needs assessment selection process**

This sets the stage for the selection of appropriate personal amplification that can be used with assistive technology. The actual selection of assistive technology may occur during the counseling session preceding the hearing-aid/assistive-device evaluation or during or following the hearing aid trial. If possible, it is best to ascertain whether hearing assistance technologies (ALDs) are needed *before* the hearing aid is ordered. This will allow you to order the appropriate type of hearing aid circuitry necessary for interfacing to ALDs and may avoid the need for re-ordering. Follow-up is essential to successful use of assistive technology and formal aural rehabilitation may be required as well. Let's examine each of these points as they involve issues and decisions that have direct impact on our goal—improving a client's ability to communicate in everyday life.

AUDIOLOGIC/COMMUNICATION NEEDS ASSESSMENT

Undoubtedly, the most important part of the needs assessment process is the time spent with a client taking a case history. Thorough assessment of a client's communicative difficulties with respect to his or her specific lifestyle needs is essential, as this will determine not only whether a hearing aid and/or assistive device is necessary, but what specific type of technology should be recommended. Analysis of face-to-face, media, telephone, and alerting communication needs should be carried out in every situation the person may encounter. These situations commonly include communication at home, at work, at school, and while recreating and traveling. Let's take a look at these situations individually as technology requirements frequently vary with each situation.

Communication Needs at Home

Communication needs at home include:

- One-to-one conversation
- Group conversation (family, relatives, friend, associates)
- TV, radio, stereo reception
- Telephone communication
- Reception of warning signals (e.g., telephone ring, doorbell/doorknock, fire alarm, wake-up alarm, appliance signals, monitoring of children's or mate's activities from another room, security signals, etc.)

Communication at home will necessitate technologies that are compatible with the client's as well as his or her family's habits. One-to-one and group conversation at home can be facilitated through the use of inexpensive hardwired remote microphone personal amplification systems. If the client has a hearing aid equipped with a direct audio input circuit, then a remote microphone can simply be plugged into the hearing aid. If not, then the telecoil circuit could be used in conjunction with a stand-alone amplification system (e.g., Williams Sound PockeTalker™). A wireless FM system, while more expensive, provides communication at greater distances as well as enhanced mobility.

Hardwired devices for television and stereo listening might be fine in a home without young children or pets, but could be hazardous in homes where children or pets could trip over or bite into wires connecting the television or stereo to the listener.

When choosing assistive listening devices, it is important to ask whether or not the client's family wants to be able to hear the stereo or television at the same time. Most stereo systems have A/B switches that allow the assistive listening device user to plug his or her system into the headphone jack without turning off the loudspeakers for other family members. For television listening, the solution may not be so easy. Some televisions have only earphone jacks; others have audio output jacks in located in the back of the set. When a device is plugged into the former, the television's loudspeaker is deactivated. This does not usually happen with the latter arrangement. If it is not possible to plug in a direct audio input cord or headset without turning off the loudspeaker (e.g., via use of audio output jacks in the back of the television), then microphone pickup should be used instead, or the television should be modified.

An amplified handset that turns itself down upon hangup might prove to be a judicious recommendation when normal hearing family members also use the amplifier-equipped telephone. A rotary volume control amplifier would be the best choice in a client's home office that is off limits to other family members as this would allow the user to maintain the volume level at a favorite setting.

Teletext[2] devices for the home should also be chosen with care. If the family can afford it, a four-row keyboard with a printer is a convenient option, allowing for faster typing and hard copies of messages. If the entire family uses teletext machines, then direct-connect models that function as phone and teletext device in one unit would make the most sense. However, availability of a voice telephone might be needed for visitors. Combination voice/teletext units are also now available. When choosing a teletext device, each make and model should be compared carefully, taking into consideration all standard and optional features and their respective prices.

Wireless alerting devices for various sounds around the home can be monitored from any room in the house having a receiver, but would be unnecessarily expensive in a one-room studio apartment where a simple hardwired system could be used. Introducing hearing-impaired children to the use of alerting devices at an early age helps them learn cause and effect (e.g., a light flashing five times means someone is at the door) as well as independence (e.g., young children can learn to wake up by

---

[2]"Teletext (TT)" is a new term for Telecommunication Device for the Deaf (TDD), also known as Teletypewriter (TTY). Although the Federal Communications Commission (FCC) has suggested that TT be used, as of this writing, the Department of Justice did not adopt this term in the Americans With Disabilities Act (ADA) legislation. For now, any of the terms is acceptable, although TTY is more accepted within the culturally deaf community.

themselves using visual or vibrotactile wakeup systems). Specialized systems can be designed to warn deaf or hard-of-hearing parents of the status of their children. For example, a wireless transmitter can be connected to a device that monitors a sick child's breathing patterns. This system would then send an FM radio wave to a body-worn receiver that would vibrate and alert a sleeping parent (or hearing-impaired nurse). Other wireless paging devices are helpful for calling family members. For example, a pushbutton FM transmitter can be attached to a family member's wheelchair with velcro. A wrist- or waist-worn receiver can be used by a deaf or hard-of-hearing caretaker. Finally, visual and vibrotactile fire signaling systems are available for the private home or apartment.

Group Home (retirement home, nursing home, halfway house, etc.)

Communication needs in a group home situation may be similar to those in the home with the addition of:

- Receptive conversation in common dining areas, game rooms, media rooms, chapel, conferring with medical personnel and other caregivers, etc.
- Telephone amplification systems and teletext machines in patient rooms, at nursing stations, on pay phones, etc.
- Reception of warning signals also apply unless under 24-hour supervision (wherein group home personnel would be responsible for client's safety, security, and for admission of visitors to client's room or apartment).
- In addition to hearing aids and assistive listening devices, acoustical treatment of common area, especially dining rooms, can do much to reduce the negative effects of noise and reverberation on communication.

Receptive conversation in dining areas and game rooms might best be enhanced with FM technology, whereas reception of television in a common area could be easily improved through the use of any of the wireless technologies. If most or all hearing-aid users have telecoils, then a room loop would be the most economical choice as a minimal number of external receivers would be needed. As with any group listening system, rules for communication must be adopted. For example, only one person should talk into the microphone at a time. Careful installation of the loop (under a carpet or along a wall or ceiling) is necessary to prevent people from tripping over the loop wire as well as to protect it from potential damage from walkers or wheelchairs. One-to-one conferences with medical personnel could be carried out economically with a battery-powered, stand-alone hardwired amplification system equipped with earphones, direct audio input, or inductive transducer.

Telephone amplifiers should be considered for residents' rooms. Pay phones should also be equipped with amplifiers with the understanding that residents, employees and visitors may require these devices.

Teletext devices should also be available to residents and their families as well as to staff. Again, four-row keyboards and printers are recommended.

Alerting devices may be needed in each resident's private quarters to warn of a doorbell, doorknock, or phone ring. In 24-hour care situations, these alerting devices would not be necessary. Visual and vibrotactile fire alarms must be installed in each room, all restrooms, and storage areas, and must be linked to a central monitoring system that will indicate where the problem originated. Visual and body-worn vibrotactile paging systems can be used to alert deaf or hard-of-hearing employees of pages (from patients or supervisors) or emergencies such as fire. Specialized wireless systems also can be designed to alert deaf or hard-of-hearing employees of the status of equipment that monitors vital biological signs as well as general building support equipment such as heating and cooling systems.

Communication Needs at Work

When querying a client about communication on his or her job, the following areas must be examined:

- Office conversation (one-to-one, meetings within office)
- Lectures/seminars within or outside of office
- Casual conversation with colleagues and/or clients (office, car, restaurants, etc.)
- Telephone communication (in office, while traveling)
- Speech recognition from a dictaphone or telephone answering machine
- Reception of important warning signals in the office and while traveling (e.g., fire alarm, telephone ring, pager, doorbell/doorknock, computer prompts)

Wireless listening devices such as FM, infrared, and induction loop systems are more appropriate for long-distance listening (e.g., seminars and group meetings) than are hardwired systems that limit movement and distance from the sound source. Hardwired devices are fine for one-to-one discussions between colleagues or between employees and customers. Computer-assisted notetaking with projection of the notes onto a screen or wall can be useful in meeting rooms to supplement what is received auditorally or manually. It can also be used as a substitute for either mode of communication. Discussions can then be saved to a disk for further reference. For one-to-one conversations between colleagues or between a supervisor and an employee, a computer or TDD can be used as a method of back-and-forth notewriting.

Selecting an amplifier for an office telephone can be more difficult than selecting one for a home phone. Numerous types of office telephones are available. Just because a telephone is modular, does not mean that its handset can be exchanged for just any brand of amplified handset. For example, an AT&T telephone cannot be used with a GTE handset due to an impedance mismatch. One must be aware of which handsets will work with which phones, as well the availability of externally powered in-line amplifiers that do work with most office phones. Further, the use of a hearing aid's telecoil with the telephone might prove to be impossible in an office beset with electromagnetic interference from computers and fluorescent lighting. In this case, it might be more appropriate to couple the hearing aid to the phone acoustically (if possible) and use a noise canceling handset. Or, special assistive listening devices can be used. Phonak's TC-1 direct audio input microphone system readily attaches to a telephone handset, providing an acoustic to electric transfer of the telephone signal. Several hardwired, FM, and infrared assistive listening devices are also available that can be connected to the telephone (Williams Sound, Audex, Oticon, Comtek, Sennheiser).

The need to listen to a dictation machine may point out the need for direct audio input- or telecoil-equipped hearing aids that would enable the listener to plug monaural or binaural direct audio input cords or a neckloop into the machine. Difficulty hearing incoming messages on an answering machine (even with a hearing aid) may point out the need for an answering machine retrofitted with a hearing-aid compatible telephone receiver. Or, a remote microphone can be held next to the answering machine's loudspeaker. Finally, a voice messaging system may be employed, since it can be used with any amplified telephone.

Four-row keyboard teletext devices with printers are recommended for the workplace. If the employee uses only a teletext device and has his or her own private telephone line, then a direct connect teletext device is recommended. However, if the office has a telephone system with link buttons for transferring and holding calls, then a voice phone will be needed. The teletext device can be interfaced to the voice phone in either of two ways. First, instead of direct connect, a teletext device with an acoustic coupler can be used. Second, a 3-way adapter can be connected to the phone jack and the voice phone, teletext device, and flashing light can be connected to the adapter. The teletext device can be answered in the usual way but calls can be transferred using the voice phone's link button.

Computers can also be equipped to function as teletext devices. Teletext device users who use computers may like this option. Software programs are available that provide answering machine capability (like many regular teletext devices) as well as directories for phone numbers and addresses that can be easily accessed and sent over telephone lines. The computer must be left on if the employee wants to be able to receive telephone calls. Most software programs (e.g., DOS Shell, Windows) allow the user to move in and out of programs to answer the telephone without having to log out.

Employees may need to hear the doorbell, a doorknock, the telephone ring, a page, or a fire alarm. Various hardwired and wireless alerting devices can be used to alert the employee to these sounds. If hardwired, then the employee must be in the same room with the device. There are exceptions to this. For example, many buildings now have hardwired visual fire notification devices that connect to the electrical system of the auditory alarm system. This installation is expensive and must be done professionally, using UL-listed strobe lights and following appropriate installation standards and codes.

A simple flashing light can be connected to a telephone outlet using a twin adapter. This device will flash a light at the employee's desk when the phone rings. This is perfect for a person who sits at his or her desk most of the day. But, if the person must be mobile, then a wireless line carrier system would be more appropriate. A system like this consists of a transmitter attached to the phone jack and remote receivers placed in rooms visited by the employee. Similar systems are commonly used in private homes.

Paging systems also may be needed on the job. Radio transmission systems such as the Personal Pager System™ by Silent Call consist of hand-held, neckworn, or table top transmitters and waist-worn receivers that pick up signals from up to 100 feet away. Potential users of these systems need to be aware of conditions that can disrupt signal transmission. For example, a building with a high content of metal support beams can cut down and even totally obliterate radio transmission. Newer systems are on the horizon that will transmit stronger signals over hundreds of feet, under optimal conditions. These systems should, therefore, perform better in buildings with metal content and other sources of interference (Elwell, 1994).

If an employee must be reached as great distances within or outside a building, then a cellular pager might be a better choice as these systems use radio frequencies that have significantly better "penetration"—that is, they transmit over a vast range and can penetrate walls and ceilings better than the previously mentioned pagers. Numeric and alphanumeric cellular pagers are available that beep or vibrate and can receive messages from great distances. These systems function like one-way cellular phones and several companies offer various pricing options. As of this writing, only one company (Mobilemedia) can be accessed via voice phone or teletext device. Unlike numeric pages, alphanumeric pagers allow a typed message to appear on a screen. Up to two and one-half pages of text can be scrolled across the screen, allowing the recipient to read the message directly, without having to search for a teletext device to call the office. Both types of pagers also can be tied into emergency broadcast systems. For example, in large businesses, security guards can be trained to perform a speed-dial group call to all pager wearers to alert them to a fire or other emergency.

Finally, hardwired or wireless enhanced auditory, visual, or vibratory signal systems may be installed as status monitors for equipment. For example, an FM transmitter connected to an automatic cooking device's timer could send a signal to a vibrating pager thus warning its user that the food is done.

School/College

Communication needs here may include:

- Speech recognition in classrooms, lecture halls
- Speech-language therapy
- Auditory training
- Meetings with teachers and other personnel
- One-to-one or group conversation in dormitory, apartment, etc.
- Telecommunications in dormitory, apartment, on and off campus

- Reception of warning signals as mentioned previously, including local (client's room, apartment) and general (hallway, common areas) fire alarm systems in dormitory and/or apartment

Traditionally, FM systems have been employed from kindergarten through high school in the United States for the education of children who are hearing-impaired. Now, this technology is finding popularity in higher education, as well as in the education of children with central auditory processing problems and fluctuating hearing loss. FM systems lend themselves nicely to classroom usage in a college setting, allowing the listener complete freedom of movement and the added advantage of being able to simultaneously tape record the lecture. The recording can later be reviewed and compared to class notes.

An exciting addition to the FM family of products is the BTE/FM system. This system employs the usual body-worn FM transmitter. However, the student uses a BTE hearing aid that contains a built-in FM receiver. As of this writing, two such products are on the market, one employing wideband and the other using narrowband transmission. This type of FM system is popular among older students due to its appealing cosmetics.

Induction loop systems are also becoming more popular in schools due to their low maintenance, comparatively low cost, and cosmetic acceptability.

Sound reinforced classrooms are also gaining favor with educators. Several systems are available in the marketplace. Most of these systems allow the teacher to wear a wireless FM transmitter that transmits his or her voice to a basestation receiver that is connected to several loudspeakers. These systems are enjoyed by children who must contend with acoustically poor classrooms. These children have fluctuating hearing loss, central auditory processing problems, attention deficit disorders, or the like. For those children who use hearing aids, body-worn receivers can also be employed. One model by Comtek (Omni Petite™) is totally wireless, consisting of a body-worn transmitter and a combination basestation receiver/loudspeaker. This can be used, for example, in a section of a large open classroom while other activities are going on. This system's frequency of transmission does not allow it to be used with body-worn receivers.

Large-area listening systems should be used not only to receive the teacher's voice, but also the signals from televisions and stereo systems.

All schools and colleges should be equipped with hearing-aid compatible, amplified telephones as well as teletext devices so that students have access to each other, to their parents, and others. It is also important that parents and others be able to contact the students. Telephone relay systems can also be used.

The same alerting needs exist in educational settings as were discussed relative to private homes and offices. However, educational settings also may have their own distinct communication needs. For example, visual and vibrotactile systems can be used to time deaf and hard of hearing students when taking tests. Alerting devices can also be useful in shop classes as equipment status monitors, in cooking classes, or for the timing of chemical or other experiments.

Recreation and Travel

Recreational and travel activities include:

- One-to-one, small or large group conversations in hotels, lecture halls, restaurants.
- Speech recognition while on indoor and outdoor tours (bus, train, plane, boat, on foot, bicycles, horses, skis, etc.)
- Instruction (any type of hobby or activity where the hearing-impaired person must be able to hear instructor/guide)
- Television reception in hotels, museums, airports, etc.
- Telephone conversation (pay phone, hotel, car)
- Portable wake-up devices and time reminders
- Warning devices for fires and other emergencies

As more and more theaters, movie houses, houses of worship, and other large areas install wireless listening systems, accessibility to these locations becomes increased. However, it becomes even more important that hearing-aid users be fitted with hearing aids that can be used in conjunction with these large-area systems. Regardless of how well a hearing aid is fitted, if it does not contain a telecoil, it cannot be used with a large area listening system unless (1) it can be coupled acoustically, or (2) it can be removed and the listener can successfully use earphones. This is not to say that all clients will need telecoils in their hearing aids. Nevertheless, when fitting personal amplification, one must insure that the client can benefit from large area listening systems in his or her community—either via a telecoil circuitry or by removing the hearing aid and using a headset. Failure to do this serves neither the client nor the profession.

Many hearing-impaired people can benefit from assistive listening devices when engaging in recreational activities. The listening device of choice can simply be determined by the type of activity. For example, skiing, horseback riding, hiking, and golfing occur outdoors and are mobile activities. Therefore, a personal FM system would be the most appropriate choice for the transmission of an instructor's voice to the hearing-impaired student (or vice versa). On the other hand, piano playing, usually an indoor and stationary activity, could be instructed with any of the wireless systems. One-to-one instruction in a foreign language might be handled with a less expensive hardwired system, since the activity could occur across a table and the student's hands would not be in danger of becoming tangled in the cord connecting the teacher's microphone to the student's personal amplifier (as might occur with piano playing).

Closed- and/or open-captioning of television and films is beneficial to deaf or hard-of-hearing persons staying at a hotels, traveling through airports, or enjoying parks, museums, and other services. For specific information on the Americans With Disabilities Act scoping requirements, see Chapter 1 by Williams and Carey.

Access to the telephone while traveling can be provided through the use of portable amplifiers and small, portable teletext devices that fit into a briefcase. More and more airports are equipped with pay phone teletext devices and facsimile machines.

Portable wake-up devices are useful in hotels, recreational vehicles, boats, and other recreational/travel situations. Some hotels are already supplying their customers with alerting systems that can be checked out at the front desk or are permanently installed in specially designated rooms. Some of these systems alert the user to the telephone ring (useful also for wake-up calls), a doorknock, and the fire alarm. Americans With Disabilities Act legislation also requires hotels to have built-in visual fire alarm systems.

Alerting devices can be used in sports competition to signal the beginning or a competition or to warn players of fouls and other penalties.

FIRE SIGNALING DEVICE STANDARDS

Alerting stimuli (enhanced auditory, visual, or vibrotactile stimuli—or a combination thereof) must be selected which meet the needs of occupants. These stimuli must be effective whether the person is sleeping or awake, and must be detected regardless of where the person is located. For example, a flashing strobe light, no matter how bright, will not alert a deaf-blind person to danger. Accordingly, a sighted deaf person would not be able to detect a bright strobe light if he is in a restroom of an office, hotel, or home, but the flashing signal is located in another room. Appropriately placed remote signalers must be installed in all locations where building occupants could possibly be—or occupants must use effective body-worn emergency pagers.

Alerting technology that meets National Fire Protection Association (NFPA) criteria is available to warn people who are deaf and hard-of-hearing in the event of a fire or other emergency. This life-saving protection is accomplished using strobe lights for both awake and asleep modes, often combined with compatible smoke detectors.

Two types of standards must be met when recommending fire alerting technology: (1) Installation standards and (2) performance standards.

NFPA's National Fire Alarm Code provides installation standards that are used by the local authorities, and provides information as to the proper use and installation of these products. Fire marshals inspect buildings to ensure that proper NFPA installation procedures and local codes have been followed, before they will allow the building to be used by the public. In the case of new construction or renovation, installation of signaling devices for people who are deaf or hard-of-hearing may also be required according to American National Standards Institute (ANSI) A117.1 - 1992 accessibility standards which have been adopted by the nation's three model building codes (Sievers, 1993).

Underwriters Laboratories (UL) evaluates products for their performance (i.e., applicable safety requirements, signal intensity rating, light pattern distribution, flashrate, etc.). All strobe lights and other devices designated for use with individuals who are deaf and hard-of-hearing must comply with UL Standard 1971 for Signaling Devices for the Hearing Impaired. If a product is found to comply with the standard, the company name and product identification is "Listed" in one of UL's Product Directories. In the case of fire alarm signaling equipment, UL has a Fire Protection Equipment Directory (the "Brown Book") that lists the different product categories and the products listed within them. The directory is used by inspection authorities to confirm that the product has been evaluated in the category that addresses its intended use (DeVoss, 1993).

By reviewing the installation standard (NFPA) and the listing information provided in the UL products directory, an inspection authority can determine the acceptability of the final field installation.

For more information on performance standards for fire notification devices for people with hearing problems, the reader is referred to UL 1971, the Underwriters Laboratories, Inc. Standard for Signaling Devices for the Hearing Impaired. To order this document, call (708) 272-8800. For further information on installation standards for fire notification devices, the reader is referred to the National Fire Protection Association (617) 984-7056. Ask for a copy of the National Fire Alarm Code. For further assistance in this area, two resources are provided at the end of this chapter.

COUNSELING

Following a thorough communication and audiologic assessment, the clinician should have a good foundation on which to base specific decisions concerning the need for personal amplification, assistive devices, and aural rehabilitation. Unfortunately, there is currently no empirical data related to degree of hearing loss, speech recognition scores, or other pertinent information on which to base decisions concerning personal hearing aids and assistive technology. However, some clinical observations are offered which might be helpful in the decision-making process:

- Often, clients with pure-tone averages of 40 or 50 dB HL may require telecoil circuitry. Telephone listening is probably the biggest concern of clients, next to one-to-one contacts and TV listening. To decide on whether to install a telecoil, observe how well the client performs on the telephone, both without and with an amplifier. If the client experiences difficulty without one, install a telecoil. If the client does not experience difficulty, then chances are good that he or she will be able to couple the hearing aid acoustically (possibly using an amplifier and an acoustic coupler designed to reduce feedback) or simply remove it (which many clients prefer not to do).
- There is not always a positive correlation between degree of hearing impairment and the need for assistive listening devices. While this is generally true, lifestyle often determines the need for an assistive listening device. For example, clients with very mild hearing impairment who work may need the assistance of a remote microphone in staff meetings or in other difficult listening situations. On the other hand, a retired person with a very mild hearing impairment and a quiet lifestyle may not even require a hearing aid. If your client can use an FM system or other assistive listening device successfully with earphones or earbuds only, then a telecoil-equipped hearing aid may not be necessary.
- In general, there is a negative correlation between the need for assistive listening devices and speech recognition ability. But, lifestyle plays an important role

here, too. An active lifestyle seems to call for assistive listening devices more often, even for people with better speech recognition scores. Clients with mild high frequency hearing impairment with good aided speech recognition scores can sometimes benefit from the use of a hearing aid coupled to a remote microphone system in staff meetings. Furthermore, clients who use hearing aids for speech awareness only can sometimes find assistive listening devices beneficial, as in the case of deaf clients who use direct audio input and neckloop interfaces with portable tape players to enjoy music.

• In general, there is a positive correlation between degree of hearing impairment and the need for alerting devices. However, even people with mild hearing impairment may need enhanced auditory or visual signaling systems when their hearing aids are not being worn or when they are using an assistive listening device to listen to media (TV, stereo, etc.).

HEARING AID/ASSISTIVE DEVICES EVALUATION

If a hearing aid is to be recommended, a decision has to be made as to whether it should be used with assistive devices. This determination will be based on the communication needs assessment as well as the performance of the hearing aid. While final decisions do not necessarily need to be made during the hearing-aid evaluation, it is a good place to decide what type of hearing aid to fit. The client should be shown models of behind-the-ear, in-the-ear, and in-the-canal hearing aids with the pros and cons of each type explained. If there seems to be a need for assistive listening devices, then they should be discussed at this time. It is also important to address the fact that telecoil circuitry and DAI can be readily incorporated into some types of hearing aids but not others. We have found that clients are often willing to sacrifice cosmetics for better hearing, once they understand the advantages and disadvantages of the various hearing aid technologies.

Selection of Appropriate Hearing Aid(s)

Although solutions to all of the client's communications difficulties are not always possible to achieve, obviously, hearing aids should be selected with the goal of filling as many of the client's needs as possible so that additional technologies are NOT required. One of the most common difficulties experienced by hearing-aid users is listening amidst background noise. This problem may be solved using state-of-the-art hearing-aid circuitry and earmold plumbing. If this technology is not used, then the hearing aid should be equipped with features to allow it to be coupled to assistive listening devices. Telecoil circuitry may also be needed specifically for telephone communication.

USE OF HEARING AID(S) WITH THE TELEPHONE

A client's ability to recognize speech through a telephone should be a major concern of the clinician during the hearing-aid selection process. For many people, the telecoil is the single most important hearing-aid option, allowing access to not only the telephone but also to interpersonal assistive listening devices and large-area assistive listening devices. Some considerations for each type of hearing aid include:

1. Behind-the-ear hearing aids offer stronger telecoil circuits and more sophisticated switching systems than do other hearing aids. They are therefore easier to use with assistive listening devices and the telephone, and provide many more listening options than do in-the-ear hearing aids.

2. In-the-ear hearing aids may be more cosmetically acceptable and may be the only hearing aid of choice in certain cases due to pinna malformation, activity level (e.g., sports), etc. If an in-the-ear hearing aid is chosen, the clinician must decide whether to install a telecoil circuit. Depending upon the degree of the hearing impairment, the in-the-ear hearing aid may be coupled to the telephone in one of two ways, inductively or acoustically.

  A. Inductive Coupling

   Inductive coupling is recommended for clients with moderate-to-severe hearing impairment, due to the occurrence of feedback with acoustic coupling and because the installation of a telecoil circuit will allow for assistive listening device interface in large areas such as theaters. When installing a telecoil, one must ensure that it has sufficient sensitivity, and that it is oriented appropriately within the hearing aid case.

   Telecoil sensitivity in in-the-ear hearing aids can be improved by asking for a pre-amplifier circuit and by orienting the telecoil perpendicular to the room or neckloop or to the telephone receiver. If the hearing aid is to be used with an assistive listening device, the telecoil should be mounted vertically (one end toward the ground and the other pointing skyward) to allow for best reception from a room loop, neckloop, or silhouette inductors. If the hearing aid's telecoil is to be used to pick up electromagnetic leakage from the telephone, then the telecoil should be mounted horizontally (one end facing the hearing-aid faceplate and the other facing the canal). If the client desires to use the telecoil with the telephone receiver as well as with a neck or room loop, then a good, vertically mounted, pre-amped telecoil should do the job, especially if the client compensates by angling telephone receiver slightly for the best reception.

   One must also consider whether switch modifications are necessary (e.g., does client need combination microphone/telecoil switch?). The client must also be instructed on proper use of the telecoil.

  B. Acoustic Coupling

   Acoustic coupling may be necessary due to ear size or client preference for an in-the-canal hearing aid. To eliminate feedback when the hearing-aid microphone is held next to the telephone handset, a foam telepad, plastic acoustic coupler, or handset amplifier (amplifier turned up; hearing-aid microphone turned down) can be tried. Completely in the cord (CIC) fittings may also facilitate acoustic coupling. It also may be possible for the client to simply remove the hearing aid and use a telephone amplifier.

If acoustic coupling (with or without a hearing aid) does not result in satisfactory telephone performance, then a hearing aid with an appropriate telecoil must be considered.

C. Direct Audio Input

It is also possible to install a direct audio input circuit on some in-the-ear hearing aids, allowing them to be coupled to assistive listening devices which can then be interfaced to the telephone. This might be warranted in the rare case of a cosmetics-conscious in-the-ear hearing aid user who cannot couple his or her hearing aid to the telephone—either inductively (due to magnetic interference) or acoustically (due to feedback, etc.)—and who cannot use the naked ear with the telephone.

Figure 12-2 illustrates the various ways the ear can be coupled to the telephone. Note that the use of a hearing-aid telecoil increases one's telephone listening options.

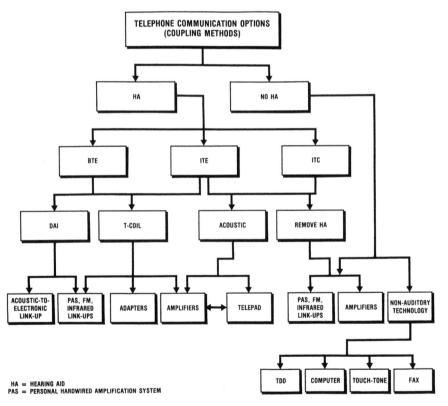

HA = HEARING AID
PAS = PERSONAL HARDWIRED AMPLIFICATION SYSTEM

FIGURE 12-2 **Telephone communication options**

© 1989, Assistive Devices Center, Department of Audiology and Speech-Language Pathology, School of Communication, Gallaudet University.

USE OF HEARING AID(S) WITH ASSISTIVE LISTENING DEVICES

If it appears that a client's interpersonal communication difficulties will not be solved through the use of a personal hearing aid only, consider interfacing the hearing aid with an assistive listening device. For some clients, communication needs may be best met through the use of an assistive listening device only as in the case of an elderly, hospital-bound person. Figure 12-3 illustrates the communication options provided by using an assistive listening device with and without a hearing aid.

Some issues to consider are as follows:

1. Behind-the-ear hearing aids provide the most flexibility with assistive listening devices. Switching systems offer various modes for control of the hearing-aid environmental microphone. Due to the larger hearing-aid case, stronger telecoils are available for use with large area induction loops, neck loops, and silhouette inductors.

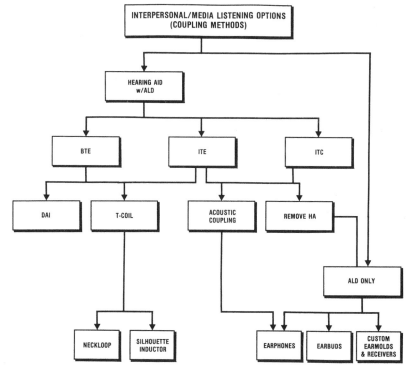

ALD = ASSISTIVE LISTENING DEVICE

FIGURE 12-3 **Interpersonal/media listening options**

© 1989, Assistive Devices Center, Department of Audiology and Speech-Language Pathology, School of Communication, Gallaudet University.

2. If an in-the-ear hearing aid is chosen, it should be equipped with a proper telecoil. If not, the client should also be counseled concerning his or her future ability to hear and understand speech in face-to-face and electronic media listening situations. The following questions must be considered:

- If the client continues to have difficulty listening in noise and from a distance, how will he or she use the hearing aid with an assistive listening device?
- Will it be possible for the person to *remove* the hearing aid and use a hardwired assistive listening device or wireless assistive listening device receiver with earphones, earbuds, or custom earmold receivers?

3. Does the client need a way of controlling the hearing aid's external microphone? Behind-the-ear hearing aids allow for more flexible manipulation of the hearing aid's external microphone. A combination microphone/telecoil mode might be desired for people who want to maintain contact with outside world while using assistive listening devices. Telecoil and direct audio input-only modes are desired for especially noisy situations, or for people whose speech recognition ability deteriorates significantly in presence of any background competition. ITE hearing aids can be ordered with microphone or telecoil toggle switches or combination microphone/telecoil switches. As mentioned previously, telecoil performance in in-the-ear hearing aids *can* be improved. Adjustments must be done on a case-by-case basis by tenaciously consulting with each manufacturer's engineering department.

Finally, as mentioned in the section on using hearing aids with the telephone, direct audio input is also available from some ITE manufacturers.

Selection of Appropriate Assistive Devices

Often, the hearing aid is fitted and the client is given an opportunity to use it in the real world prior to a final decision being made concerning the need for assistive devices. During the hearing aid trial, the needs assessment process can be repeated. If the client continues to have difficulty in certain listening situations, then assistive devices may be indicated. In addition to the lifestyle considerations already discussed, several other issues need to be weighed when selecting appropriate assistive technology. Each issue is listed below and is accompanied by several examples.

Effectiveness
Clients should be fitted with effective technology. While this may seem obvious, all too often technology is recommended that is too complicated for the client to use. Or, the client has not received sufficient instruction in the use of the technology to make it effective.

Affordability
Affordability of technology will always be an issue, especially if the client has been instructed to purchase hearing aids in addition to assistive devices. It is important to

present the assistive device(s) and the hearing aid(s) as a "total communication system." If the client understands that, for example, the hearing aid by itself cannot be expected to meet the four basic communication needs, then he or she will be more accepting of the need to purchase additional technology. Sometimes it is helpful to have the client prioritize his or her communication needs. This helps in selecting the most versatile system, and also effectively involves the client as an active participant in the solution of his or her communication problems. Funding for assistive technology is available through several sources, including vocational rehabilitation, crippled children's services, employee benefits plans, and service clubs. The Americans With Disabilities Act (P.L. 101-336) and Section 504 of the Rehabilitation Act of 1973 (29 U.S.C. §794, as amended) also require that government and private employers provide communication technology and interpreters if requested.

Operability

Is the system too complicated for the client to manage? Will additional training/counseling be needed? If so, this service and the time it commands must be built into the audiologist's fee structure. Again, third party reimbursement is possible for this service. Physical design of the device is also important. Are the batteries easy to remove/replace? Is a raised volume control wheel needed? Can the device be recharged without removing the batteries?

Reliability

Clients demand and deserve technology that will perform when needed and that will last. Prices for technology vary, and each client should be counseled regarding which is the most reliable technology for the money. In this day and age of slick advertising, clients need to understand that, in most cases, reliable technology will cost more. This becomes an even more important issue in the area of emergency alerting systems such as smoke detectors. The reliability (and safety) of alerting devices can be determined by checking to see that the device is labeled with the UL listing appropriate for its intended use. As mentioned previously, appropriate installation is also needed for fire notification devices.

Although we do yet have ANSI standards for assistive listening devices, these technologies can be judged in the same way we judge hearing aids—by company reputation, by word of mouth, and by experience. Performing electroacoustic measurements (even without ANSI guidelines) can yield valuable information, although long-term usage is really the only way to test reliability.

Portability

Some systems are easier to carry around than others. For example, a direct audio input remote microphone system is lighter in weight and easier to set up than is an FM system (although an FM system is more versatile). A battery-powered portable telephone amplifier is easier to put in one's pocket or purse than is a replacement handset amplifier (which can be used only with a modular telephone).

Versatility

Some systems are more versatile than others. While they may cost more, they avoid the need for a different system for each application—and the training that goes it. For example, FM is more versatile than other interpersonal listening systems. It works well indoors or outdoors, can be used for TV or telephone listening, or for listening to a lecture or meeting. If, however, a client has only TV listening needs, then an inexpensive hardwired system might be the system of choice. All interpersonal listening systems can be equipped with various types of microphones, making them applicable to a variety of listening situations. Similarly, some alerting systems allow the user to select the most effective way of alerting him or her to the sound.

Mobility

Distance and mobility needs will often determine the choice between hardwired and wireless systems (Figure 12-4). For example, short distance and immobile activities (e.g., TV listening, one-to-one, small group conversation) can be met with both hardwired or wireless systems. Short distance, mobile, indoor and outdoor activities (e.g., sports, hobbies) can best be met with FM technology, although some short distance, mobile activities, such as "working a room" at a party can be met via a hardwired remote microphone system (e.g., direct audio input directional boom microphone).

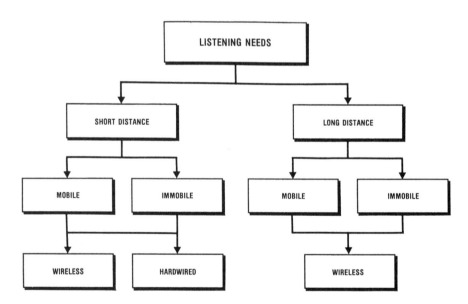

FIGURE 12-4 **Distance and mobility needs often determine the choice between hardwired and wireless systems.**

Long distance, immobile, indoor or outdoor (e.g., lectures) needs can best be met with FM or loop technology (although infrared technology would be appropriate for indoor activities). A wireless system such as FM would be most appropriate for a person with both mobile and immobile receptive communication needs. A person with a limited budget and mostly indoor, immobile needs, might be best served with hardwired technology, provided that his or her large-area listening needs can be met with wireless systems available in the community.

Durability
Clients want technology that will last, especially if they have paid a significant amount of money for it.

Compatibility
If a person must wear a hearing aid all the time, care should be taken to assure its compatibility with telephones as well as with personal assistive listening device receivers in the home and community. This is most easily accomplished by including a telecoil circuit, although direct audio input circuitry can be added if necessary. In some cases, acoustic coupling of the hearing aid to the telephone can be successfully carried out, and use of assistive listening devices can be accomplished by removing the hearing aid and using earphones or earbuds.

Compatibility of teletext devices with each other and with computers is also an important issue. Traditional teletext devices operate in a Baudot code at a baud rate of 45.5. ASCII-compatible teletext devices operate in an ASCII code at a baud rate of 300. Computers work in ASCII language and at much faster rates than 45.5 or 300. To use a computer as a TDD, it must be equipped with a "smart modem" that can switch baud rates upon demand. For more information on using computers as teletext devices call Gallaudet's Technology Assessment Center at (202) 651-5257. For general information on teletext devices, call Gallaudet's National Information Center on Deafness at (202) 651-5051.

Cosmetics
Clients may require reassurance and possibly assertiveness training to use certain assistive listening devices. In general, it is best to first demonstrate the equipment before discussing cosmetics. Often the client is so impressed with the assistance provided by the technology that the issue of cosmetics becomes less important. Sometimes "more is less"—that is, equipment such as an FM system can be less obvious than a small, hardwired direct audio input remote microphone, since the FM receiver and neckloop can be hidden under clothing. Audio loop systems are particularly cosmetically acceptable since they allow the listener to use his or her hearing-aid telecoil as the assistive listening device receiver. Some people may associate hardwired amplifiers and wireless receivers with portable radios or tape players and may therefore not be adverse to using assistive listening technology.

Previous Experience

Previous experience with technology and/or hearing health care professionals can have a positive, negative, or neutral effect. It is important to find out where the patient is "coming from" so that his or her preconceptions can be understood and handled in a positive way.

Need for Nonauditory Telecommunications Systems

Teletext devices, computers, fax machines, and decoders may be needed to augment or even replace auditory devices. One must consider standard and optional features in light of the client's communication needs in the various living situations.

Need for Alerting Devices

Alerting devices can augment or replace hearing aids. Alerting devices might be needed in the home or office while the client is using an assistive listening device to couple to a desired sound source (e.g., dictation machine or television). They can also be indicated when a hearing aid is used in noise, reverberation, from a distance, in another room, or is not being used at all (e.g., while sleeping). While vibrotactile devices can maintain privacy, some people may, at first, consider them an intrusion into their physical space.

Alerting devices should not be recommended unless they have appropriate UL listing and meet safety and housing codes. When selecting a device for a client's home, office, or other setting, a floor plan is helpful. Coverage and mobility needs must be addressed (e.g., if sender and receiver must be mobile, then a phone-activated alphanumeric pager might be best; if both sender and receiver are confined to a particular building, then an AC- or battery-powered interoffice paging system might work, depending upon the transmission range required and the amount of metal support beams in the building). Alerting devices offer various options in terms of the way they monitor, transmit, and signal. The advantages and disadvantages of hardwired and wireless systems should be considered and explained.

Cultural Issues

Although hearing impairment is often treated from a medical model point of view, many hearing-impaired people view it from a cultural perspective. Cultural orientation can have an important impact on a person's acceptance or rejection of technology. Clients who have lost their hearing gradually, usually consider themselves "hard-of-hearing" and from an auditory world. Consequently, they may be reticent, and even fearful, to use nonauditory technologies representative of deaf culture (teletext devices, decoders, and visual and vibrotactile alerting devices). Similarly, clients who, despite their significant auditory skills, identify themselves with the deaf culture, are often fearful of using auditory technologies. This may be due to negative past experiences as well as current conceptions that the use of auditory technology will cause them to be labeled by their peers as "hearing-minded".

It is critical to provide clients with a comfortable, supportive, and nonjudgmental atmosphere in which a client can examine his or her technology options. It is important to communicate to the client that assistive devices are simply tools for communication access and that the use of these tools does not suggest that the client must abandon his or her cultural identity.

The support of the client's family, friends, and colleagues is often instrumental in the successful use of assistive devices. As such, it is important to involve them in counseling sessions. Introduction of clients to support groups such as Self Help for Hard of Hearing People is also helpful.

Demonstration/Evaluation of Equipment

Behavioral Evaluation

When demonstrating assistive technology, it is important to provide the client with "ears on" and "hands on" experience so he or she can gain an appreciation and a comfort level for it. The demonstration should be made as relevant as possible to the client's real life communication needs. Some examples:

1. If a client is experiencing difficulty on the telephone, then the hearing aid telecoil, telephone amplifier, or other device should be demonstrated using telephone recordings or actual telephone conversations.

2. A client desiring to once again enjoy music can be shown how to connect his or her hearing aid to a portable stereo tape player via a binaural, stereo DAI cord, or a neckloop connected to a stereo-to-mono adapter.

3. Demonstration of television as played through an assistive listening device or closed captioned decoder can be made using recordings of interesting programs. A library of relevant audio- and videotapes can be developed—for example, music: classical to jazz; television: Sesame Street for kids, music videos for teens, health news for elders, Wall Street Week for bankers.

4. If desired, a hardwired or wireless remote microphone system can be demonstrated in a test booth in background noise or in a room set aside for assistive device demonstrations. This room might be equipped with a loudspeaker system through which various types of background noise could be played.

5. A small display of selected alerting devices is helpful in explaining their set up and use.

Objective Measurement

Choosing an assistive listening device for a client involves an analysis of that client's hearing impairment and listening needs in a variety of relevant everyday situations. Once the type of device is determined, then a brand must be selected. A serious impediment to the objective selection of assistive listening devices is the lack of standardized protocols for electroacoustic and probe tube measurement.

Although electroacoustic measurement procedures have been suggested (Sinclair, Freeman, & Riggs, 1981; Hawkins & Van Tasell, 1982; Van Tasell & Landin, 1980; Gravel & Konkle, 1982; Thibodeau, 1990a; Lewis, Feigin, Karasek, & Stelmachowicz, 1989), until there is a national standard[3], we will not see unity of measurement across the various brands of products, making it difficult to judge the quality of the various types of systems. Clinical test equipment and protocols are also needed for electroacoustic evaluation of telephone amplifiers, adapters and specialty telephones. Finally, although there is a standard for the electroacoustic measurement of telecoils (ANSI 53.22, 1987), it uses only one frequency (1000 Hz) for measurement, which may misrepresent the overall telecoil gain across frequencies of the hearing aid. Additionally, the standard uses an input field strength of 10 ma/m which is significantly weaker than that provided by many telephones and assistive listening devices. Finally, 2 cm³ measures often do not accurately reflect the telecoil response that is present in the real ear when the hearing aid is being worn.

If probe tube measurement is considered a crucial step in the hearing-aid fitting process, then a comparable protocol must be developed for the evaluation of assistive listening devices. Assistive listening devices can be used alone or in conjunction with a personal hearing aid. Either way, objective measurement of the system (assistive listening device and/or hearing-aid telecoil) must be made if one is to ascertain that an appropriate frequency response, without the risk of excessive harmonic distortion, uncomfortable and/or overamplification, or underamplification is being provided.

Research has shown that when hearing aids are coupled to FM systems, the hearing-aid characteristics are not necessarily maintained (Hawkins & Schum, 1985; Thibodeau, McCaffrey, & Abrahamson, 1988; Thibodeau, 1990b). Currently, there are very limited assessment techniques being developed to look at the real ear performance of assistive listening devices (Hawkins, 1987; Lewis et al., 1989; Thibodeau, 1990a; Grimes & Mueller, 1991). The establishment of a national measurement protocol is essential for clients to be fitted in a scientific and safe manner. This is particularly important for young children or others who cannot provide subjective feedback regarding potentially inappropriate fittings.

Speech Perception Testing

Once appropriate coupling method and settings have been chosen, speech recognition or discrimination testing may be carried out to determine the performance of the assistive listening device, or to compare performance between the personal hearing aid and the assistive listening device. Lewis et. al. (1989) provide a step-by-step method for documenting the advantage of an FM system. This protocol could also be adapted for other assistive listening devices as well. Holmes and Frank (1984) and Wallber, MacKenzie, and Clyme (1987) have developed formalized behavioral assessment procedures for documenting telecoil performance with the telephone.

---

[3]In May of 1991, the American National Standards Institute (ANSI) S3 Committee on Acoustics authorized the establishment of a new writing group on assistive listening devices. One of the tasks of this group is to develop a national measurement standard for ALDs.

Documentation of the assistive listening device performance may be needed for educational purposes, for third party and/or employer financial support, or to simply prove to a client that he or she can be assisted by the technology.

FOLLOW-UP/AURAL REHABILITATION

Just as with personal hearing-aid fittings, follow-up counseling and evaluation is essential following the recommendation of assistive technology. Additional orientation and training may also be necessary. For example, some clients may require repeated instruction on how to use their hearing aid telecoil circuit with the telephone and assistive listening devices. Others may need intensive practice in setting up, using, troubleshooting, and maintaining auditory and nonauditory assistive devices. Speech reading, auditory training (face-to-face and telephone), training in the use of communication/environmental strategies, and counseling may also be needed. Furthermore, assertiveness training may be required as the use of assistive technology often requires the cooperation of others. For example, it can be especially anxiety-producing to have to ask a lecturer to wear an FM transmitter, to request that colleagues at a staff meeting take turns talking into a microphone, or to ask a speaker to slow down for the real-time captioner. For these reasons, it is important to assist the client, via instruction and role playing, in developing the skills and psychological strength necessary to assure successful, long-term assistive device usage.

THE ROLE OF THE PROFESSIONAL

In the last decade, the area of assistive technology has matured from an academic curiosity to a legitimate clinical specialty. Several forces have contributed to this transformation, with two being the most influential—consumer activism and legislative mandates. Consumers who are hearing-impaired are becoming increasingly aware of their rights to communication access. Third-party providers are beginning to recognize and pay for this technology. What does all this mean to our field?

Although each professional's role will differ slightly, it is critical that future audiologists be able to recognize when assistive technology is needed, be able to evaluate it, to recommend it, to advocate for it, to secure funding for it, and to train clients to use it. This training will extend to school officials, employers, and others who impact on the lives of people with reception communication problems. Work in the area of assistive technology will also demand excellent networking skills. Audiologists must be able to work effectively with consumers, acoustical engineers, attorneys, employers, teachers, state and local government officials, and with managers of public accommodations.

Basically, the popularity of assistive technology is expanding the role of the audiologist from diagnostician and hearing-aid fitter to that of communication access specialist. Increasing numbers of us will be asked to perform communication needs assessments for our clients and help them, via technology and behavioral strategies, find ways of communicating on the job as well as in other settings

SUMMARY

A broad assortment of auditory and nonauditory technology is available to assist in removing the communication barriers that can prevent deaf and hearing-impaired people of all ages from leading independent and productive lifestyles.

By carefully evaluating our clients' communication needs and by having a good working knowledge of today's hearing aids and other equally important assistive technologies, we can select systems to effectively meet these needs and can incorporate them into appropriate and comprehensive rehabilitative programs that will improve our clients' communication skills and empower them to function in today's society with independence and dignity. To do less would be a disservice to our patients as well as to our profession.

REFERENCES

Compton, C. (1992). Assistive listening devices: Videotext displays. *American Journal of Audiology, 1(2)*, 19–20.

Compton, C.L. (1991). *Assistive devices: Doorways to independence.* Annapolis, MD: VanComp Associates.

Compton, C.L. (1991). *Assistive devices: Doorways to independence.* (videotape) Washington, DC: Gallaudet University. Available through VanComp Associates.

DeVoss, F. (1993). Underwriters Laboratories, Northbrook, IL, personal communication.

Elwell, G. (1994). Silent Call Corporation, Clarkson, MI, personal communication.

Gravel, J., & Konkle, D. (1982). Electroacoustic hearing aid performance with neckloop inductive coupling. Presented at the American Speech-Language-Hearing Association Convention, Toronto, Canada.

Grimes, A.M., & Mueller, H.G. (1991). Using probe-microphone measures to assess telecoils and assistive listening devices. *The Hearing Journal, 44(6)*, 16–21.

Harkins, J. E. (1991). Visual devices for deaf and hard of hearing people: State-of-the-art. *GRI Monograph Series*, Series A, No. 2. Washington, DC: Gallaudet Research Institute.

Hawkins, D.B. (1987). Assessment of FM systems with an ear canal probe tube microphone system. *Ear and Hearing, 8*, 301–303.

Hawkins, D.B., & Schum, D.J. (1985). Some effects of FM coupling on hearing aid characteristics. *Journal of Speech and Hearing Disorders, 50*, 132–141.

Hawkins, D., & Van Tasell, D. (1982). Some effects of FM-system coupling on hearing aid characteristics. *Journal of Speech and Hearing Disorders, 47*, 355–362.

Holmes, A., & Frank, T. (1984). Telephone listening ability for hearing impaired individuals. *Ear and Hearing, 5*, 96–100.

Lewis, D., Feigin, J., Karasek, A., & Stelmachowicz, P. (1989). Evaluation and assessment of FM systems. *Ear and Hearing, 12(4)*, 268–280.

Sinclair, J.S., Freeman, B.A., & Riggs, D.E. (1981). Appendix: The use of the hearing aid test box to assess the performance of FM auditory training units. In F.H. Bess, B.A. Freeman, & J.S. Sinclair (Eds.), *Amplification in Education*, pp. 381–383. Washington, DC: A.G. Bell Association, Inc.

Sievers, D. E. (1993). Donald E. Sievers & Associates, LTD, Bethesda, MD (Fire Safety consultant to the National Association of the Deaf), personal communication.

Thibodeau, L. (1990a). Clinical considerations in using classroom amplification systems. Paper read at the Second Annual Meeting of the American Academy of Audiology, New Orleans, LA, April.

Thibodeau, L. (1990b). Electroacoustic performance of direct-input hearing aids with FM amplification systems. *Language, Speech and Hearing Services in the Schools, 21*, 49–56.

Thibodeau, L., McCaffrey, H., & Abrahamson, J. (1988). Effects of coupling hearing aids to FM systems via neckloops. *Journal of the Academy of Rehabilitative Audiology, 21*, 49–56.

Wallber, M., MacKenzie, D., & Clyme, E. (1987). Telecoil evaluation procedure. *National Technical Institute for the Deaf, RIT*, Rochester, New York, by agreement with the U.S. Department of Education. Auditec of St. Louis.

Van Tasell, D., & Landin, D. (1980). Frequency response characteristics of FM mini-loop auditory trainers. *Journal of Speech and Hearing Disorders, 45*, 247–258.

APPENDIX 12-1: RESOURCES

Suggested Professional Library

✓ ASSISTIVE DEVICES: DOORWAYS TO INDEPENDENCE

Compton, C.L., *Assistive Devices: Doorways to Independence* (videotape and companion book). Book: Annapolis, MD: VanComp Associates. (1991) Videotape: Washington, DC: Gallaudet University. (1991) Available from VanComp Associates, 2740 Gingerview Lane, Annapolis, MD. (202) 651-5326 or (410) 266-0028

> This 65-minute open-captioned videotape and booklet discuss assistive devices in depth at the consumer level. It is also appropriate for professionals interested in learning about the various auditory, visual, and vibrotactile technologies for receptive communication. Designed to be used in waiting rooms, professional libraries, graduate training programs, senior centers, nursing homes, etc., the extensively illustrated booklet serves as a detailed reference for topics discussed in the video and contains a comprehensive section on large-area assistive listening device applications and nonauditory technologies, topics often overlooked.

✓ LEGAL RIGHTS: THE GUIDE FOR DEAF AND HARD OF HEARING PEOPLE

DuBow, S., Geer, S., Peltz Strauss, K., *Legal Rights: The Guide for Deaf and Hard of Hearing People*. Washington, DC: Gallaudet Press. (1992).

Authored by Gallaudet's National Center for Law Deafness, this excellent book features complete information of the Americans With Disabilities Act, the Television Decoder Circuitry Act, and full updates on all other laws that affect deaf and hard-of-hearing people. Written for the lay person, it is an excellent guide for compliance with federal legislation requiring removal of communication barriers in all aspects of our society.

RESOURCES FOR FIRE SAFETY ISSUES

Donald E. Sievers & Associates, LTD
6309 Bradley Blvd.
Bethesda, MD 20817-3243
(301) 469-0278
(301) 469-7541 FAX

Ferdinand DeVoss
Engineering Group Leader
Engineering Services, Dept. 417C
Underwriters Laboratories
333 Pfingsten Road
Northbrook, IL 60062
(708) 272-8800
(708) 272-3846 FAX

Increasing Consumer Acceptance of Assistive Devices

GLEN SUTHERLAND
The Canadian Hearing Society

INTRODUCTION

Deaf, deafened, and hard-of-hearing people currently have a wide variety of excellent technical devices. These devices include telecommunication devices for the deaf (TDDs), visual alert systems, television devices, assistive listening systems, and new high tech communications devices (such as TDD modems and alphanumeric pagers). Given such a comprehensive range of available products, consumers need to be well-informed about their options. Detailed information about the wide variety of available devices is discussed in other chapters.

This chapter highlights the following strategies for increasing consumer and public acceptance of technical devices:

- Educating consumers about technical devices, including their limitations
- Training consumers to use technical devices
- Helping consumers make informed decisions
- Providing consumers with support
- Encouraging more experienced consumers to help those who are learning about technical devices
- Empowering consumers by working closely with them as part of a team or partnership
- Aligning with consumers to advocate for better laws and services, and for universal accessibility for people with hearing loss

For the purpose of this chapter, individual consumers include any potential users of assistive devices. Some consumers may be deaf, deafened, or hard-of-hearing. Others may be family members or caregivers in hospitals or homes for seniors. In order to help individuals with hearing losses, support people should also be knowledgeable about assistive devices.

Consumers may also be members of the general population, such as government, corporate, and business employees who provide services and facilities that should be rendered accessible through the installation and use of technical devices; educators; and granting agencies/funders who are committed to accessibility.

Hearing health care professionals should keep in mind that many consumers are more likely to receive maximum benefit from technical devices if they receive the required information and training gradually and in stages. Potential users may not be experienced in dealing with electronic equipment; they may be apprehensive about wearing devices, setting them up properly in their homes, or how to troubleshoot these "electronic gizmos". Mastering the successful use of technical devices takes time, patience, and practice.

MEETING CONSUMER NEEDS

Information/Training

The provision of easy-to-understand information and client training is one of the most important ways to increase consumer acceptance of technical devices. The goal of information and training sessions is to ensure that the clients 1) understand the devices thoroughly, including their limitations, 2) understand their options, 3) make informed decisions, and 4) are empowered to take responsibility for the management of their hearing loss.

The information and training sessions may be offered on an individual basis, in the form of specialized counseling sessions, individual training sessions, home visiting programs, or training of family members or caregivers. They may be offered to groups of consumers, in the form of training sessions to self-help groups, training sessions in aural rehabilitation classes, or in-service training to family members or other caregivers. These different forms of training and instruction are explained in greater detail below. Figure 13-1 shows the components of group and individual training sessions.

INDIVIDUAL INFORMATION/TRAINING SESSIONS

Specialized Counseling Services

People who are expected to accept a new "gadget" designed to facilitate communication must first be both comfortable with, and knowledgeable about, the nature, degree, and implications of having a hearing loss; if hearing aids are involved, clients

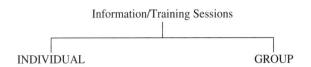

Information/Training Sessions

INDIVIDUAL	GROUP
a) specialized counseling sessions	a) training sessions of self-help groups
b) individual training sessions	b) training sessions in aural rehabilitation classes
c) home visiting programs	c) in-service training to groups to family members or other caregivers (e.g., staff in-service at hospitals or seniors' homes)
d) training of a family member or caregiver	

FIGURE 13–1   **Classifications of Information/Training Sessions**

need the relevant information. Individuals incorporate information in different ways and over varying timespans. Some people catch on quickly, while others require several specialized counseling sessions to bring them to the point where they are able to appreciate the fact that a technical device may help them to communicate better.

The hearing health care professional must be sensitive to the individual's unique needs. Initially, some people are not comfortable with the thought of having some electronic device strapped to their bodies. Many deaf, deafened, and hard-of-hearing individuals require specialized individual counseling sessions/needs assessments to help them gradually become more accepting of an assistive device.

Such specialized sessions will include the following information to prepare clients to use hearing aids and technical devices:

- A review of the individual's audiogram
- A discussion of the nature and degree of hearing loss
- A discussion and demonstration of hearing aids, including what they can and cannot do for the client
- A discussion about the acceptance one's hearing loss

In the majority of cases, a series of these sessions is required. However, once clients feel more comfortable with and knowledgeable about their hearing loss, their acceptance and incorporation of assistive devices in daily living will be more successful.

In certain situations, when clients demonstrate a high level of anxiety about their hearing loss, the hearing health care professional should refer them to other counselors (such as psychiatrists, psychologists, or social workers). These professionals may help such clients deal with their feelings about living with a hearing loss and, when the time is right, may refer them for further training sessions with the hearing health care professionals. Where appropriate, the two professionals may work together with the client and family members.

Individualized Training Sessions

By the time many people are ready to acquire an assistive device, they have accepted their hearing loss. Most hard-of-hearing people will have worn a hearing aid, become familiar with it, and have a basic understanding of batteries, volume controls, microphones, and receivers. Most culturally deaf people will be familiar with basic TDDs and alert/warning systems.

People receiving a new device need training in its use. The goal of individualized training sessions is to teach consumers how to use the device(s) and to inform them about all available applications and options.

These sessions will include the following information:

- A description of the device, how it works, and any available options
- An explanation of the device's capabilities and limitations
- Where applicable, installation instructions for devices such as visual alert systems, which convert sound energy (from doorbells, telephones, etc.) to visual energy (lamps). Occasionally, an electrician should come to the home at the same time as the hearing health care professional, in order to ensure proper installation
- Instruction by the hearing health care professional in how to use the device
- A demonstration on the correct use of the device by the consumer to the professional (for example, the consumer demonstrating his or her ability to set up the device as it would be done in the home)
- An overview of troubleshooting techniques by the hearing health care professional
- An explanation of troubleshooting techniques by the client
- An opportunity for a question-and-answer session

If instruction on more than one device is being given during a single session, the hearing health care professional should complete instruction on the first device before moving to the next one. Some consumers may require more than one session before they are able to demonstrate and use the device successfully. The time and patience taken in the initial stages of the learning process will ensure less need for follow-ups and will reduce the occurrence of complaints.

Once the client has demonstrated the effective use of each device, a review of all available options should follow, to ensure that the consumer chooses the device best suited to his or her needs and capabilities.

Products are accompanied by instructional manuals and pamphlets. Consumers should be encouraged to read them carefully, in order to reinforce their hearing health care professional's teaching.

Home Visiting Programs and Individual Training of a Family Member/Caregiver

On occasion, the hearing health care professional may be required to visit a client's home to help install a device and demonstrate its use. Individuals who are unable to leave their residences (for example, those who are bedridden, frail, or elderly) are appropriate candidates for home visits. An additional benefit of the home visit is that a family member or caregiver will often be present to learn about the device.

The goal of the home visit or family member/caregiver training is similar to that of individual training sessions; to install the assistive device and to train the consumer in its effective use.

GROUP INFORMATION/TRAINING SESSIONS

Self-Help and Aural (Re)Habilitation Groups

Much of the information and training vital to increasing consumer acceptance can be effectively conveyed in groups, such as self-help and aural rehabilitation groups.

The difference between self-help groups and aural rehabilitation groups relates to leadership. Self-help groups are usually initiated by deaf, deafened, or hard-of-hearing people who organize and coordinate the group themselves. The group coordinator contacts guest speakers to participate, at the group's request. In contrast, aural rehabilitation groups are typically organized and coordinated by hearing health care professionals, who contact clients they think will benefit from a group setting and provide classes according to a pre-established curriculum. With regard to technical devices instruction, the general format for both groups is very similar:

- A specialist in technical devices is invited to speak to the class
- The presentation includes information about and demonstration of technical devices
- The group is given an opportunity to examine and use the devices as they would in their own homes
- A question-and-answer period follows

A demonstration of one device should be completed before the group moves on to the next device. Often, the demonstrator will be required to make one or two return visits. After the devices have been demonstrated to participating individuals, the group should discuss various options.

In-Service Training to Groups of Family Members or Other Caregivers

In some cases, it is appropriate to provide information sharing and training for caregivers, including family members or staff in facilities such as hospitals and seniors' homes. Although the "customer" is the caregiver, rather than the person with hearing loss, the information/training sessions call upon the hearing health care professional to educate the caregiver about all aspects of hearing loss, as well as technical devices. This instruction may require several sessions. The key components of such sessions include:

- Hearing and hearing loss
- Communication difficulties resulting from hearing loss
- Psychology of hearing loss
- Hearing aids
- Assistive devices

Family members should always be encouraged to attend aural rehabilitation classes in order to learn about hearing loss, hearing aids, and technical devices. In facilities, a series of in-service training sessions should be set up with the caregivers to acquaint them with the use, troubleshooting, and care of a client's hearing aid and other technical devices.

Experience shows that once a facility has obtained technical devices (such as large-room systems to assist hard-of-hearing people to hear better in a group setting), the most frequently expressed complaint is that the staff of the facility do not know how to use or troubleshoot the equipment. This is also true for caregivers of individuals with hearing loss who use assistive listening devices. Well-informed caregivers ensure increased consumer acceptance of technical devices.

USE OF VOLUNTEERS AS TRAINERS

Informed consumers who have experience with the devices can help increase consumer acceptance. Many people with hearing loss are willing to volunteer their time to help other people who have hearing loss. These volunteers may act as guest speakers to self-help groups and aural rehabilitation classes, to staff in-services, or they may participate in home visits. They can talk about their experiences with technical devices, highlighting how the devices have helped them, discuss what limitations the devices may have, and what options are available. Because of their empathy for the potential users, volunteers often can help consumers to accept technical devices more readily.

In summary, the key elements of individual and group training sessions about technical devices include:

- A description of the device
- A simple explanation of what the device is designed to do
- A demonstration on how the device works
- An opportunity for the potential user to practice using the device
- An explanation/demonstration of troubleshooting techniques
- An opportunity for potential users to ask questions

If this process is carefully managed, consumers will learn all about the devices and are likely to become much more accepting of them as aids to daily communication.

EDUCATIONAL MATERIALS

Educational materials are addressed to clients' needs and to increasing consumer acceptance. They should be presented in a user friendly format, be clear, concise, and informative, with key points emphasized. It is a good idea to target them to a variety of uses, such as aural rehabilitation classes, presentations to individuals, potential funders and service clubs, and public education forums. The person giving the presentation determines which materials are appropriate to a particular audience.

Educational materials designed to increase consumer acceptance include audiovisual materials, written materials (such as pamphlets on related topics and relevant publications), and instructional/therapy materials.

Audiovisual Materials

A wide variety of audiovisual tapes on many topics related to issues of concern to deaf and hard-of-hearing people are now available. These materials have been produced by many organizations that provide services to people with hearing loss. The Canadian Hearing Society, for example, recently published a series of twelve videos which are particularly useful in aural rehabilitation classes. Four of these tapes focus on technical devices.

The series covers the following topics:

1. Hearing Loss: Recognizing It
2. Hearing Loss: There's Help
3. Hearing Loss: Identifying It
4. Communication is a Two-Way Process
5. Improving Communication
6. Hearing Aids: Time, Practice, and Patience
7. Hearing Aids: They've Come a Long Way
8. Hearing Aids: Care and Maintenance Techniques
9. Help With the Telephone
10. Help With the Television
11. Signalling Devices
12. Public Listening Systems

These videos are open captioned and available in five languages (English, French, Italian, Chinese, and Portuguese), and are packaged with pertinent written materials. They (and many other videos) are available from Information Services, The Canadian Hearing Society, 271 Spadina Road, Toronto, Ontario, Canada, M5R 2V3. If you live in an area that has an organization which provides a variety of services to deaf and hard-of-hearing people, you may wish to contact it to find out if it distributes audiovisual materials, or knows of other regional facilities that do.

Written Materials

Numerous books, pamphlets, bookmarks, bumper stickers, posters, and professional and consumer magazines are available. Many are intended to teach people with hearing loss about its implications, and to inform them about hearing aids, and other technical devices. I have appended an instructional example, entitled *Recommendations to Make Public Places Accessible to Deaf and Hard of Hearing People*, to the end of this chapter. Hearing health care professionals should have on hand a good selection of pamphlets and articles for their consumers, who can read them while they wait for an appointment, or take them home to look over, as they adjust to their hearing aid or other new device.

Instructional/Therapy Materials

Many hearing-aid manufacturers, associations that work with deaf and hard-of-hearing people, and consumer groups, publish instructional/therapy materials of benefit to consumers. They may take the form of children's coloring books, workbooks on a variety of topics related to hearing loss, hearing aids and technical devices; and other helpful materials, such as tent cards, which can be placed in an accessible location to serve as quick and easy references. Tent cards placed at bedside, for example, might contain information about how use of a device: One side of the tent card can explain how to turn on the device and wear it in the morning; the second side can detail how to turn it off and put it away at the end of the day. Communication tips to assist the person with a hearing loss can be printed on the third panel.

There is no need to reinvent the wheel. Many excellent materials are currently available. Hearing health care professionals and people who sell devices should do some research to find helpful materials for increasing awareness and acceptance of technical devices. Here are some self-help groups that are valuable sources of information:

Self-Help for Hard of Hearing People (SHHH)
7800 Wisconsin Avenue
Bethesda, MD, 20814

Association of Late Deafened Adults (ALDA)
P.O. Box 641763
Chicago, IL, 60644-1763

Canadian Hard of Hearing Association (CHHA)
P.O. Box 3176, Station "D"
Ottawa, Ontario, Canada K1P 6H8

Canadian Association of the Deaf (CAD)
205-2435 Holly Lane
Ottawa, Ontario, Canada K1V 7P2

These groups keep up-to-date lists of available materials for their members. If they publish a magazine, helpful materials will often be highlighted in articles or advertised for sale.

Your search should also involve:

- Contacting other professionals in your area to see if they are aware of any helpful materials
- Reading the advertisements in related publications, where you may find some useful materials
- Contacting associations that deal with issues and services related to deaf, deafened, and hard-of-hearing people; for example, the A.G. Bell Association, 3417 Volta Place Northwest, Washington, DC 20007, telephone (202) 337-5220; the Bicultural Centre, 5506 Kennelworth Avenue, Suite 105, Lower Level, Riverdale, MD, 20737-3106, telephone (310) 277-3945
- If your research reveals that certain materials you deem to be important don't exist, sharing your ideas with self-help groups or associations, which may be able to assist you in producing your materials
- Contacting professional speech-language and hearing associations such as: The American Speech and Hearing Association (ASHA), 10801 Rockville Pike, Rockville, MD 20852; The Canadian Association of Speech-Language Pathologists and Audiologists (CASLPA) 1215-25 Main Street West, Hamilton, Ontario, Canada L8P 1H1; or your state or provincial professional association.

Because the quality of materials varies, and some meet your needs better than others, you must determine which materials are best suited to your audience. Make sure that you carefully study your market and then use the most helpful materials.

PUBLIC AWARENESS AND PUBLIC ACCESSIBILITY

When accessibility for people with hearing loss becomes a global reality, consumer acceptance of technical devices will increase. Achieving universal accessibility requires strong advocacy on the part of consumers and hearing health care professionals, in order to educate the public and ensure that public facilities are rendered barrier-free for people with hearing loss.

Consumer involvement is a key part of this strategy. People with hearing loss make the best advocates for hearing health care issues. Consumers who live with its daily consequences are often eager to volunteer for involvement in public education and advocacy forums.

Public Education

Public awareness of hearing loss, technical devices, and accessibility issues can be heightened through:

- 800 number information lines: These phone lines could be advertised as special lines for information about hearing loss, hearing aids, and technical devices. Consumers simply call the number and ask a question related to technical devices; information is provided instantly by computer response. At the end of the message, the consumer is directed to an appropriate source for more detailed information.
- Open forums on related topics: Hearing health care professionals and consumers can organize public forums on current issues or demonstrations of communications technology. Guest speakers can be invited. People attend free of charge or for a nominal fee. The audience may include deaf, deafened, or hard-of-hearing people, their families and friends, interested professionals, and any other interested parties.
- Conferences for consumers, their families and the public: These could include poster sessions, presentations by professionals and consumers, and exhibit areas where manufacturers display the latest technology. Social activities for everyone attending the conference would be organized to give delegates an opportunity to meet and share information and ideas.
- Exciting, innovative consumer-driven programs should be created and implemented to enhance people's knowledge of assistive devices and the importance of them to improve communication. For example, ACCESS 2000 is a bold and exciting innovation that draws new sectors into an old, but good, cause. ACCESS 2000 provides a national framework within which consumer groups and service agencies for deaf, deafened, or hard-of-hearing people can promote accessibility among local companies, hospitals, and other public facilities. The goal of the program is nationwide accessibility for deaf, deafened, and hard-of-hearing people in major public facilities and service industries by the year 2000.

Making Public Facilities Accessible to People with Hearing Loss

All public facilities should be required to obtain any system or device necessary to ensure accessibility to persons with hearing loss. This mandate includes devices such as theater FM and infrared systems, emergency alerting devices, and TDDs, as well as such structural considerations as carpeting, sound dampers in the ceiling, appropriate signs to ease communications, and well-informed, helpful staff.

Programs to make public facilities accessible should include:

- Meeting with the facility to determine accessibility needs
- Installing the necessary devices
- Providing staff in-services to explain the devices and train staff to use and troubleshoot them
- Ongoing device monitoring and staff in-services

Advocacy

There are many issues of concern to deaf and hard-of-hearing people, to parents of hearing-impaired children, and to those involved in hearing health care delivery that point to the need for changes in public policy and government legislation/regulations. The term *advocacy* is often used to describe the educational and political initiatives that promote such progressive changes. The following are examples of advocacy issues relevant to deaf and hard of hearing people:

- Message relay services
- Public telephone accessibility
- Access to public facilities

To ensure better laws, services, and funding for these programs, consumers and professionals must lobby their government. Government awareness of the necessary programs, the need for global accessibility, and other related issues must be raised. Consumers and professionals should arrange to get themselves seated on government advisory committees and barrier-free design and public access committees.

Consumers, professionals, and government must form partnerships to meet the needs of people with hearing loss. With all three groups cooperating to achieve common goals, we can look forward to better education, heightened understanding and global accessibility for deaf, deafened, and hard-of-hearing people.

SUMMARY

This chapter has highlighted a number of important ways to increase consumer and public acceptance of technical devices:

- Educating consumers about technical devices, including their limitations
- Training consumers to use technical devices
- Helping consumers make informed decisions
- Providing consumer support
- Using experienced consumers to help those who are learning about technical devices
- Empowering consumers by working in close partnership with them
- Joining consumers in their fight for better laws and services and for global accessibility for people with hearing loss

Every day of their lives, deaf and hard-of-hearing people are obliged to contend with barriers to communication. These barriers materialize in a world in which much of our business is conducted on the telephone, in which emergency systems depend solely upon sound, in which security systems make buildings inaccessible for those unable to use an intercom, in which paging systems and most public announcements in terminals and on board public transit vehicles depend solely on sound, in which few public places make provisions for hearing-aid users, and in which even such mundane matters as ordering a pizza become complicated for persons with hearing loss. Although they comprise 10 percent of the population, deaf and hard-of-hearing people are denied participation in worship, lectures, meetings, classes, and enjoyment at theaters, films, and concerts. The solution to their exclusion is special devices that have been designed to improve the social and professional functioning of people with almost any type and degree of hearing loss. As public awareness rises, more institutions are installing these devices to ensure that deaf and hard-of-hearing people have access to many of the services, functions, and enjoyments previously denied them.

Services to deaf and hard-of-hearing people will continue to improve with heightened consumer acceptance, public education, and advocacy for better laws and services. Partnerships of informed consumers, hearing health care professionals and representatives from various government agencies will ensure that deaf, deafened, and hard-of-hearing people are enabled to function at their full communication—and human—potential.

APPENDIX 13-1

Recommendations to Make Public Places Accessible to Deaf and Hard of Hearing People

The Canadian Hearing Society is committed to ensuring that hard-of-hearing and deaf people, who make up 10 percent of the population, have access to public functions, buildings, and services. It is our belief that all public buildings and offices dealing with the public should have the proper type of equipment to help make them accessible for deaf and hard-of-hearing staff and clients. Listed below you will find many suggestions that will assist you in making your facility accessible to people with a hearing loss.

1. **Volume Controls and Compatible Telephones:**

   Many hearing aid users find that they can hear better over the telephone by using the T-switch on their hearing aids. The T-switch picks up the magnetic field produced by the receivers of many telephones. Unfortunately, not all modern telephones produce a magnetic field and are, therefore, not compatible with hearing aids.

   Bell Telephone will provide compatible receivers on request. Many other telephone companies do not have compatible telephones at all. There are, however, devices that can be added to phones to make them compatible with hearing aids.

Volume controls can be added to the receivers of many telephones to assist hard-of-hearing people. It should be noted that a phone with a volume control will not necessarily be compatible with hearing aids. Volume controls are often used by people with normal hearing who work in noisy environments.

All public telephones should be hearing-aid compatible, and every bank of telephones should have at least one telephone with a volume control handset. If only one public telephone is available, it should have a volume control. This service can be arranged upon request from Bell Canada at no charge.

Employees who are hard-of-hearing should be provided with telephones that are compatible with hearing aids and have volume controls. Business telephones that are used by clients should also be so equipped.

2. Telecommunication Devices for the Deaf (TDDs):

Deaf people rely on TDDs to communicate over the telephone. These devices use the regular telephone and allow people to type back and forth over the phone lines. There must be a TDD at each end of the call.

Any business that relies on the telephone to reach its customers and to receive orders from the public should invest in a TDD. TDDs should also be available in all public buildings for deaf individuals who need them. If you provide public information of any sort, you should have a trained staff person who will use the TDD to communicate with deaf customers.

Transportation terminals, department stores, hospitals, and many businesses have purchased TDDs, and they note that deaf people are using more of their services because they are able to communicate with the use of the TDD.

3. Visual Announcement:

Public announcements should be augmented with visual displays, much like the ones used in the subway stations or like the TV screens used in airports. The visual announcements will complement the spoken message and will be appreciated by hearing people as well as people with a hearing loss.

If a facility uses a cash register, it is necessary that a visual display be provided for hard-of-hearing and deaf people. Many frustrations can be alleviated if a display is provided for the customer. Without an easily visible display, your customers have to rely on hearing the sales clerk to give them the total.

4. Signage:

All public buildings should have clearly printed directions so that deaf or hard-of-hearing individuals do not have to struggle to ask for directions. Clearly printed directions would include floor plan layouts, signs on walls indicating directions to various offices, and maps with helpful notes to assist the deaf and hard-of-hearing individual find the way. Good signage is a boon to everyone.

5. Printed Information:

Information such as schedules, price of admission, hours when open, etc. should be readily available in written form for deaf and hard-of-hearing people. The written form could be pamphlets, posters, or billboards. Good visual information is always useful for hearing people as well.

6. Sign Language Interpreters:

Sign language interpreters are fluent in American Sign Language and English. They function as a communication bridge between deaf and hearing people who need to communicate. Sign language interpreters should be provided at public meetings of all kinds.

7. Oral Interpreters:

Oral interpreters are necessary to facilitate communication in group situations where the deaf or hard-of-hearing individual uses lipreading to understand conversation. The oral interpreter silently mouths the words of the speaker, changing them where necessary to synonyms that are more visible on the lips. Oral interpreters should be provided at public meetings of all kinds.

8. FM and Infrared Systems:

Public functions can be made accessible to hard-of-hearing people by installing assistive listening systems, such as FM and infrared systems. Both these systems assist hard-of-hearing people by bringing the sound right to the individual's ear and thus overcoming the problems of distance and noise which hearing aids cannot cope with.

In the FM system the transmitter sends signals to the user receivers by way of wireless, designated radio waves. The speaker uses the transmitter or it can be jacked into the amplifier of an existing PA system. The receiver, which the hard-of-hearing person wears, is the size of a deck of cards, and allows the hard-of-hearing person to adjust the volume of the sound. These systems can be used with or without a hearing aid.

The infrared system is similar to the FM system, but uses light energy to transmit the signal from the transmitter to the hard-of-hearing person's receiver.

Theaters, lecture halls, and other places of assembly can have FM or infrared systems installed on a permanent basis. The receivers can be made available to hard-of-hearing people as needed.

There are also smaller FM and infrared systems which can be used to facilitate communication with hard-of-hearing people particularly in places such as ticket or information booths, where communication is important and which may well be in noisy areas.

9. Smoke and Fire Alarms:

Fire alarms and smoke detectors and other audible warnings in all public places should be equipped with flashing lights. Visual alarms should be installed particularly in areas such as washrooms where people are in isolation. These devices would ensure that people with any degree of hearing loss would be aware of any emergency when it happens.

10. Lighting:

Good lighting is essential to facilitate lipreading and signing.

11. Electrical Interference:

Anti-static treatment of carpets and increased humidity will help reduce electrical interference which can adversely affect hearing aids.

12. Captioning:

Many TV programs are now closed-captioned. This means that if a closed captioned decoder is attached to the TV, those programs will print out the spoken word in the form of captions on the screen. Places that have TVs such as hotels/ motels, libraries, trade shows, and the like, should provide decoders. Informational or promotional material presented at conferences, trade shows, etc., should include open captioning. With open captioning the spoken word is printed on a screen without the use of a "decoder."

13. Staff Training:

All of the above suggestions would be greatly enhanced with staff training to develop awareness of the problems of hearing impaired people and some understanding of their areas of difficulty. The Canadian Hearing Society has a video, "One to One," which can assist with staff training.

14. The International Access Symbol—Hearing Impairment:

It is suggested that this symbol be used to identify any building that is accessible, as well as any special areas inside the building. This will ensure easy identification so that deaf and hard-of-hearing people know where assistance is available.

Special accessible areas in a building may include telephone stations, booths, reservation/information counters, announcement areas, places of assembly, and any other areas in the building that are accessible to deaf and hard-of-hearing people. The type of service provided should be indicated below the access symbol.

For more information about accessibility for deaf and hard-of-hearing people, please feel free to contact

The Canadian Hearing Society

Access 2000 Program
271 Spadina Road
Toronto, Ontario
M5R 2V3

Telephone number	(416) 964-9595
TDD number	(416) 964-0023
Fax number	(416) 964-2066

▶ 14

Assistive Device Research Needs

DEAN C. GARSTECKI
Northwestern University

The Americans With Disabilities Act (ADA) is expected to impact on society in ways that are unprecedented in the history of our country. The ADA (PL 101-336) is intended to eliminate discrimination against all disabled individuals, including those with hearing loss. It provides federally enforceable standards for accessing employment, public accommodations, transportation services, government services, and telecommunication services. These targeted areas are addressed in the law's four major titles. Assurances under each title have implications for audiologists and other professionals concerned with evaluation, selection and use of assistive devices, and concerns requiring new clinical investigations.

Title I (Employment) guards against discrimination in job-related matters such as hiring, orientation, advancement and dismissal (EEOC, 1991). Under Title I, employers are required to make existing facilities and equipment accessible and usable by disabled individuals. To this end, employers of hearing-disabled individuals will need to consider factors relating to selection and use of signaling devices, interpersonal communication aids, telephone amplifiers, and text telephones in the work setting. Job applicants will need to know what devices are available in a particular setting, what additional devices may need to be acquired or made available by an employer, and their potential for benefiting from use of assistive devices.

Title II (Public Services) protects hearing-disabled individuals from exclusion or denial of services, programs, or activities sponsored by any public entity (DOJ, 1991). Under Title II the right to communication access is protected. This will require knowledge of factors to consider in selection and use of telephone amplifiers, per-

267

sonal communication systems (e.g., pocket amplifiers), hearing-aid-compatible telephones, text telephones, and captioning devices by hearing-disabled individuals.

Title III (Public Accommodations) ensures nondiscrimination toward hearing-disabled individuals in the employment of goods, services, and accommodations of any public entity unless undue burden would result (DOJ, 1991). Under Title III, hearing-disabled individuals will need to know about the availability, use, and ability to benefit from devices that enhance communication access in such diverse places as lodging, exhibition or entertainment centers; public gathering places; sales or rental establishments; stations used for public transportation; places of public display, recreation, exercise, and education; and social service establishments. They will need knowledge of factors to consider in usage of personal amplification systems, telephone amplifying or decoding devices, television amplifying or captioning devices, and alerting devices.

Finally, under Title IV (Telecommunications), the hearing-disabled individual's right to inter- and intrastate telephone communication is ensured. Beyond what is covered in earlier components of the law in regard to specialized telephone equipment, this section of the law focuses on use of telephone relay services (FCC, 1991).

In all, the ADA mandates provision and guarantees opportunity for use of "accessibility aids" by hearing-disabled individuals. The problem at present is that there are no international standards for measurement of assistive devices and no established guidelines for clinical practice in their selection and use. As such, assistive devices are not likely to be evaluated uniformly in clinical settings or fitted objectively in clinical practice. They are likely to be acquired without knowledge of potential benefit. Nevertheless, armed by the ADA, hearing-disabled individuals and their employers will demand these products. It is incumbent upon technical researchers and skilled clinical practitioners, therefore, to attempt to bring necessary and appropriate new knowledge to those responsible for device management and to hearing-disabled consumers.

To this end, the purpose of this chapter is to identify fundamental areas of research in regard to assistive device performance (product research) as well as in regard to consumers of these devices (people research). Each of these needs is addressed below. Applied research findings should not only guide future investigation, they should eventually lead to maximizing quality of clinical care. Without such information, consumers risk being ill-served in spite of the hearing professional's and device manufacturer's best intentions.

PRODUCT RESEARCH

Essentially three types of devices are available expressly to assist hearing-impaired individuals in compensating for hearing loss. These include *amplifying*, *decoding*, and *alerting devices*. Amplifying device research needs can be categorized into three broadly encompassing areas: *electroacoustic characteristics, microphone transducer characteristics and microphone usage*, and *device interactions*.

Amplifying Device Research

Electroacoustic Characteristics
In regard to research relating to electroacoustic measures, published reports suggest that American National Standards Institute—ANSI S3.22 (1987) is inadequate for measuring nonlinear amplifying devices (Revit, 1991). For example, instead of using swept sinusoids as the test signal, speech-shaped noise may more closely match the signal/listening task of interest to the device-user. Use of speech noise allows for study of the relationship between complex signal input and perceptual data output (e.g., consonant confusions).

When measuring a nonlinear system, use of complex speech noise helps avoid the problem of "blooming" or activating a device's compression circuit during a portion of the measured frequency response range. This phenomenon is likely to occur when a swept sinusoid serves as the test stimulus (Preves, Beck, Burnett, & Teder, 1989).

Kates (1991) in reviewing concerns in measurement of distortion characteristics in hearing aids acknowledged that ANSI S3.22 is limited in that it specifies harmonic distortion measures at 500 Hz, 800 Hz, and 1600 Hz. In actuality, distortion and gain factors are intertwined throughout a hearing aid's circuitry. Therefore, when measuring a high frequency-emphasis amplification system, distortion properties occurring before the frequency response shaping may disproportionately increase the gain given to distortion components. In addition, existing measures do not explain how distortion properties at the highest frequencies affect lower frequency, simultaneously occurring speech signals. Finally, existing intermodulation distortion measurements may not be sufficiently robust to reveal the true characteristics of the distortion mechanism.

To overcome these shortcomings in current measures, Kates recommended using broadband noise as the test signal instead of a simple sinusoid. With broadband noise, the effects of noise present in the amplifier's circuitry, harmonic distortion, and intermodulation distortion are combined. The same case can be made for using broadband noise in making distortion measures in assistive listening devices.

At this early stage in the process leading to routine clinical evaluation of assistive listening devices, there is a need for several types of basic information. First, there is a need to define the average spectral characteristics of everyday speech stimuli. Next, there is a need to understand the interaction between signal processing and signal characteristics. Finally, there is a need to understand the relationship between complex noise test stimuli and measures of loudness discomfort level (Stelmachowicz, Lewis, Seewald, & Hawkins, 1990). Other fundamental questions must be explored as well. For example, how do commercially available listening devices vary in power and gain functions? Are some devices more appropriate than others for a given hearing loss? How can power and gain measures be efficiently conducted in the clinical setting? What are the volume control characteristics of commercially available devices? Are some more linear than others? Are there practical benefits to using nonlinear systems in everyday communication? If so, what are they?

Distortion characteristics of available assistive listening devices also must be able to be measured clinically. The range and limits of all adjustable controls such as gain controls, tone/frequency shaping/frequency limiting controls, and "sound enhancer" controls must be measurable. How should this be done? What is the cost/benefit ratio in conducting such measures as part of a routine clinical service? On measured devices, what is the expected relationships between control setting adjustment and labeling? How closely do low, mid, and high control settings relate to device performance characteristics? These questions need to be answered in order to effectively manage device evaluation and selection.

A possible scheme for clinical evaluation of listening devices may incorporate the following steps. First, it is helpful to establish a theoretical premise (Beck, 1991). For example, it can be reasoned that pocket and telephone amplifier user benefit will relate directly to device performance characteristics. Devices demonstrating minimal gain and high harmonic distortion levels would be expected to be of lesser benefit than devices providing more gain and less distortion. Frequency response, gain, output limiting, and volume control characteristics are important factors to weigh in selecting and fitting assistive listening devices. By measuring these product characteristics, it should be possible to objectively differentiate among available devices and to predict how beneficial a particular device might be in compensating for a given hearing loss.

The second step is to measure the physical properties of the device. It is important to be able to measure an amplifying device's range of function in a clinical setting. Performance specification data have prescriptive value and, as a result, they are critical to the selection process. This information may include descriptions of evaluation equipment, equipment set up, equipment and device control settings, and stimulus signal type and presentation level. After device performance characteristics have been measured, clinical trials should be conducted. Clinical trial data should specify device performance, define user candidacy, and describe appropriate use of a given device. Finally, to address questions of reliability, durability, and appearance, field trials should be conducted. Field trials should address questions of device quality, dispenser practices, and consumer satisfaction in using devices. Field trials would answer questions relating to how well a particular device performs under selected conditions. User-perceived differences across technologies could be noted. User surveys also would provide data regarding field experiences that may be helpful in dealing with future device selection decisions.

When critical performance characteristics can be measured and representative products can be identified and/or developed, a benchmark will have been established against which to weigh the quality of all other devices. Through such systematic and orderly clinical investigation, it will be possible to bring control over the selection and use of available devices, including those created by user-assembled components.

Microphones

Another important area of investigation centers on microphone technology and use. Microphone characteristics are important, yet are often ignored in listening device selection and use. Microphones used in assistive listening devices are relatively inefficient in that there is considerable loss of energy from acoustic signal input to electrical signal output. Microphone properties vary considerably and physical characteristics influence performance. Ideally, a microphone's frequency response characteristics will be uniform or flat so that it does not contribute its unique artifacts to an amplified output signal. In addition, microphone impedance characteristics should match the impedance load of the amplifying device. Ultimately, a microphone should be highly sensitive to the acoustical energy it transduces.

Microphone varieties include dynamic (magnetic), ceramic (semiconductor), electrostatic (condenser), and carbon types. In selecting a microphone for use with an assistive listening device, Brandt (1989) recommended an electret condenser microphone for its superior sound clarity over alternative types. For best performance, input impedance should match output impedance. Where performance is a key factor, Brandt recommended a microphone with a low output impedance (50 to 500 ohms). He warned that inexpensive microphones generally demonstrate high impedance.

In regard to microphone pickup, omnidirectional patterns are most often used in assistive listening devices, because they are less expensive than other types and most accommodating under everyday listening conditions. For large group or distance listening, cardioid microphone pickup patterns are preferred in that they focus on capturing signals directed toward the microphone from the front.

While considerable information exists in regard to performance characteristics and pickup patterns of microphones in general, comparatively little is known about the practical application of this information. There is a need for study of microphone construction/performance differences in assistive listening devices. This research would also help those inclined to enhance existing systems with higher quality microphones to know the advantages and limitations of available microphones.

A concern that is unique to assistive listening devices is the relationship between microphone-amplifier impedance characteristics and microphone wire length. A clear advantage to using a pocket amplifier is to improve the signal-to-noise ratio by locating the microphone nearer the sound source than would be possible with a personal hearing aid. It is important, therefore, to understand the influence of increasing microphone wire length on device performance.

Finally, it would be helpful to know the relationship between microphone pickup pattern and performance characteristics under a variety of everyday listening conditions. Which microphone options are best suited to common, yet different listening experiences (e.g, listening in a large lecture hall vs. listening in a party situation)? Is it better to use an omnidirectional microphone than a cardioid microphone in selected settings? Performance data would improve clinical decision making.

Interfacing Amplification Systems

Listening device users accept amplification because of self-perceived benefit in everyday communication. While some may not readily accept hearing aids, many hearing-aid wearers use listening devices as alternate amplification systems or to enhance benefits from hearing-aid use. For example, it is not uncommon for hearing-aid wearers to simultaneously use telephone, television, or pocket amplifiers, as well as an array of room amplification systems. Hearing-aid users may be coupled to other systems inductively (e.g., neck loops) by means of a hardwired connection, or by acoustic coupling as when amplifiers are linked in series (e.g., hearing aid with microphone input and a standard telephone amplifier). Since it is well-documented that electroacoustic characteristics of hearing aids are influenced differently by microphone, telecoil, and direct audio input (DAI) conditions, it behooves the audiologist to determine the effect of interfacing amplification systems on signal output and user performance.

Inductive coupling technology enables hearing aids equipped with telecoils to pick up magnetic field leakage generated by hearing-aid-compatible telephones and loop amplification systems. In order to function effectively, the induction coil must have sufficient energy to attract the magnetic field (Beck & Nance, 1989). Induction coil pickup strength is proportional to its size; the larger the coil, the greater the strength. Small hearing aids can accommodate small telecoils (if any), reducing the likelihood of device interfacing by induction. Unfortunately, it is not possible to characterize the functional adequacy of an induction coil from procedures described in the present standard.

Clinical studies are necessary to provide *in situ* data on induction coil performance. For example, currently there are no specifications for telephone handset performance with telecoils even though the Americans With Disabilities Act ensures telephone accessibility for hearing-disabled individuals. There also is a need for information on the influence of power lines, transformers, and fluorescent lights on telecoil performance. Hearing-aid-compatible telephones may be rendered useless because of their placement near interfering sources, interference which may cancel the benefit of using an amplifying system.

Direct audio input (DAI) coupling provides a direct electrical connection between a hearing aid and an attached accessory (e.g., external microphone, television, or radio). Care must be taken to ensure a proper impedance match between interfacing systems. When there is an impedance mismatch, audio signal output may be weakened or overdriven and distorted. Clinical investigations are needed to define changes in hearing-aid performance associated with use of direct electrical coupling. Whenever practical, device evaluation protocols should include measures of performance with and without common interfacing units (Beck & Nance, 1989).

Acoustic coupling provides an open-field connection between two or more amplifying devices. The most common contraindication to such an arrangement is acoustic feedback. If feedback can be successfully controlled, the amplified signal from the initial system (i.e., hearing aid) may be boosted by the second amplifier (e.g., telephone amplifier). While the result could be additive, it may also be that the second system is overdriven by the first which will distort the end product. The effect of acoustic coupling on signal output remains to be quantified.

Alerting Device Research

Alerting devices monitor sound using sensor microphones, inductive pickup, or direct electrical connection. They transmit signals using either hardwired or wireless technology and by visual (e.g., strobe light), auditory (e.g., low pitched signals), or tactile (e.g., bed shaker) stimulation (Compton, 1991). These systems can be used to monitor sound in small areas, homes, and office buildings. They are used for wake-up and telephone alerting purposes, as well as for fire and emergency alarms.

There is a need for more study of the relative effectiveness of auditory, visual, and tactile signal transmitting technologies. Auditory alerting devices lose their impact with increasing hearing loss. Research is needed to determine the interaction between alerting signal intensity and frequency and hearing loss characteristics. Logically, visual alerting devices (e.g., flashing light systems) lose their impact as alerting light contrast lessens in comparison with environmental conditions. Studies are needed to determine alerting light threshold levels and the effectiveness of lights varying in candlepower and on-off signaling rate. In addition, vibrotactile aids succeed in alerting their users in proportion to the strength of their signal as it may be influenced by the size, method of placement, and location of the vibrating transducer. Studies are needed to examine the effectiveness of existing systems and to foster development of continually improving systems. In this way, user capabilities and device performance characteristics can be defined and behavioral differences within and across user groups can be identified.

Decoding Device Research

Decoding devices provide telephone and television access for hearing-impaired individuals. The term Telecommunication Device for the Deaf (TDD) or Text Telephone (TT) applies to a typewriter-like device that translates keyboard input into an acoustic (Baudot) code. This code is transmitted by telephone line to a compatible receiver (another TDD/TT). The device then displays the message as printed text. Alternate printed message systems include personal computers equipped with modems and used with telecommunication software and facsimile machines. Closed-caption television decoders enable viewers to read text accompanying televised programming. While the printed text is not a verbatim reiteration of the spoken text, it does relay the intent of the spoken message. This enables hearing-impaired individuals to receive the gist of the message and mentally fill in what is not perceived through listening or viewing.

There is a need to address the relative advantages of all decoding systems. Judging from clinical observation, only the most severely hearing-impaired individuals rely on a caption system for television viewing. Nevertheless, questions regarding the legibility and visibility of printed word displays should be formally addressed. Advantages of text telephone technology as compared with personal computer and facsimile equipment used for telephone communication remain to be defined. In addition, from the consumer's standpoint, there are questions about how decoding equipment compares in availability, cost, performance, ease of use, and repair? How easy is it to see, read, and understand printed instructions and warranties accompanying various devices? How do consumers rate quality of product construction, design, appearance, portability, durability, and other features? Answers to these questions may define behavioral differences within the hearing-impaired population as well as quality differences across systems.

PEOPLE RESEARCH

Demographic data are useful for developing clinical service and marketing plans. Kochkin (1993) reviewed factors considered to impact on hearing-aid consumption, and these may just as well relate to assistive device consumption. Barcham and Stephens (1980) reported that individuals were embarrassed by the visibility of hearing aids. This was reported as the most frequently cited problem in hearing-aid acceptance and use by adults. Hearing aids suggest weakness to others. They draw attention to hearing loss and may serve as a sign that one is growing older, disabled, or handicapped (Kochkin, 1993). Blood, Blood, & Danhauer (1978) and others have reported a "hearing aid effect" among those who use hearing aids and who are perceived to be less intelligent, lower achieving, less attractive, and more likely to demonstrate negative personality traits than others.

Cost may be a deterrent to hearing-aid consumption. Kochkin (1993) reported that the results of a 1990 Hearing Industries Association's focus group survey indicated hearing aids cost more than their perceived value in compensating for hearing loss. Behavior of hearing professionals is another factor to consider (Goldstein, 1984). Some hearing professionals may be skeptical of the degree of assistance provided by an aid in comparison with its cost. Examples from clinic files suggest a conservative attitude toward hearing-aid dispensing, according to Goldstein. Hearing-aid marketing tactics may help explain low consumption. The hearing aid dispenser risks being regarded as a high-pressure salesperson. Elderly adults, in particular, tend to be skeptical of high-pressure sales techniques, and this may manifest itself in a negative attitude toward hearing-aid use. Another factor is the medical funnel (Kochkin, 1993). The purchaser of a hearing-aid in the United States must first receive a medical examination from a physician (United States Food and Drug Administration, 1977) or sign a waiver. This process may create a bottleneck in the flow of services to potential hearing-aid users. Finally, hearing-aid sales practices must be considered. The hearing-aid industry's response to low sales has been to persuade the consumer to purchase the aid through promises of improved products, free hearing exams, and discounted prices. Little attempt has been made to understand the underlying motivational differences between users and nonusers. Emphasis is directed toward dispensing the product. This may explain why some aging adults do not use their hearing aids (Smedley & Schow, 1990). Because of this, data estimating the low consumption of hearing aids may actually overestimate the number of hearing-aid users.

Concerns relating to acceptance of hearing aids potentially apply to acceptance and use of all assistive devices: listening, alerting, and decoding devices. This supports a need for survey data to better define candidates for using assistive devices. There is a need for information describing the potential consumer's age. This may help identify consumer preferences and describe concerns in acceptance and use. Consumer gender differences may explain potential differences in device selection preferences influenced by device size, weight, and appearance. Consumer hearing loss differences may relate to amplifier versus decoder decisions. Hearing handicap differences may explain preferences toward use of selected devices in various environmental and situational conditions. Information relating to history of device ownership may be useful in predicting success and failure with new devices. Device familiarity may also impact on replacement preferences. Assistive device consumers, more than hearing aid consumers, appear to be more prone toward the use of devices to help compensate for hearing loss. They may be driven by known or expected product features. Finally, lifestyle, education level, and discretionary income differences also may be expected to influence device selection and use.

From this information, underserved hearing-impaired individuals can be identified. For example, if personal amplification systems are not purchased by those with mild hearing loss, the advantages of using these devices in selected situations should be made known. If the consumption of television captioning devices is low among potential user groups (e.g., severely hearing-impaired minorities or elderly adults), these individuals should be targeted for receipt of informational literature and participation in educational programs.

Once it is known that consumers within certain age, hearing loss, and income levels prefer multifunction to single-purpose equipment, one sound transmission technology over others, and selected product brands over others, then prospective consumers with similar pedigrees can be approached more efficiently and managed more effectively.

Survey data may be used to develop user profiles describing hearing loss and handicap characteristics for individuals who elect to use various types of devices. Success factors may be identified and the effect on life quality and lifestyle may be defined. Differences between hearing aid users and nonusers in their decisions to use listening devices should be investigated. Answers to all of these questions are important in making in assistive device management decisions.

SUMMARY

Assistive devices are critical tools available to hearing-disabled individuals in their management of listening, decoding, and alerting needs. Assistive device popularity and use is expected to increase with new federal legislation mandating public access for hearing-impaired individuals. However, currently little is understood about available products or potential consumers. Studies are needed to determine the performance characteristics of available devices and changes in behavior with their use. In addition there is a need to identify individuals who demonstrate the best potential for benefiting from their use.

REFERENCES

American National Standards Institute. (1987). *American National Standard for the Specification of Hearing Aid Characteristics* (ANSI S 3.22-1987). New York: American National Standards Institute.

Barcham, L.J., & Stephens, S.D.G. (1980). The use of an open-ended problem questionnaire in auditory rehabilitation. *British Journal of Audiology, 14*, 49–54.

Beck, L.B. (1991). Chapter 1. Amplification needs: Where do we go from here? In G.A. Studebaker, F. Bess, & L.B. Beck (Eds.), *The Vanderbilt hearing-aid report II*, pp. 1–9. Parkton, MD: York Press, Inc.

Beck, L.B., & Nance, G.C. (1989). Hearing aids, assistive listening devices, and telephones: Issues to consider. In C.L. Compton (Ed.), Assistive devices. *Seminars in Hearing, 10*, 1, 78–89.

Blood, G.W., Blood, I.M., & Danhauer, J.L. (1978). Listeners' impressions of normal-hearing and hearing-impaired children. *Journal of Communication Disorders, 11*, 513–518.

Brandt, F.D. (1989). Microphones and assistive listening devices: A tutorial. In C.L. Compton (Ed.), Assistive devices. *Seminars in Hearing, 10*, 1, 31–41.

Compton, C.L. (1991). Chapter 26. Clinical management of assistive technology users: Issues to consider. In G.A. Studebaker, F. Bess, & L.B. Beck (Eds.), *The Vanderbilt hearing-aid report II*, pp. 301–318. Parkton, MD: York Press, Inc.

Department of Justice (DOJ). (1991). 28 CFR Part 35. Non-discrimination on the basis of disability in state and local government services: Final rule. *Federal Register, 56*, 144, July 26, 35544–35604.

Equal Employment Opportunity Commission (EEOC). (1991). 29 CFR Part 1630. Equal employment opportunity for individuals with disabilities: Final rule. *Federal Register, 56*, 144, July 26, 35726–35755.

Federal Communications Commission (FCC). (1991). 47 CFR Parts 0 and 64. Telecommunications services for hearing and speech disabled: Final rule. *Federal Register, 56*, 148, August 1, 36729–36733.

Goldstein, D.P.(1984). Hearing impairment, hearing aids, and audiology. *Journal of the American Speech-Language-Hearing Association, 9*, 24–35, 38.

Kates, J.M. (1991). Chapter 12. New developments in hearing aid measurements. In G.A. Studebaker, F. Bess, & L.B. Beck (Eds.), *The Vanderbilt hearing-aid report II*, pp. 149–163. Parkton, MD: York Press, Inc.

Kochkin, S. (1993). MarkeTrak III: Why 20 million in US don't use hearing aids for their hearing loss—Part 1. *The Hearing Journal, 46*, 1, 20–27.

Preves, D., Beck, L., Burnett, E., & Teder, H. (1989). Input stimuli for obtaining frequency responses of automatic gain control hearing aids. *Journal of Speech and Hearing Research, 32*, 189–194.

Revit, L. (1991). New tests for signal-processing and multi-channel hearing instruments. *The Hearing Journal, 44*, 5.

Smedley, T.C., & Schow, R.L. (1990). Frustrations with hearing aid use: Candid observations from the elderly. *The Hearing Journal, 43*, 21–27.

Stelmachowicz, P.G., Lewis, D.E., Seewald, R.C., & Hawkins, D.B. (1990). Complex and pure-tone signals in the evaluation of hearing-aid characteristics. *Journal of Speech and Hearing Research, 33*, 380–385.

United States Food and Drug Administration, 21. (1977). *Code of Federal Regulations 801. 1*, 420–421.

Index

A

Abrahamson, J., 176, 246
Accessibility of public facilities, 260, 262-266
A.G. Bell Association, 259
Alerting, assistive listening, and visual support systems checklist, 121-122
Alerting methods, 202-205
    acoustic, 202, 203, 203
    light, 202, 204
    vibratory, 202, 203, 204, 205
American National Standards Institute (ANSI), 241
    A117.1-1992, 234
    S3 Committee on Acoustics, 246
    S3.22, 246, 269
American Speech-Language-Hearing Association (ASHA), 9, 259
American Telephone & Telegraph (AT&T), 26
Americans with Disabilities Act (ADA; P.L. 101-336), 1-9, 62, 66, 135, 136, 185, 197, 208, 221, 234, 241, 250, 267, 272
    glossary, 21-23
    role of assistive technology, 3-7
        communication barriers, 6-7
        implications for audiologists, 7-9
        in employment, 4-5
        in private facilities and public programs, 5-6
        telecommunications access, 7

statutory deadlines and responsible agencies, 3
    Title I (Employment), 3, 267
    Title II (Public Accommodations), 3, 4, 5, 267
    Title III (Transportation), 3, 4, 5, 197-198, 202, 268
    Title IV (Telecommunications), 3, 268
    Title V (Miscellaneous), 3
Anderson, C., 207
Anderson, K., 159
Ankermann, H.A., 131
ASCII, 60, 243
Assistive listening devices
    definitions, 15-16, 17
Association of Late Deafened Adults (ALDA), 258
Automatic Gain Control (AGC), 170, 172

B

"Baby Bell," 27
Bagwell, C., 159
Balkany, T., 88
Ball, K., 148
Bally, S.J., 104
Bamford-Koval-Bench (BKB) Standard Sentence test, 148
Barcham, L.J., 274
Barras, B., 138
Baudot (acoustic) code, 60, 273
Beck, L.B., 269, 270, 272

Bell, Alexander Graham, 25
  first hearing aid, 25
Benafield, N., 179
Bennett, R.L., 124, 146
Bentler, R., 158
Beranek, L., 146, 150, 157
Berg, F., 159, 169, 179
Berger, K., 169
Bergquist, L., 207
Berliner, K.I., 89
Bess, F., 144, 146, 147, 151, 153, 154, 155,
  156, 159, 165, *166*, 168, 169
Bicultural Centre, 259
Bilger, R.C., 74, 145
Black, R.C., 89
Blair, J., 146, 147, 179, 180
Blamey, P., 76
Blood, G.W., 274
Blood, I.M., 274
Bolt, R., 143, 148
Boney, S., 165
Boothroyd, A., 165, 168, 169, 170, 172, 176
Borrild, K., 143, 150
Boyd, J., 138
Boyd, M., 207
Brackett, D., 165, 169
Bradley, J., 143
Brandt, F.D., 271
Brown, L., 159, 179
Burger, J., 143
Burnett, E., 269
Burton-Koch, D., 89
Byers, C.L., 89

C
Campos, C.T., 88
Canadian Association of the Deaf (CAD),
  258
Canadian Association of Speech-Language
  Pathologists and
  Audiologists (CASLPA), 259
Canadian Hard of Hearing Association
  (CHHA), 258
Canadian Hearing Society, 257, 262-266
Caption Center of WGBH, 137, 139
Captioned Films/Videos Service, 138

Captioning, 125, 136-138
  closed, 136, 137
  open, 138-139
  real-time, 138
Carbon bell telephone, 29, 30, 36, 45
Carlin, N.F., 214
Carter Phone Decision, 26, 64
Casey, D.E., 89
Castle, D.L., 71, 72
Cats, pet, 97
Clark, G.M., 76, 89
Classroom acoustics
  methods to improve, 155-160
Client assessment, 8
Closed-set testing, 71
Clyme, E., 246
Cochlear Corporation, 72, 81, 91
Cochlear Implant Club International, 93
Cochlear implant users
  alerting systems for, 95-99
  assistive listening and visual support
    systems, 99-104
  needs assessment and counseling, 89-95
Cohen, N.L., 67-74
Cole, C.A., 124
Communication needs
  at group home, 228-229
  at home, 226-228
  at school/college, 231-232
  at work, 229-231
  during recreation/travel, 232-234
Computers and telecommunication devices,
  60-62, 101
Compton, C.L., 88, 89, 96, 136, 137, 138,
  197, 198, 224, 249, 273
Conners, S., 148
Cooper Committee, 11
Cooper, J., 145
Cox, R., *166*
Crandell, C., 143, 144, 146, 148, 150, 151,
  153, 154, 155, 156, 157, 158, 159,
  165
Critical distance, 153
Cronin, B.J., 137
Crosstalk, 195
Cutts, B., 145

D

Daly, C., 89
Danhauer, J.L., 274
Dankowski, K., 67
Davis, D., 159, 180
Davis, J., 158
Demonstration/evaluation of equipment, 245-247
Department of Justice (DOJ), 197, 267, 268
Devens, J., 143, 144, 146, 150
DeVoss, F., 234
Digital key system, 30-32, 31, 32
    interfaces, 32, 33
    modems, 32, 33
    switches, 32
Dirks, D., 144, 147
Division of Small Manufacturers Assistance, 14
Dogs
    pet, 97, 98
    trained hearing ear, 97, 98, 99
Dorman, M.F., 67
Dove, H., 67
Dowell, R., 76
Downs, M., 144
Dubno, J., 147
DuBow, S., 249

E

Eaton, B., 179
Eddington, D.K., 89
Edwards, H.T., 214
Equal Employment Opportunity Commission (EEOC), 267
Ekhaml, L., 133, 136
Electronic interference, 128
Elfenbein, J., 158
Elliott, L.L., 74, 148, 154, 155
English as a Second Language learners, 139
English, B., 88
Erber, N., 67, 71, 74, 82-85, 104, 165
Evaluation
    formal, 68-78
    informal, 67
Everly-Myers, D.S., 214

F

Fabry, D., 166, *166*, 167, *167*, 168
Facsimile transmission, 63, *63*, 101
Federal Communications Commission (FCC), 168, 268
Feigin, J., 172, 246
Fidell, S., 124, 146
Fikret-Pasa, S., 72, 79
Finitzo-Hieber, T., 143, 144, 146, 147, 148, 150, 151, 155, 157, 165
Fire Protection Equipment Directory, 234
Fire safety
    fire signaling device standards, 234-235
    resources, 250
Fisher, B., 154
Flexer, C., 154, 159, 167, 168, 179, 180
FM systems, 127, 133, 135, 136, 157, 165-181
    design features, 169-179
    in classrooms, 165-181
Fong, M.M., 89
Food and Drug Administration (FDA), 274
    Medical Device Amendments, 11-14
        advisory panels, 13-14
Food, Drug, and Cosmetic Act, 11, 14
Food and Drugs Act of 1906, 11
Forster, I.C., 89
Fourcin, A., 150
Frank, T., 246
Freeburg, J., 123, 210
Freeman, B.A., 246
Friedman, B., 177
Functional assessment, 8

G

Gallaudet University, 139
Garrettson, C., 104
Garstecki, D.C., 72, 79, 92, 206
Geer, S., 249
Gengel, R., 150, 165
Gerhardt, K., 176
Gelfand, S., 144
Gibson, G.C., 214
Giolas, T.G., 146, 154, 165, 215
Glasberg, B., 149
Godfrey, J., 142

Goldstein, D.P., 274
Goldstein, W., 132
Good manufacturing practices (GMPs), 12
Gorga, M., 158
Gravel, J., 168, 169, 177, 246
Gray, R.F., 89
Grimes, A.M., 246

H
Hammond, L.B., 169
Harford, E., 177
Harkins, J.E., 224
Harris, C., 143, 146
Harris, J., 151, 157
Hassall, J., 143
Hawkins, D.B., 149, 165, 169, 170, 172, 177, 246, 269
Haynes, H., 151
Hearing aid regulation, 18-19
Hearing Industries Association, 274
Hermanson, C., 207
Hochberg, I., 144
Holmes, A., 176, 246
House, W.F., 89
Houston, M.J., 124
Houtgast, T., 143
Hull, R.H., 133

I
Induction, 129-130, 185-186
Induction loop system, 129, 129, 133, 185-195
Infrared, 131-132, *132*, 133, 135
Interpersonal/media listening options, *239*
International Electrotechnical Commission (IEC) Standard 118-4, 195

J
Jackler, R.K., 89
Jackson, W., 137
Jared, C., 210
Jenkins, J., 142
Jensema, C.J., 136, 138
Jensen, G., 207
Jerger, J., 167
John, J., 146, 154
Johnson, C.E., 214

Jones, J., 179
Joy, D., 150

K
Kalikow, D.N., 74, 154
Kallail, K.J., 214
Kaplan, H., 104
Karasek, A., 172, 246
Kates, J.M., 269
Katz, D., 148
Keiser, H., 179
Keith, R., 147
KEMAR manikin, 154
Kennedy, M., 150
Kessler, D.K., 89
Khal, G., 207
Kille, E., 148
King, C.M., 139
Klein, W., 153
Knight, J., 150
Knowles, S., 150
Knox, E., 150
Knudsen, V., 143, 146, 157
Kochkin, S., 274
Kodaras, M., 143
Konkle, D., 177, 246
Kopun, J., 179
Kraemer, K.B., 210
Kuk, F., 166, 167
Kurtovic, H., 143

L
Landin, D., 177, 246
Larsen, D., 167
LaSasso, C.J., 139
Lass, N.J., 214
Leavitt, R.J., 90, 123 139, 154, 166, 167, 168, 180, 210
Leder, S., 88
Lee, F.S., 215
Lehiste, I., 142
Levin, S., 148
Lewis, D., 170, 172, *172*, 174, *174*, *175*, *176*, 177, *177*, *178*, 246, 269
Lind, C., 104
Liss, M.B., 123, 138

Lochner, J., 143
Loeb, G.E., 89
Logan, S., 169
Longhurst, T.M., 215
Long-term average speech spectrum, 175
Loop system standards, 195

M
MacDonald, A., 143
MacKenzie, D., 246
Madell, J., 169
Mahon, W.J., 110
Markides, A., 146, 147
Martin, M., 150
Matkin, N., 144, 150
Matthews, L.J., 215
Maxon, A., 165, 169
McCaffrey, H., 176, 246
McCarthy, P.A., 88, 110
McCroskey, F., 143, 144, 146, 150
Medical device, definition, 11-12
    classification of, 12-13
Medwetsky, L., 172, 176
Merzenich, M.M., 88
Message relay systems, 62-63
Middleton, R.A., 133, 136
Millar, J.B., 89
Miller, G., 145, 146
Millin, J., 159, 169, 179
Mills, J.H., 215
Mims, L., 165
Moncur, J., 144
Moore, B., 149
Moore, J., *166*
Morgan, D., 147
Mort, J., 150
Moss, S., 205
Mueller, H.G., 246
Multiplicative hypotheses, 151
Murray, M., 88
Myers, C., 151
Myrup, C., 179, 180

N
Nabelek, A., 143, 144, 145, 146, 147, 148,
    151, 153, 155, 157

Nabelek, I., 143, 144, 148, 151, 153, 155, 157
Nance, G.C., 272
National Captioning Institute, 137, 138
National Fire Alarm Code, 234
National Fire Protection Association
    (NFPA), 234
Needs assessment selection process, 225-
    234, *225*
Neuman, A., 144
Neuss, D., 179
Nicely, P., 145
Niemoeller, A., 144, 150, 155
Nober, E.H., 146, 205
Nober, L., 146
Noise, 145-150, 151-152
    ambient, 146-147, 150
    external, 146
    internal, 146
Northern, J., 144

O
O'Loughlin, B.J., 89
Olsen, W., 143, 144, 146, 150, 152, 155,
    157
Open-set testing, 71
Owens, E., 145

P
Palmer, C.V., 90, 92, 140, 209
Pannbacker, M.D., 214
Parkin, J., 67
Parmiter-Jacobs, L., 210
Patrick, J.F., 89
Paul, R., 146, 147
Pearsons, K.S., 124, 146
Pehringer, J.L., 125, 132
Peltz Strauss, K., 249
Penton, J., 150
People research, 274-275
Perkins, R., 137
Peutz, V., 153, 154
Pickett, J., 143, 144, 145, 146, 147, 151
Plomp, R., 147
Poole, D., 150
Powell, C., 150
Preves, D., 269

Price, D., 123, 138
Product research, 268-273
  alerting devices, 272-273
  amplifying devices, 269-272
  decoding devices, 273
Pruitt, J.B., 216

Q
QUEST?AR exercise, 74, *76*, 83

R
Ramsdell, D.A., 87
Rapid Speech Transmission Index (RASTI),
  155, 167
Rauterkas, M., 92
Ray, H., 159
Rebscher, S.J., 89
Reed, C., 145
Rehabilitation Act of 1973, 1-2
  Section 504, 241
Reverberation, 143-145, 151-152, *145*
Revit, L., 269
Richardson, F., 88
Riggs, D., 146, 147, 156, 165
Riggs, D.E., 246
Ring equivalents, 36, *37*
Robinson, P., 144, 148
Rodriguez, G., 176
Room acoustics, 142-160
Ross, M., 125, 143, 146, 147, 154, 155, 157,
  165, 168, 169

S
Sabine, W., 143
Safe Medical Devices Act of 1990, 15
  Medical Device Reporting (MDR), 15
Sanders, D., 142, 146, 147
Saniga, R.D., 214
Sarff, L., 159, 179
Saucedo, K., 179
Scherz, J.W., 214
Schindler, R.A., 89
Schmitt, J.F., 214
Schow, R.L., 215, 274
Schum, D., 158, 170, 172, 177, 207, 215, 246
Schum, L., 78, 86, 88, 89, 90, 91, 92, 96,
  100, 104, 105, 106

Searls, L., 207
Seewald, R.C., 269
Selection of assistive devices, 240-245
Self Help for Hard of Hearing People
  (SHHH), 90, 93, 207, 258
Seligman, P., 76, 89
Sensing mechanisms, 198-201
  acoustic, 198, 199, *199*
  electronic, 198, 199, *200*
  inductive, 198, 200, *201*
Shapiro, W.H., 67
Shaver, J.P., 214
Shepard, N., 158
Sher, A., 145
Side-tone, 30
Siemens, Werner von, 26
Signal-to-noise ratio, 125, 147, 155, 165,
  168-170, 174, 180
Silman, S., 144
Sinclair, J.S., 146, 147, 156, 165, 246
Smaldino, J., 144, 147, 150, 157, 159, 165
Smedley, T.C., 215, 274
Smith, L., 165
Sound propagation and reflections, 152
  counseling, 139-140
Speaker-listener distance, 152-155, *154*
Speech Perception in Noise (SPIN) test, 74,
  148, 154
Speerschneider, J., 166
Spitzer, J., 88
Stach, B., 166
Standard for Signaling Devices for the
  Hearing Impaired, 235
Stein, R.L., 214
Stelmachowicz, P., 158, 172, 246, 269
Stephens, S.D.G., 274
Stevens, K.N., 74, 154
Strange, W., 142
Strategies for increasing consumer and
  public acceptance of
  devices, 251-261
Strong, C.J., 214
Summerwill, J., 207
Survey of assistive listening, visual support,
  and alerting
  system use, 110-121
Suter, A., 147

T
Talis, H., 147
Tecca, J.E., 214
Teder, H., 269
Telecoils, consumer's guide, 191
Telecommunications devices for the deaf
     (TDDs), 26, 58-63, 79, 101, 227,
     228, 273
Telephone assistive devices, 33-58
     alerting devices, 33-44
     amplification devices, 45-58
     communication options, *238*
Telephone Compatibility Act, 185
Telephone transmission system, 27-32
     multiline systems, 30-32
     signal distribution, 28-29
     speech network, 29-30
     telephone subassemblies, 27
Television band radios, 130, *131*
Television Bureau of Advertising, 123
Television Decoder Circuitry Act, 136-137,
     250
Television viewing
     assisted listening for, 125-136
     captioning, 136-139
     the problem, 124-135
Test site, 80
Thibodeau, L., 170, 176, 177, 178, 179, 246
Thomas, H., 146, 154
Thompson, C., 179
Tillman, T., 144, 147, 148, 150, 151, 155, 165
Title 21 of the Code of Federal Regulations,
     13, 16
Tong, Y.C., 89
Transmission technologies, 201-202
     hardwired, 201
     wireless, 201, 202
Tye-Murray, N., 76, 78, 86, 88, 89, 90, 91,
     92, 96, 100, 104, 105, 106
Tyler, R.S., 166, 167, 207

U
Underwriters Laboratories (UL), 234
Urban, J., 89
U.S. Department of Commerce, 123, 137
U.S. Department of Justice, 9
U.S. Office of Special Education, 139

V
Vader, E.A., 138
Van Tasell, D.J., 124, 167, 177, 246
Viehweg, S., 179, 180

W
Wallber, M., 246
Waltzman, S.B., 67
Wang, M., 145
Warning signals
     basic environmental, 87, 94
     lifestyle-specific, 87, 92, 94, 99
Washington Post, 137
Watson, T., 150, 154
Weatherton, M., 179
Weinstein, B.E., 214
Well, A.D., 205
Whitford, L., 89
Wiley, Dr. Harvey W., 10
Wolfe, S., 207
Wolinsky, S., 167
Woodford, C.M., 214

Y
Yacullo, W., 149
Yanda, J.L., 89

Z
Zacharchuk, S., 67
Zaveri, K., 143

3-D Loop, *186-188*, 194-195
911 emergency services, 2, 62